Gut Solutions

By Brenda Watson, N.D. and Leonard Smith, M.D.
with Susan Stockton, M.A.
Foreword by Stephen Holt, M.D.

Copyright© 2003 by Brenda Watson, N.D.
All Rights Reserved

Printed in the United States of America

No part of this book may be reproduced, stored in retrieval system or transmitted in any form or by any means, either electronic, mechanical, through photocopying, microfilming, recording or otherwise, without written permission from the publisher.

ISBN 0-9719309-2-9

Library of Congress Catalog Card Number: 2003096214

This book is for educational purposes. It is not intended as a substitute for medical advice. Please consult a qualified health care professional for individual health and medical advice. Neither Renew Life Press nor the authors shall have any responsibility for any adverse effects arising directly or indirectly as a result of the information provided in this book.

Throughout this book, trademarked names are used. Rather than put a trademark symbol after every occurrence of a trademarked name, we use names in an editorial fashion only, and to the benefit of the trademark owner, with no intention of infringement of the trademark. Where such designations appear in this book, they have been printed with initial caps.

First Printing 2003
Second Printing 2004
Renew Life Press and Information Services
2076 Sunnydale Drive
Clearwater, FL 33765
1-800-830-4778

Acknowledgements

It is the ongoing crusade to contribute naturally to the digestive health of millions of people that inspired the creation of our second book, *Gut Solutions*. Thanks to the tens of thousands of people that allowed us to "renew" their lives through better digestion and detoxification by purchasing our first best selling digestive care book, *Renew Your Life*.

For the creation of *Gut Solutions*, we wish to give a special acknowledgement to the following folks, both inside and outside of the Renew Your Life Press family, for their valued contribution to this book. Without the skill, commitment and hard work of the Renew Your Life Press staff, this book would not be a reality. Thanks to:

Bobby and Kerrie Broe, for their insightful input into the Digestive Care Diet.

Brian Ferraci, for his dynamic cover design and talented illustrations throughout the book.

Kelly McKnight, for managing and keeping everyone on task, and skillfully handling the printing and PR aspects of this project.

Kathi Murray, for her creativity, outstanding book design talent and her patient acceptance of our various project revisions.

Thomas Pendleton, for his vast industry knowledge and his keen editorial input.

Susan Stockton, for providing research, and guidance in creating this book. Her knowledge of natural digestive care and writing contributed greatly to the completion of this book.

Stan Watson, my husband, for his loving strength and endurance of our second book project. His endless support and encouragement have been one of the main reasons for my continued success.

Brenda Watson

Brenda Watson, N.D.
Clearwater, FL
2003

Preface

By Dr. Leonard Smith, M.D.

For the purpose of education, this book is divided according to conditions, using both medical and common lay names. These common names have been included because most people, through various media pronouncements, have come to know them to some extent. While these labels – both common and technical - can be useful in identifying different aspects of what can happen to the esophagus, stomach, intestinal tract, liver and gallbladder, it can be even more important to understand the common ground that ties these conditions together. It will become apparent throughout this book that we have the option to focus on labels and details as they relate to symptoms or to see the bigger picture of what is the underlying cause before symptoms manifest. This is essentially the difference between the focus of allopathic medicine (symptom and disease oriented) and naturopathic medicine (primary cause and prevention oriented).

It should be obvious that both the allopathic and naturopathic approaches are of great value. Tumors, bleeding or obstruction in the intestinal tract usually require direct outside intervention to save and or restore health. On the other hand, in our era of skyrocketing health costs (well over a trillion dollars spent annually in the US), prevention through a deeper understanding of cellular function is of paramount importance.

This book has been created in a particular format to help the reader understand what the condition is, what causes it, who gets it, what are the signs and symptoms, how it is traditionally diagnosed, what are some of the standard medical treatments and, finally, what are some of the optional nutritional approaches and lifestyle changes that can be implemented to entirely avoid the condition. These same optional nutritional approaches and lifestlyle changes can be profoundly helpful when combined with more invasive allopathic treatments, as well.

A variety of tools are needed in every toolbox to accomplish any task, and so it is with health. The simple principles of drinking pure filtered water, eating more organic vegetables, fruits, seeds and nuts, exercise, high quality sleep, efficient bowel function, stress modification (including psycho-emotional and spiritual rejuvenation) and appropriate dietary supplementation are "tools" that will help maintain or restore lost health.

Too often, health care practitioners give such vague, generalized (and often inaccurate) advice as: "Just eat your standard, balanced diet," and "You can take supplements, but they really don't matter and won't be helpful," or "A bowel movement every two or three days is okay." These are examples of arcane attitudes being espoused by some who are not even reading their own literature. It is statements like these that we would like to address with further clarity and documentation from the medical literature.

Finally, there will be notable repetition in the Optional Nutritional Approaches section at the conclusion of each condition in the book. This repetition underscores the fact that all of these conditions arise from common grounds of cellular dysfunction. We have even created a simple acronym, which is weaved throughout the book: AAA-HOPE. Antioxidants, Anti-inflammatories, Alkaline Diet, High-fiber diet, Oils (essential fats), Probiotics and Prebiotics, and Enzymes. These are the diet and supplement "tools" that, along with life style changes, form a firm foundation of good health. Solid foundations last longer, resist destructive forces and are generally easier to reconstruct in the face of disaster. In the same fashion, humans who maintain a healthy foundation recover and survive stress and illness better than the less healthy. This book is about educating and helping restore foundational health.

Foreword

By Dr. Stephen Holt, M.D.

It is a great pleasure to write an introduction to this excellent book on Natural Ways to Digestive Health. "Gut Solutions" fills a major gap in health care consumer information about the use of remedies of natural origin for the promotion of digestive comfort. In my own writings, I have stressed the need for education among consumers of digestive aids. Many people with digestive upset purchase over-the-counter (OTC) pharmaceuticals without a complete knowledge of their benefits, disadvantages and limitations. I believe in the treatment power of patient education – a concept that I have termed "edutherapies." This well written book is an example of valuable "edutherapy."

In the mid-1980s, I published several articles on the therapeutics of common digestive disorders such as heartburn, gastroesophageal reflux disease and functional gastrointestinal disturbance, such as irritable bowel syndrome. My research work on the clinical development of drugs that block acid secretion, such as cimetidine, famotidine, ranitidine and omeprazole led me to uncover some of the disadvantages of these short-term treatments. While acid-suppressing drugs often melt symptoms of heartburn or dyspepsia, these symptoms return rapidly upon cessation of these types of medications. Thus, drugs that merely suppress stomach acid exert a "band-aid effect" because they do not go to the root cause of many digestive diseases. The vast majority of upper digestive discomfort is caused by adverse lifestyle, such as poor nutrition, the use of a variety of medications and substance abuse. Thus, common digestive disorders that do not involve serious forms of tissue inflammation or disease are better managed by simple, gentle, natural first-line options. This message is clear in "Gut Solutions."

The switching of H2 receptor antagonists from prescription to over-the-counter status triggered many questions about the effectiveness and safety of these drugs; and some of these questions remained unanswered. Recently, the self-treatment of digestive disease has been expanded by the availability of the drug omeprazole, which is a potent inhibitor of acid secretion by the stomach. Proponents of natural medicine are concerned about the elimination of acid from the stomach in terms of its potential negative impact on health and well-being in the long term.

Drugs that block acid secretion were initially labeled for short-term use, but patients now use them for extended periods of time. The ability of acid-suppressing drugs to cause rapid symptom relief in several upper digestive disorders is both a blessing and concern. Since many symptoms related to stomach hyperacidity are caused by poor lifestyle, the mere symptomatic improvement experienced with drugs can act as a way of reinforcing the adverse lifestyle that causes the problems in the first instance. For example, my colleagues and I estimated that as many as 45% of all males in North America, between the ages of 18 and 40 drank alcohol excessively, at one time or another. Many young people have learned that popping an OTC, acid-lowering drug can partially diminish the digestive components of a hangover. I present this as a common example of the misuse of medication in a manner that promotes unhealthy lifestyle.

This book "Gut Solutions" focuses on natural alternatives to standard drug treatments for digestive disorders. It is known that almost three-quarters of all digestive upset occur from digestive disorders not associated with severe disease, such as cancer or inflammation in the digestive tract. Many consumers are hoodwinked into believing that there is a "techno-fix" out there for many diseases, but this is self-styled deception. At best, many medicines are merely quick-fixes.

Marketing research of OTC and prescription drugs seems to indicate that it is symptom relief that drives the sales of medications. Incidentally, evidence suggests that quick-fixes drive the prescription of drugs by doctors. However, after awhile the quick-fix just won't satisfy the individual with a recurrent problem. The patient's inevitable disenchantment will drive him or her to look for alternative options that may help go to the root of the problem.

The increasing emergence of alternative and complementary medicine in the twenty-first century has more to do with health care consumers than with any revolution in thought among physicians. While alternative medicine remains somewhat lacking in research and development strategies, a practicing physician can expect that about two-thirds of his or her clientele will have used or sought non-conventional medical therapies. Given our increasing knowledge about the potential interactions between alternative and conventional medicine, a major dilemma presents itself in modern medicine.

This book is well written and up-to-date in its discussion of remedies of natural origin for digestive disorders. Many people with digestive upset will find simple answers to their problems within the pages of "Gut Solutions." I believe that the information provided within this book can enrich the doctor-patient relationship, and it takes a hard look at the value of natural medicine and lifestyle strategies in the management of digestive diseases. I commend the authors on their lucid delivery of complicated information that can help patients take control of their own health initiatives. We are experiencing a change in treatment paradigms where health care consumers are much more self-reliant and willing to engage preventive medicine. The quick stroke of the prescription pen and the flash of the surgeon's knife are less popular than they used to be, as we rediscover the secrets of natural medicine and traditional medical disciplines that have been overshadowed by the unfulfilled promises of the "pharmaceutical revolution."

Stephen Holt, MD, gastroenterologist, best selling author.

Author, "Natural Ways to Digestive Health", M. Evans Publishers, Inc., NY, NY, 2000; and "Digestion," Wellness Publishing, Newark, New Jersey, 2003

Table of Contents

Healthy Digestive System

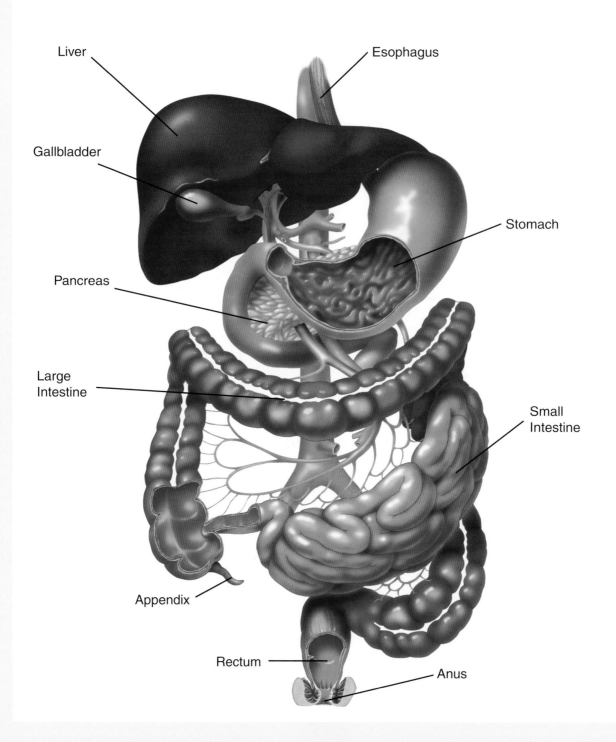

Liver

Esophagus

Gallbladder

Stomach

Pancreas

Large
Intestine

Small
Intestine

Appendix

Rectum

Anus

Unhealthy Digestive System

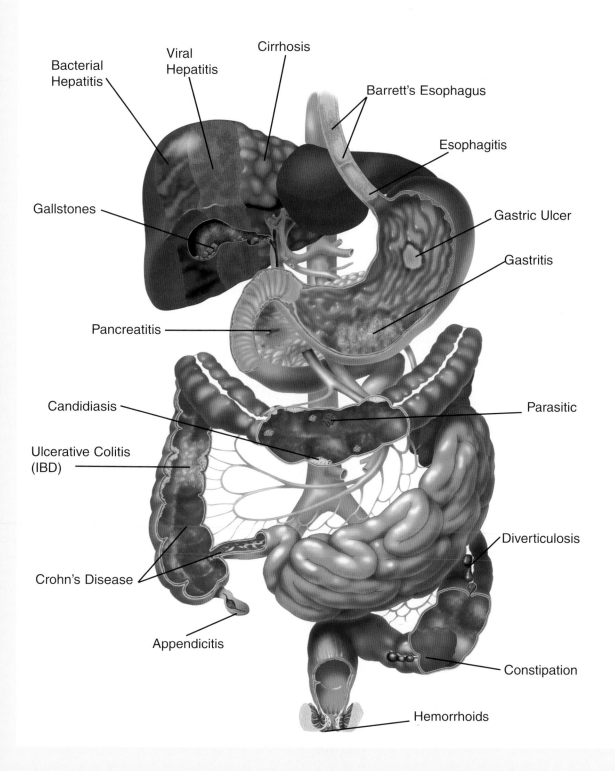

Gut Solutions Introduction

If you have bought this book because you are one of the millions of Americans with digestive problems, you're on the right track. You've made an intelligent choice to take control of your health and well being, and we're going to be with you every step of the way.

Digestive problems cost Americans more than $100 billion dollars annually. That is more money than we spend on books, movies, music and videos combined ($82 billion); it is more money than we spend on new automobiles ($65 billion); it is more money than we spend on vacations ($10 billion); it is more money than we spend on higher education or computers ($62 billion); it is even more money than we spend on weight loss ($33 billion)! What is more interesting is how we allocate expenditures on digestive care:

- $25 billion on physician visits
- $21 billion on medical procedures
- $10 billion on prescription medications
- $3 billion on over-the-counter medications
- $0.3 billion on dietary supplements

The media doesn't help. We are overwhelmed with TV commercials and magazine articles that urge us to see a physician for prescription drugs or to purchase over-the-counter medications for heartburn, gas, bloating, constipation and irritable bowel syndrome. There are certainly some acute and serious digestive conditions that require immediate medical attention. However, the reality is that most digestive problems are the result of a long term and chronic "poor digestive lifestyle." We do not wake up one day with heartburn. We do not "catch" constipation. These digestive problems are the result of years of digestive abuse. We eat too much, drink too much, fail to chew our foods thorough-

ly and do not eat high quality, properly combined foods. Prescription drugs and physician visits are often expensive and unnecessary options that we employ to mask the pain or other symptoms of our chronic digestive problems.

A good example of this is how we treat heartburn. If you have heartburn or gastro-esophageal reflux disease (GERD), it is likely that your physician will give you a drug (Nexium® or Prilosec®) to stop or reduce the secretion of hydrochloric acid in your stomach. The problem with this approach is that heartburn is common in people with *low* stomach acid production. In fact, low stomach acid can *cause* heartburn! Giving a person with low stomach acid a pill to further decrease stomach acid production may reduce the short-term symptoms of heartburn, but it can lead to long-term digestive problems. It is easy to take a pill to stop the pain of heartburn, but what are we doing to our digestive systems and our overall health when we disrupt our natural digestive processes? Unless your physician is giving you a hydrochloric acid challenge test, s/he cannot properly assess your acid production levels. You may say that your physician knows best. Well, if you had seen a physician for a peptic ulcer in 1985 s/he would likely have diagnosed the cause as over production of hydrochloric acid. Ten years later (in 1995), that same physician would most likely conclude that your ulcer is caused by H. pylori, a common bacterium that is easily, quickly and inexpensively treated.

The key point is that the human body is one big digestive machine. Our health and vitality are determined by how well that machine functions. If the engine of our car is running great, but we fill the fuel tank with sodas and beer, how long will it take for the car to start running badly? Not very long. If we go to a mechanic and he says, "Let's drop this pill in the gas tank every day," will this solve the problem? If the car does run better even though we continue to fill the tank with beer and sodas, have we really solved the long-term problem? Of course, not. In order to get the engine running properly without the necessity for pills, the engine needs to be cleaned and maintained with the proper fuel. The solution to chronic digestive problems ultimately can be found through an understanding of how our digestive systems were designed to function and by creating a healthy digestive lifestyle that maximizes our digestive processes.

The purpose of this book is to help all of you with digestive problems learn more about your particular condition and to provide you with information on the various therapeutic options available. The book is divided into five sections. The first section provides an overview on the properly functioning digestive system. The most common digestive problems are discussed in the next three sections (2, 3 and 4); these deal respectively with the three primary divisions of the digestive tract – esophagus, stomach, and intestines. Section 5 discusses the diseases of the accessory organs – liver, pancreas gallbladder. In each section, you will find these sub-sections:

- **What is it? (overview of the disease)**

- **What causes it?**

- **Who gets it?**

- **What are the signs and symptoms?**

- **How is it diagnosed?**

- **What is the standard medical treatment?**

- **Optional Nutritional Approaches, – natural therapies, diet & lifestyle and supplements**

With this information, you have the necessary data to fully understand the causes and therapeutic options available to assist in dealing with your particular digestive condition. You will be empowered to ask your physician intelligent and focused questions about your gut problems. You will have the option of trying diet and lifestyle changes before you are given a prescription or surgical procedure to treat your digestive disease. And finally, you will have the opportunity to make informed decisions and play an active role in your Gut Solutions.

Healthy regards,

Brenda Watson

Brenda Watson, N.D., C.T.
President of International Colon Therapy (IACT)

Some Basics

A QUICK TRIP DOWN THE DIGESTIVE TRACT

> **"The digestive system is like the roots of a tree. When the roots are diseased, the whole tree is affected. Nutrition, digestion, absorption, bacterial balance and intestinal permeability all play interdependent functions in the health of the gastrointestinal tract and the health of the whole body."**
>
> *Author Unknown*

The "gut" is also known as the gastrointestinal (GI) tract or the digestive tract. It is essentially a long tube made up of layers of muscle lined by cells and glands imbedded in a mucous lining. The job of the gut is to ingest food, digest and absorb it and to excrete waste products. The digestive system works hard. It is pressed into service every time we eat. In fact, over the course of a lifetime, it will digest some 23,000 pounds of solid food.[1]

There are numerous organs involved in the digestive process – mouth, esophagus, stomach, large and small intestines, anus, gallbladder, liver and pancreas. These last three organs are located outside the digestive "tube" or tract but none-the-less play an important role in digestion. Should something go wrong with any of the digestive organs, the process of digestion becomes impaired. Nutritional status and overall health are then adversely affected. This happens more often than we might suspect. More people are hospitalized for GI disorders than for any other,[2] and some 80 million Americans are reported to have digestive problems.[3]

In the process of digestion, food is converted into fuel to run the body. Large pieces of food are broken down physically (through chewing) and chemically (through enzyme activity) into microscopic particles so that they are small enough to cross the cell membranes of the gut and enter the bloodstream. Any glitch in the digestive conversion process short-circuits our energy supply and robs us of vitality.

Before looking at what can go wrong in the process, let's look at what a properly functioning system does and how it works.

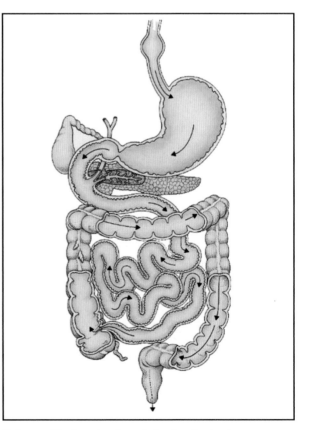

Pathway of food moving through the digestive tract

Peristalsis

From the time food is put into the mouth until its waste products are excreted, it is propelled through the body by a series of muscular contractions known as peristalsis. Along the way, digestive juices break down food products so that nutrients can enter and travel through the bloodstream.

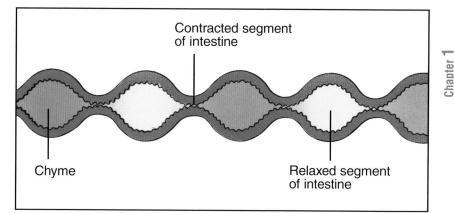

Intestinal Movement: *Short segments of the intestine contract for a few seconds, while others segments relax. This action mixes the chyme with digestive enzymes.*

Swallowed food is pushed by peristaltic waves into the esophagus, the tube that connects throat to stomach. When the food reaches the bottom of the esophagus, a ring-like valve, known as the lower esophageal sphincter (LES), opens to allow its passage. The LES is normally closed, but as food approaches, the surrounding muscles relax, allowing a temporary opening through which food may enter the stomach. As the LES opens, the muscle of the upper part of the stomach relaxes, permitting large volumes of food to enter. Here food is stored and broken down. In this way, the stomach acts like a large blender, churning and mixing food and liquid with its own digestive juices. Finally, the stomach empties its contents into the small intestine. By the time food enters the first section of the small intestine (the duodenum), it has already changed significantly. What enters the duodenum is called chyme, which is a mixture of food, hydrochloric acid (HCl) and mucus. The small intestine secretes digestive juices that act upon and dissolve the food once it enters the small intestine. The liver and pancreas also empty secretions into the small intestine to assist in digestion.

The next step is the absorption of digested nutrients through the wall of the small intestine into the bloodstream. That part of the food that is not digestible (fiber), along with worn out cells shed from the mucosa (mucus lining of the GI tract), constitute waste products. These products are propelled by peristalsis into the large intestine, colon, where they are dehydrated, turned into stool and expelled from the body in the form of a bowel movement.

In this sequence of events, we see the importance of peristalsis. The muscles in the GI tract work in harmony with hormones and nerves to control motility (spontaneous movement) throughout the digestive system. Most GI problems are functional (rather than structural) and involve defects in motility, absorption or secretion.[4]

Beneficial Bacteria

Trillions of bacteria, yeasts and parasites live in the intestines, primarily in the colon, where over 400 different species of microorganisms typically reside. In the healthy person, the bulk of intestinal bacteria will be of the beneficial variety – primarily Lactobacillus acidophilus and Bifido bifidus – with a minority being potentially pathogenic (disease-causing). An ideal ratio of "good/ neutral" to "bad" bacteria would be approximately 80% to 20%. In the presence of many digestive disorders, however, a state of dysbiosis exists, where this ratio is distorted, even reversed. Restoring the optimal bacterial balance in the GI tract is vital to full recovery of health.

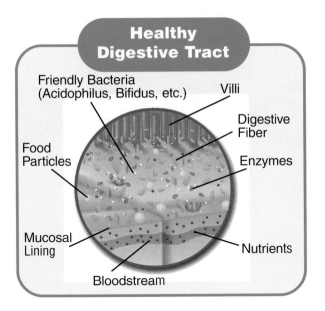

Healthy Digestive Tract

Friendly Bacteria
(Acidophilus, Bifidus, etc.)

Villi

Food
Particles

Digestive
Fiber

Enzymes

Mucosal
Lining

Nutrients

Bloodstream

Beneficial bacteria in the GI tract serve many vital functions. In the colon, they produce certain B vitamins, including B12 and biotin, as well as vitamin K. They also control the growth of harmful microorganisms, break down toxins and stimulate the immune system. Additionally, bacteria ferment dietary fiber into short-chain fatty acids, which have a healing effect on the intestine.

Secretion

Glands in the GI tract produce digestive juices that break food down into its component parts (fat into fatty acids, protein into amino acids and carbohydrates into simple sugars). These same glands produce hormones that assist in controlling the digestive process. We'll cover hormones shortly, but for now will focus on the digestive secretions. These secretions begin in the mouth where saliva is produced by the salivary glands. These glands contain the enzyme amylase, which begins to break down starch. Thus the digestive process begins in the mouth. Actually, it begins before food enters the mouth. You've heard the term "mouth watering"? It relates to a very real physiological reaction, because the very thought of food is sufficient to trigger salivary gland activity.

Glands in the stomach lining produce hydrochloric acid (HCl) and the enzyme pepsin. Both of these secretions are essential for protein digestion.

Secretions from the pancreas and the liver act upon ingested food once it enters the small intestine. Pancreatic juice contains enzymes that will break down fats (the enzyme lipase), carbohydrates (amylase) and proteins (protease). The small intestine itself secretes juices (from glands inside its walls) that assist in the digestive process. The liver produces bile, a digestive secretion that is stored in the gallbladder. When food is eaten, the bile is released from the gallbladder into the small intestine (via bile ducts) where it emulsifies or

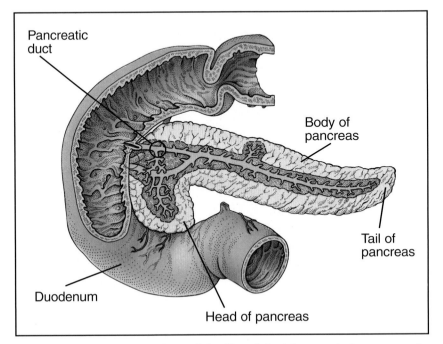

Pancreatic
duct

Body of
pancreas

Tail of
pancreas

Duodenum

Head of pancreas

Pancreas: *The pancreas is an elongated gland lying behind the stomach. In response to the entry of food into the upper digestive tract, the pancreas secretes digestive juice containing enzymes that break down fats, nucleic acids, proteins and carbohydrates. The juice also contains sodium bicarbonate to neutralize stomach acid. The enzymes are secreted into ducts that converge to form the pancreatic duct, which transports the enzymes to the duodenum.*

dissolves fat. The fat is then digested by pancreatic enzymes and enzymes that line the intestine.

Absorption

Absorption takes place in the small intestine. Here macronutrients (fats, carbohydrates and protein) are broken down into smaller units and then carried throughout the body along with micronutrients (water, vitamins and minerals) via the bloodstream. These materials will either be stored for later use or undergo further chemical change.

The surface of the duodenum, the first section of the small intestine, is smooth for the first few inches, but quickly changes to a surface with many folds and small finger-like projections called villi and microvilli. These threadlike projections cover the surface of the mucous membrane lining the small intestine and serve as the site of absorption of fluids and nutrients, actually sucking up small particles of digested food.

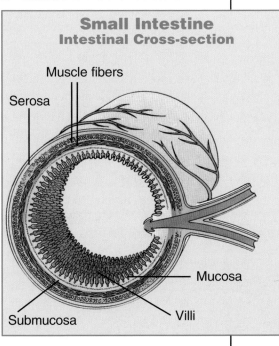

Small Intestine
Intestinal Cross-section

Muscle fibers

Serosa

Mucosa

Submucosa

Villi

The walls of the small intestine consist of four layers of muscle. The innermost layer of the small intestine is called the mucosa. This mucous lining serves two vital functions: It allows nutrients of the proper size to pass through and to enter the bloodstream, and it blocks the passage of undigested food particles, pathogens and toxins into the bloodstream. The surface of the mucosa is thick and slippery. Much of the mucus here consists of

the amino sugar N-acetyl-glucosamine (NAG), which the body makes from L-glutamine, one of its most abundant amino acids. An adequate amount of glutamine must be present in the body to manufacture NAG (N-aceytl-glucosamine), which is vital to the health of the mucosa.

The mucosa is normally shed and rebuilt every

three to five days. In the presence of some inflammatory bowel conditions, it appears to be sloughed off at a higher rate, however, possibly due to an inability of the body to convert L-glutamine to NAG.

Hormones

Hormones within the digestive system control its functions by regulating secretions and movement of digestive organs. Cells within the mucosa of the stomach and small intestine produce and release the major hormones that control GI activity. These hormones, their sources and functions[5] are:

Gastrin – released by the antral cells in the stomach:

• Strongly stimulates stomach to produce HCl (regulates its release from parietal cells in stomach)
• Strongly stimulates stomach to produce pepsin
• Weakly stimulates secretion of pancreatic enzymes
• Weakly stimulates gallbladder contraction
• Stimulates secretion of histamine by special cells (ECL cells) in the stomach lining
• Controls gastric motility

Secretin – secreted by mucosa in the upper two thirds of the small intestine in response to the presence of acid chyme:

• Stimulates secretion of bicarbonate-containing pancreatic juice
• Stimulates, to a

lesser extent, bile and intestinal secretion

Cholecystokinin (CCK) – secreted by the small intestine:

• Stimulates gallbladder contraction
• Stimulates secretion of pancreatic enzymes

The Two Nervous Systems

While the digestive process is under the control of the hormonal system, hormone release is under the control of the nervous system. We're all familiar with the central nervous system (CNS), made up of the brain and spinal column. Not so familiar to most is the enteric nervous system (ENS). The word "enteric" means "pertaining to the small intestine," and you might be surprised to know that half of the body's nerve cells are located in the gut.[6]

The central nervous system and the enteric nervous system connect through the vagus nerve, which is the longest of the cranial nerves. There is therefore a direct and literal brain-gut connection. Or, we might say that the gut has a mind of its own. The ENS is the gut's brain, and it runs the length of the GI tract.

Much of what we know about "the second brain" was revealed by Dr. Michael Gershon in his 1998 book of the same name. Gershon, a professor of anatomy and cell biology at Columbia Presbyterian Medical

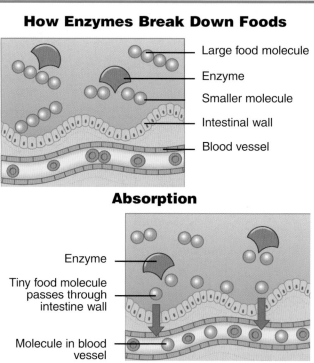

How Enzymes Break Down Foods

— Large food molecule
— Enzyme
— Smaller molecule
— Intestinal wall
— Blood vessel

Absorption

Enzyme
Tiny food molecule passes through intestine wall
Molecule in blood vessel

Center in New York City, proposed in the 1960s that the neurotransmitter serotonin was produced in and targeted to the ENS. (A neurotransmitter is a chemical substance – that facilitates communication among nerve cells, as well as from nerves to muscles, glands and vessels.[7])

It has since been verified that not only is serotonin found in the ENS, but that every class of neurotransmitter found in the brain is also found in the ENS.[8] Interestingly, we have more nerve cells in the bowel than in the spine![9] Additionally, the gut has approximately the same number of neurotransmitters as the brain – some hundred million.[10] Major cells of the immune system are also found in the gut, as well as a couple of dozen neuropeptides (small brain proteins).[11] All this new information about the gut-brain connection is profoundly altering our understanding of how the digestive system works.

There are two types of nerves that control all activity in the digestive system. They are extrinsic and intrinsic nerves. The extrinsic nerves enter the digestive organs from the outside, from the spinal cord or from the brain, while the intrinsic nerves are embedded in the walls of the digestive organs and so are inherent within the ENS. The extrinsic nerves release the neurotransmitters acetylcholine and adrenaline that cause the muscles of the digestive organs to contract and relax respectively (peristalsis). The intrinsic nerves go into action when food enters the digestive organs. They release a variety of substances to regulate the speed

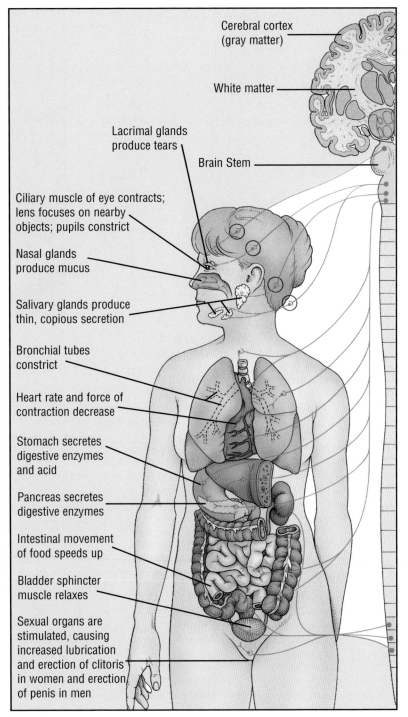

Cerebral cortex (gray matter)

White matter

Lacrimal glands produce tears

Brain Stem

Ciliary muscle of eye contracts; lens focuses on nearby objects; pupils constrict

Nasal glands produce mucus

Salivary glands produce thin, copious secretion

Bronchial tubes constrict

Heart rate and force of contraction decrease

Stomach secretes digestive enzymes and acid

Pancreas secretes digestive enzymes

Intestinal movement of food speeds up

Bladder sphincter muscle relaxes

Sexual organs are stimulated, causing increased lubrication and erection of clitoris in women and erection of penis in men

Parasympathetic nerves: *The parasympathetic division of the autonomic nervous system (ANS) usually has an opposing effect to the sympathetic division. It operates mainly in quiet, non-stressful conditions, and its activity predominates during sleep. The parasympathetic nerves arise in the brain stem and the lower spinal cord, and their axions are very long.*

with which food moves through the system and the production of digestive juices.

The Mind-Gut Connection

As stated, we know today that there is a "brain," or inherent nervous system, in the bowel. This nervous system is able to mediate reflexes in the digestive system without input from the brain or spinal cord. As a result, the "nervous system in the gut" is able to accomplish some very important jobs without conscious thought. One such job is warning us when our digestive systems are in trouble. Most people know something is wrong in the gut when they experience such symptoms as pain, heartburn, gas or diarrhea; these are the gut's way of making us aware that we do have feelings there and that something is amiss.

As many studies have shown, stress, anger and fear have a profound effect upon the digestive tract – even a greater effect, in fact, than food. It is of utmost importance that we get in touch with our "gut feelings" and sort these feelings out as part of the process of healing. If there are unresolved conflicts with relationships, enduring sorrow from loss of loved ones or residual effects of childhood traumas, these hidden issues can have a negative effect on our health. This often creates digestive problems.

Many people turn to traditional medicine when they begin to experience digestive problems. Unfortunately, traditional medicine is split into specialties. Specialists often do not treat the body as a whole as most holistic practitioners do. It is often necessary to look at the whole person when dealing with digestive problems; this includes consideration of the emotional and mental state of the individual. Many doctors address patients' gut problems by prescribing drugs. Often, these drugs create more problems than they solve. I believe drugs serve a constructive purpose when there is an acute problem, but most GI problems are chronic in nature and can be best solved with a non-drug approach.

Traditional doctors should consider the emotional and mental state of their patients that suffer from

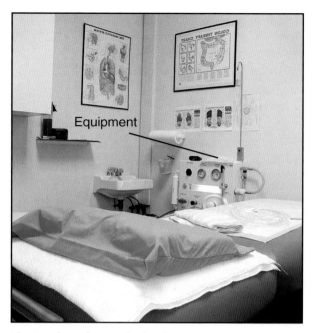

Equipment

This is a photo of a typical colon therapy room.

intestinal problems.

In my work as a colon hydrotherapist with thousands of clients over the years, I found many with emotional/gut issues. It was quite common for people to come for colon therapy and not be at all in touch with their "gut feelings." After having a few sessions of colon therapy, many would begin to process unpleasant experiences or emotions.

In the following case studies we'll look at two specific instances of emotional distress impacting digestive health. These represent only a small fraction of the patients I've seen over the years.

John

John came into the clinic one day to "experience cleansing." He had heard about it but had never had the opportunity to undergo colon therapy. John wrote on the intake form that he had irritable bowel. As we began the first therapy session, he had a lot of spasms as water was leaving the colon. It was uncomfortable, but he was enthusiastic about coming back for a second treatment. During the second session, John began to talk about his mother. His mother had committed suicide. This had no doubt hurt John immensely, and as he talked during this session and subsequent sessions, he realized that he felt responsible for her actions and had actually taken on a lot of guilt over the situation. As John went through this cleansing process, the colon therapy treatment ceased to be uncomfortable, and he realized his "irritable bowel" was due to his emotional state surrounding his mother's suicide. Imagine the breakthrough and healing John experienced by unpacking the "emotional baggage" that was the cause of most of his bowel problems!

Jill

Jill was in her thirties. She had suffered from constipation most of her life. She had a very good job, one that put her on the road a good deal of the time. But Jill could not have a bowel movement unless she was at home. This meant she went for days, and sometimes a week at a time, without bowel movements. Jill came in for colon therapy because of her constipation. Over a period of a few months, Jill became more comfortable and started to talk a lot about her childhood during her sessions. As it unfolded, Jill's mother had an obsession with cleanliness. During Jill's childhood, when the family traveled and stopped to use the restroom at a service station or rest stop, her mother would line the floors and toilet with paper towels. Jill became terrified of germs and, as a result, developed constipation that carried over into adulthood.

Over and over again, I saw real healing take place as people looked beyond diet and supplementation to handle their digestive problems. The truth is, if you are experiencing any of the conditions we address in this book, you must discover the underlying emotional, psychological or spiritual issues. The following affirmations written by one of my teachers, Bernard Jensen, can help in this regard:

• We are living in a world of cause and effect. I myself set up the causes, by thinking good or bad, for the things that happen to me. The result is that I live in cause and not effect.
• Through negative thinking, I force the power within to work against me; therefore, I will think positively.
• In each different situation, I look for new positive ideas, constructive possibilities, people who can be helpful and enterprises with new vistas.
• Success, health and happiness lie within me; they do not come from the outside.
• In each situation, I will search for positive thoughts as I would search for the pearls of a broken necklace.
• From now on, I take one step at a time.
• To all difficulties, I respond with indifference, courage and self-confidence.
• My life is what my thoughts make it.
• When I am kind to others, I am the best to myself.
• I nurture my mind with great thoughts because to believe in the heroic makes heroes.
• I will be true to myself that others may know me just as I am and know all that it is possible for me to be.
• To love others as myself is to accept them as they are, to receive them without resentment and to so live in such a way that all my actions reflect harmony, happiness, joy and serenity – in my own body and in everyone I meet.

In summary, the responsibility resides within each of us to find the right balance and work through our issues, past and present, so that we may experience good health. This requires getting in touch with ourselves and developing awareness about how stress affects us and how to begin to effectively handle it rather than letting it handle us. We will then listen to our "gut feelings" as a positive guide to lead us through life's many trials and tribulations.

Dr. Smith's Comments

Virtually every illness in the body has some psycho-emotional elements. This certainly includes the intestinal tract, ranging from swallowing difficulties,

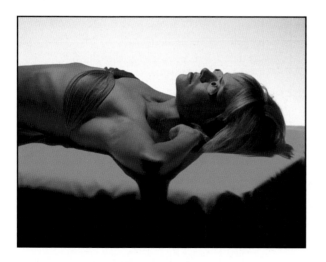

psychogenic vomiting and abdominal pain, to IBS, diarrhea and hemorrhoids. The treatment for stress of the GI tract is basically the same as for the entire body. It requires employing some new strategies and having a major shift in how we perceive our world.

One of the past presidents of the American Medical Association, in a speech years ago, stated a fundamentally important question for humankind to consider, "Is the Universe a friendly place for us to be or not?" He went on to point out that humans need not only purpose in life, but a sense of peace, security and order to deal with the challenges and stress of life. Another physician pointed out that time urgency may well be the basis of most, if not all, illnesses.

Living by the clock, meeting deadlines (this word says it all), running out of hours before the tasks are done: these are major causes of underlying chronic stress that ultimately can cause physiologic derangement and earn one a label (disease) that takes him or her into the "healthcare" system. It would be more appropriate to call it, a "sickness care" system. Few would question that we have the best "sickness care" system in the world. However, it is now time for professions dealing with health to learn more about lifestyle changes, diet and nutrition, and stress reduction and share these concepts with their patients. This is not new. Dr. Charles Mayo, at the turn of the century, stated that the physicians' real purpose was to educate their patients about health and how to eliminate the need for doctors!

Since stress seems to be the central theme to illness, it is worth pointing out some of the methods of managing it:

• Time management and learning to say "no"
• Eight to nine hours of sleep most nights and catch up on weekends, if needed
• Exercise – aerobic (30-60 minutes), five days/week; resistence training or Pilates, three times/week
• Hatha yoga, tai chi and swimming or water aerobics to balance the aerobic and resistence training, two to three times per week
• Spiritual rejuvenation of your choice, could include singing and dancing
• Meditation of your choice; according to research, the best physiologic benefits come from spending about 20 minutes twice each day in meditation, and then consciously attempting to hold the feeling of peace and joy throughout the day.

Meditation has been shown to rebalance the autonomic nervous system. With meditation, the overstimulated life with attention directed outward, becomes more inwardly centered, coherent, focused and peaceful. There can be an inner body awareness with joy in the midst of outward worldly activity. Various meditation programs have documented significant improvement in many common illnesses with regular practice.

We will mention here some of the salient features found in different meditation programs:

• Sit comfortably in a chair, with your back erect, legs uncrossed and feet flat on the floor. This tends to prevent falling asleep. It is not bad if you fall asleep; we would call that a nap. Attempting to meditate is the major diagnostic test for sleep deprivation. After the nap, if there is time, attempt again to meditate.
• Breathe slowly in through your nostrils into your abdomen (if need be, place your hands over your abdomen to see if it is expanding on inhalation). Take about 4 seconds to breathe in; hold it for 1-2 seconds, and let it out for another 4 seconds; hold it out for 1-2 seconds, and then start the cycle over.

Each in/out cycle takes about 10-12 seconds; this drops your normal unconscious breathing from 12-18 breaths/minute to 5-6 breaths/minute. Your brain tends to entrain on your slow deep breathing. It shifts from an outward oriented thinking form of consciousness known as a Beta rhythm, which is 13-30 cycles per second (cps), to an inner, still, feeling form of consciousness which is alpha (7-12 cps). In alpha, you can be in the present moment with minimal (if any) thoughts, just observing your breathing pattern.

- *Since stopping thought is a challenge, some recommend visualizing light or divine energy coming in on the in breath, and allowing any accumulated negative energy to leave on the outbreath. Alternatively, if thinking comes up, choose to focus on an "attitude of gratitude" for all of your blessings in life.*

- *As you watch the breath (and/or light) going in and out, become aware of the entire inner energy field of the body. Feel it; don't think about it. This will help reclaim conscious awareness from the always thinking mind. This technique is beautifully described in Eckhart Tolle's book Practicing the Power of Now pages 61-64. I highly recommend this to anyone.*

- *At times, with practice, as you go deeper into a state of stillness, thought stops, and the perception of time changes radically. You may think you have been sitting still for 20 minutes, only to find you have been there for over an hour! Yet, you did not sleep. This is considered by many to be the true state of meditation; you are neither sleeping, dreaming or thinking (some traditions call it Turiya, fourth state of consciousness). It is the state of present moment, choiceless awareness, or being. Isn't it strange we call ourselves human beings and yet spend so little time just being? Often feelings of joy or bliss arise from this state of expanded consciousness*

For those who are interested, this type of meditation works well with the Freeze-Framer™ technology (see biofeedback in the appendix). It is a nice way to monitor the inner body awareness that arises from this practice. Regularity is the key. With time, most stress-related conditions in the body including IBS, may improve.

What Can Go Wrong?

With aging there is a tendency for the metabolism to slow down, meaning that food is converted to energy more slowly. Enzyme production decreases with age. So does HCl production. This leads to a decrease in digestive efficiency and nutrient absorption, resulting in sluggish body functions, including digestion and elimination.

Apart from the aging process, digestion can become impaired as a result of such factors as stress, processed food consumption (which leads to nutritional deficiency), inadequate chewing, intake of fluids with meals (which dilutes digestive juices) and over-eating. When gut bacteria act upon undigested food in the intestine, toxic chemicals and gases are produced. These internally produced toxins (endotoxins) can damage the mucosal lining, increasing its permeability. Consequently, the gut will "leak," permitting toxins to enter the bloodstream. These toxins tend to settle in organs of greatest weakness, causing disease. Intestinal toxins also produce renegade chemical fragments known as "free radicals." These molecules with unpaired electrons can get the upper hand and cause toxic damage if the body is lacking in sufficient antioxidants to buffer them. The major antioxidant nutrients, vitamins A, C and E and the minerals selenium and zinc, serve as free radical scavengers. A steady diet of processed foods will create a deficiency of antioxidant (and other) nutrients. Such a diet will also provide inadequate fiber, needed by the body to absorb toxins, reduce cholesterol, increase short-chain fatty acid production and combat constipation by reducing bowel transit time, the amount of time it takes for food to pass through the body.

A toxic environment in the bowel makes it difficult for beneficial bacteria to survive. Dysbiosis sets in when the pathogenic bacteria gain the upper hand. With this condition, the stage is set for the development of parasite problems and/or proliferation of normally harmless organisms such as the yeast Candida albicans. In its fungal state, Candida grows very long roots, known as rhizoids, which actually puncture the mucous lining of the intestine, increasing the "leakiness" of the gut. A build up of toxicity results in a decrease of enzyme production by the pancreas and intestine, which in turn further impairs digestion. A vicious cycle sets in, where toxicity leads to overgrowth of pathogens, which enhances the absorption of yeast toxins and increases the "leakiness" of the gut.

As the body burden of toxins builds up, an increased load is placed on the organs of elimination – the liver, colon, kidneys, lungs and skin. We make the problem worse when we routinely ingest processed foods, junk food, alcohol, prescription drugs and over-the-counter medications and when our exposure to environmental toxins (exotoxins), such as chemicals and heavy metals, is high. Many commonly used household and personal care items have a high degree of toxicity and will add to the problem. Additionally, the mouth, the upper end of the digestive tract, frequently harbors heavy metals in the form of dental restorations and toxicity as a result of invasive dental treatments.

The bottom line is that many of us unknowingly lead a toxic lifestyle, which makes it very difficult to recover from digestive (and other) disorders that invariably have a strong toxic component to them. Toxicity, from the natural healing perspective, is the basic cause of disease. It makes sense therefore that the first step toward wellness would be detoxification.

Symptoms of Digestive Dysfunction

It is a tribute to the strength and resiliency of the human body that it can often endure years of toxic abuse before breaking down. Many who consider themselves to be in good health are, in fact, accidents waiting to happen. The deterioration of the digestive system can occur silently for some years, producing no symptoms or only minor, non-specific ones. Headaches, reduced energy,

lowered resistance to infections, gas, bloating, constipation and indigestion – these can be a prelude to the onset of chronic degenerative disease, which has its roots in the toxicity produced by digestive dysfunction.

As this dysfunction progresses and the GI tract continues to deteriorate, more serious problems may appear – anything from allergies to cancer. Autoimmune diseases such as rheumatoid arthritis, scleroderma and lupus have been linked to digestive dysfunction. Chronic digestive problems can take the form of irritable bowel syndrome or the more serious inflammatory bowel diseases, Crohn's disease and ulcerative colitis. Since the skin is a major organ of elimination, chronic skin conditions like psoriasis and eczema can result from faulty GI function. In fact, virtually any chronic disease can have its roots in poor digestion and absorption of nutrients, increased intestinal permeability and dysbiosis, the hallmarks of digestive dysfunction.

Restoration of Normal Function

Subsequent chapters will deal with specific gastrointestinal disorders and offer natural solutions. What is good for one person with one disorder may not be good for another person with another (or even the same) disorder. While it is important to tailor your health regimen to your individual needs, there is some degree of generalization possible with regard to digestive health. What follows are some general guidelines for keeping the GI tract in good health or restoring it to good health:

- Eat a well balanced diet of whole, natural, unprocessed food, preferably organic (grown without chemical fertilizers and pesticides).
- Avoid large meals.
- Avoid eating two to three hours before going to bed.
- Identify and eliminate foods to which you're allergic (see Resource Directory for information on sources for allergy testing).
- Exercise on a regular basis.

- Minimize (or eliminate) use of alcohol and caffeine.
- Take prescription drugs only as directed by your physician. Do not discontinue them without his or her consent and supervision.
- Use over-the-counter drugs with care if at all.
- Consider herbal alternatives.
- Chew thoroughly.
- Avoid drinking beverages with meals.
- Avoid carbonated drinks.
- Avoid icy cold beverages. Room temperature water is preferred.
- Avoid eating starchy carbohydrates (like bread and pasta) at the same meal with proteins (like meat and eggs).
- Do not eat fruit at the same time that other foods are eaten.
- Avoid the use of sugar and artificial sweeteners.
- Rest after meals whenever possible (to aid absorption).
- Get adequate rest at night, preferably 8 hours of sleep.
- Do not eat when upset.
- Minimize stress in your life.
- Drink 1/2 oz. of water for every pound of body weight. (Divide your weight in half, and drink that many ounces of water daily.)
- Use appropriate herbal formulas to cleanse and support digestive organs.
- Take enzymes (and HCl, if stomach acid is low) with each meal to improve digestion.
- For most digestive problems, follow the anti-Candida diet (see Candida section, chapter 4) for a minimum of one to three months.
- Reduce or eliminate exposure to environmental toxins.

Dr. Smith's Comments

Most people, including health care practitioners, are not aware of how critical it is to manage the bacteria living in your intestinal ecosystem. This is definitely not a new concept. Ancient records from Iraq from 3200 years ago indicated that fermented milk and cheese were used in the human diet. Dr. Eli Metchnikoff, who won a Nobel Prize in 1908, postulated in 1904 that friendly bacteria may be essential to human health and longevity. One hundred years later, modern day research is about to prove him correct. Throughout the cultures of the world, fermented foods such as dairy, vegetables and meat have been a mainstay of the diet. This has largely changed due to refrigeration. Before refrigeration, managing bacteria was a matter of life and death – either put the safe bacteria in the food or the disease-producing ones could kill you. I actually think this is still true today despite our improved hygiene and refrigeration.

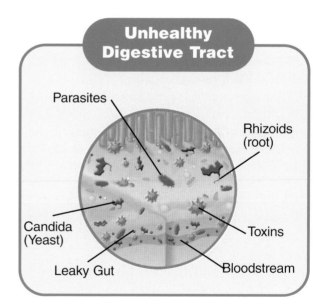

Unhealthy Digestive Tract

Parasites

Rhizoids (root)

Candida (Yeast)

Toxins

Leaky Gut

Bloodstream

There are major negative effects of not so friendly bacteria in the human intestinal tract, which have far reaching consequences. These effects are largely due to high enzyme activity of the 500 species of bacteria, 90% of which live without much oxygen (anaerobic). This is what they do:

- Deactivate enzymes made in the pancreas like trypsin and chymotrypsin (needed to digest protein)
- Consume the vitamin B12 that is in our diet
- Produce ammonia, increasing the work on the liver and kidneys
- Inactivate intestinal brush border enzymes, such as disaccaridases (that digest sugars)
- Inactivate dietary antioxidants such as flavonoids
- Destroy essential fatty acids and make them free radicals, so an essential food now becomes a poison
- Degrade the protective mucus of the intestinal lining
- Produce carcinogens (cancer producing chemicals) from ingested food
- Eat your nutrients and then produce toxins that damage the lining and cause it to leak, which creates immune imbalance, leading to autoimmune diseases like lupus and arthritis
- Produce enzymes that affect normal metabolism of hormones like estrogen; this allows estrogen, which was packaged and ready to leave the body, to be resorbed and create high estrogen levels that can lead to fibrocystic disease and cancer.
- Enter the circulation from the GI tract and travel via the blood to areas that are damaged such as wounds and injuries; in addition, the bacteria can take up residence in the lungs and urine and cause infections there as well.

These are a just some of the problems created by bad bacteria. Actually, most of this can be prevented by regular use of fermented foods with live cultures of various strains of Lactobacilli and Bifidobacteria. Supplementation here is important, as you will see throughout the book. I personally feel if a person could only take one supplement, it should be a good combination of the beneficial bacteria.

The following is the **HOPE** we can give people to keep their digestive systems well-functioning. This is recommended as a maintenance protocol for everyone:

High Fiber

Oils - Essential Fatty Acids, Flax, Fish and Borage

Probiotics - Good Bacteria

Enzymes - Taken with Meals

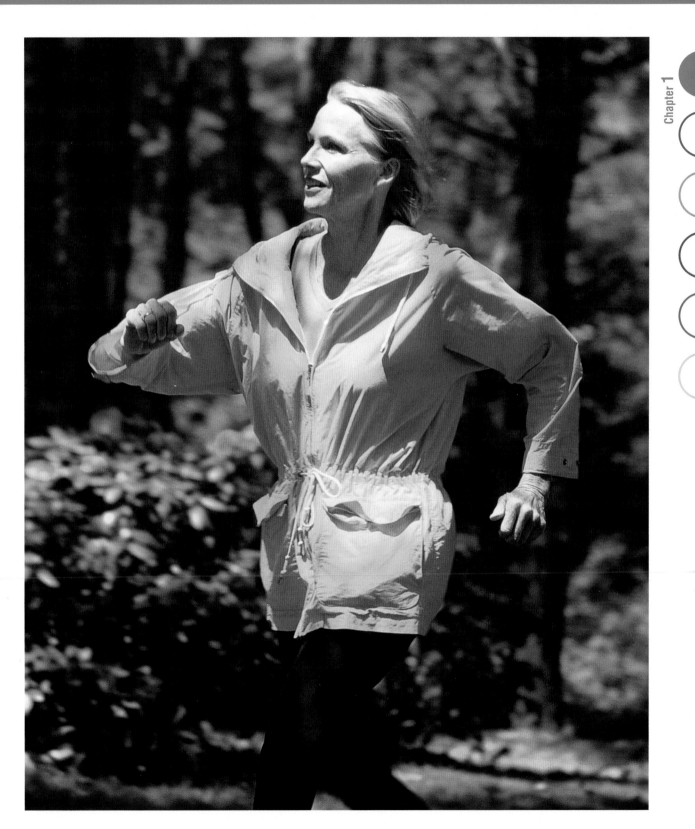

Esophageal Problems

Barrett's esophagus is three times more prevalent in males than females and predominantly affects white males with a history of chronic heartburn or GERD.

Source:
www.barrettsinfo.com

BARRETT'S ESOPHAGUS

What is it?

The esophagus is the tube that connects your throat to your stomach. Barrett's esophagus is a condition characterized by abnormal cell growth in the esophagus, marked by a dramatic discoloration of the esophagheal tissue. The lining of the esophagus is normally pinkish white but the abnormal cells of Barrett's esophagus are reddish in color. This discoloration occurs when the normal squamous (flat) cells of the esophagus are transformed into columns of cells, which can produce mucus. Three types of columnar cells have been identified. Two resemble normal stomach tissue, and the third – known as specialized intestinal metaplasia – is believed to have malignant potential. Only microscopic analysis can distinguish true Barrett's esophagus tissue from stomach lining tissue. The abnormal (Barrett's) esophageal tissue is considered to be premalignant, which is to suggest that it may develop into cancer. Patients suffering from Barrett's have a 30 to 40 fold increased risk of developing esophageal adenocarcinoma, a cancer of the lower esophagus, as compared to the general population.[1] But most patients with Barrett's will not develop cancer as a result of this disorder. Autopsies of Barrett's esophagus patients have shown that most never developed cancer, and death was attributable to other causes.[2]

What Causes it?

The presence of abnormal red tissue (Barrett's tissue) in the lining of the esophagus appears to be largely the result of stomach acid, bile, food and bacteria, all rising into the esophagus over a prolonged period of time. This abnormal "reflux," or backflow, of corrosive material from the stomach into the esophagus is characteristic of gastroesophageal reflux disease (GERD). The most common symptom of GERD is heartburn or a burning sensation that can extend from the upper abdomen behind the breastbone up into the back of the throat. After years of acid irritation, the injured cells of the esophagus lining can fail to grow back normally. Instead, they are replaced by

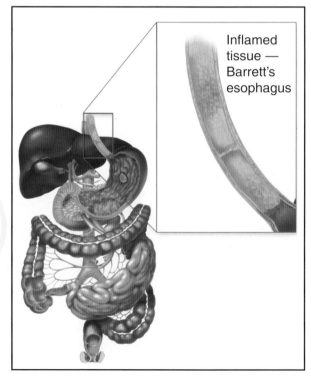

Inflamed tissue — Barrett's esophagus

the abnormal lining known as Barrett's esophagus. People who have heartburn get Barrett's esophagus three to five times more often than those without heartburn.[3]

Though long-standing acid reflux is the most prevalent cause of Barrett's esophagus, in some rare cases, the disease may be congenital (present at birth).[4] About one in ten patients with GERD are also found to have Barrett's esophagus.[5] No one knows why some GERD patients develop Barrett's esophagus and others do not. However, it seems likely that healthy functioning esophageal cells are an important factor. Intracellular nutrition, including hydration, acid-base balance, oxygenation, antioxidant levels, with optimum mitochondrial (energy-generating) function, will help to produce high quality mucus, which minimizes cellular transformation. GERD develops when the valve connecting stomach to esophagus (the lower esophageal sphincter, LES) weakens and fails to prevent backflow of stomach contents. Causes of this weakening are discussed in the GERD section of Chapter 2. The presence of stomach lining tissue along with Barrett's tissue in the esophagus appears to serve the purpose of helping to protect the esophagus from ongoing assault from gastric reflux. This may be the reason why GERD symptoms sometimes diminish in Barrett's esophagus patients. This is an example of physiologic adaptation: If the esophagus repeatedly receives stomach contents, it will begin to make more mucus and thus in some ways perform as a stomach.

Who Gets it?

Anyone with a long history of heartburn or GERD is at risk for developing Barrett's esophagus, which may progress to malignancy. However, as many as 40% of patients who are diagnosed with esophageal adenocarcinoma deny having typical symptoms of heartburn such as burning chest pain or regurgitation of acid.[6]

Barrett's esophagus is three times more prevalent in males than females[7] and predominantly affects

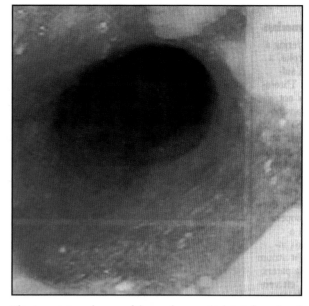

This is an internal scope of the esophagus, which is inflamed and has Barrett's esophagus.

white males[8] with a history of chronic heartburn or GERD. This fact puts white males at highest risk for development of esophageal adenocarcinoma, though the incidence of this cancer among white females has risen dramatically over the last three decades. Children rarely develop this condition. In fact, the average age at diagnosis of Barrett's esophagus is 60,[9] and one study found that Barrett's esophagus was twice as likely to be present in a patient in his 70s as compared to a patient 40 years of age or less.[10]

Risk factors for development of Barrett's esophagus include obesity, age and to a lesser and less certain degree, family history.[11] Studies indicate that a high-fat diet may also be a risk factor.[12] Increased fat deposits in the abdominal area are thought to increase pressure on the stomach, especially when lying down. As to family history, findings are inconclusive and indicate that family members of patients with Barrett's esophagus or esophageal adenocarcinoma, may be at greater risk for developing these diseases if they have a history of chronic heartburn as compared to others with

GERD-like Symptoms

- Difficulty swallowing solid foods
- A burning sensation or feeling of pressure as food travels down the esophagus
- Peristant heartburn
- Vomiting or choking
- Blood in stool or vomit
- Weight loss
- Nocturnal regurgitation that disturbs sleep

GERD.[13] See sections on GERD and heartburn for information on risk factors associated with these disorders.

What are the Signs and Symptoms?

Patients suffering from Barrett's esophagus typically suffer from GERD-like symptoms, which may include[14]:

- Heartburn (pyrosis) 70-85%
- Regurgitation – 60%
- Angina-like chest pain – 33%
- Asthma – 15-20%
- Laryngitis
- Chronic cough
- Sleep disturbance
- Loss of dental enamel
- Vomiting and weight loss

Some Barrett's patients may also suffer from other complications of GERD such as esophageal peptic ulcers, and stricture – a narrowing of the esophagus that comes from scarring,[15] – which may give rise to dysphasia (food getting stuck in the esophagus).

How is it Diagnosed?

Barrett's esophagus cannot be diagnosed solely on the basis of symptoms, as the above symptoms may have other causes. A definitive medical diagnosis can only be made through application of a special procedure called esophagogastroduodenoscopy (EGD) or upper endoscopy with biopsy. This procedure is described in the appendix of this book. If the esophagus, which is normally pinkish-white, is lined with red, Barrett's esophagus is suspected. With the aid of the endoscope, the doctor can then take a tissue sample (a biopsy) that will later be examined for the purpose of confirming the diagnosis. In addition, the endoscope may be used to stop the bleeding of an ulcer. It has been recommended that patients who have a history of GERD for at least five years and are age 50 or older should undergo upper endoscopy to look for Barrett's esophagus.[16]

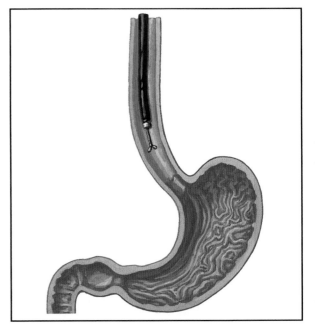

This is an example of an upper endoscopy.

What is the Standard Medical Treatment?

There is no actual cure for Barrett's esophagus short of surgical removal of the esophagus (an esophagectomy) in part or in full. An

Chapter **2**

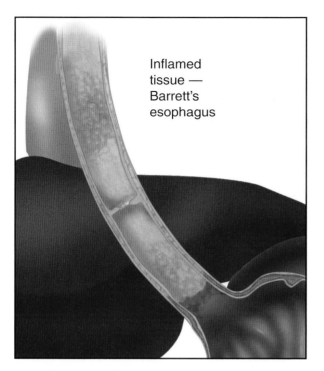

Inflamed tissue — Barrett's esophagus

Area of Barrett's esophagus

esophagectomy is a high-risk surgery with a high mortality rate, so this radical procedure is generally reserved for cancer patients and those with high-grade dysplasia (pre-cancerous cell changes).

One internet site (www.pslgroup.com) describes a new non-surgical treatment for Barrett's esophagus called Photodynamic Therapy (PDT). This procedure involves the use of a photosensitizing drug called "PHOTOFRIN®" and an argon dye laser. First, endoscopic biopsies are done to confirm the diagnosis of Barrett's esophageal tissue. Then, a photosensitizing drug is injected into the body through a vein, where it concentrates in the dysplastic (pre-cancerous) and cancerous tissue. Two to three days later, a specially designed balloon, placed next to the endoscope, delivers laser light. A chemical reaction occurs, creating intracellular free radicals that kill the abnormal cells but minimally affect normal cells.

PDT was developed by researchers at the

Thompson Cancer Survival Center in collaboration with the College of Veterinary Medicine at the University of Tennessee. For more information on this treatment, contact the Thompson Cancer Survival Center's Laser Treatment Center at 865-541-1433. PDT may be considered an experimental medical approach (one of several) to treating Barrett's esophagus.

Apart from esophagectomy and experimental approaches, medical treatment of Barrett's esophagus is generally aimed at controlling underlying GERD symptoms in an effort to slow the progress of the disease and prevent complications. There are three main approaches to doing this:

1. Use of acid-suppressing medications
2. Surgery to strengthen the LES (and thereby prevent reflux)
3. Lifestyle and dietary changes

See the subsequent section on GERD in this chapter of the book for details on these approaches.

The use of some of the most potent acid-suppressive drugs, such as the proton pump inhibitors, as well as anti-reflux surgery, can cause some of the normal esophageal lining to partially grow back inside of the Barrett's esophagus lining.[17] However, even where it appears that abnormal cells have been replaced with normal ones, it is unknown whether these effects are lasting and whether or not they result in reduced cancer risk. It is worth noting also that, in some cases, normal cells may simply mask abnormal ones rather than replace them.[18]

While acid-suppressive drugs can protect the delicate tissues of the esophagus from harm, they have a vast array of undesirable side effects, which may offset their therapeutic value. These are described in the GERD section.

Surgical repair is another approach to treating GERD. But, while it may control reflux symptoms, it does not appear to cure Barrett's esophagus.[19]

Optional Nutritional Approaches

There is no known cure for Barrett's esophagus, but the following suggestions could be helpful:

DIET

- Follow the Digestive Care Diet in the appendix of this book.
- If you are in pain, a juicing diet for 2 to 3 days may be helpful. Follow the juicing recipes in the appendix of this book, and then start the Digestive Care Diet.
- Eat small meals slowly.
- Chew your foods to mush or liquid before swallowing.
- Do not drink cold liquids with meals; have no more than 1/2 glass of room temperature water with meals.

SUPPLEMENTS

- Take digestive enzymes before and after meals. This supplement should include: high potency protease (at least 100,000 H.U.T.), amylase and lipase, cellulase, as well as papain.
- Chew DGL (deglycyrrhizinated licorice) between meals.
- Drink aloe vera juice or syrup (about 5 ounces) between meals daily. Dilute 50% with water and gradually increase strength as tolerated (see appendix).
- Take 5,000 mg. to 20,000 mg. of glutamine powder with N-acetyl-glucosamine (NAG) and gamma oryzanol once to twice daily on an empty stomach.
- Take a multivitamin/mineral supplement (see appendix).
- Take antioxidant supplements (vitamin C - 500 mg. to 3000 mg., vitamin A - 10,000 I.U. daily and zinc – 30 mg. to 60 mg. daily), selenium 200 mcg./day after meals. Other antioxidants may also be taken with these (see appendix for specification on antioxidants).
- Take EFAs (essential fatty acids). A combination of fish and flax oils (Omega-3) with borage oil (Omega-6) is good to reduce inflammation in the gastrointestinal tract. Absorption of the oils may be enhanced with the addition of lipase (a fat-digesting enzyme). Take three to six 1000 mg. capsules twice a day with food (see appendix).
- Take a probiotic (beneficial bacteria) supplement. It should contain a minimum of 2 to 6 billion cultures. A prebiotic could be helpful (see appendix).

LIFESTYLE

- Sleep on your left side to avoid heartburn.
- Do not lie down for at least 3 or 4 hours after eating.
- Elevate head of bed 4 to 8 inches when sleeping.
- Make sure you have good bowel elimination daily.
- Exercise daily (at the least, take a walk).

COMPLEMENTARY MIND/BODY THERAPIES

- Yoga
- Massage
- Biofeedback
- Music therapy
- Meditation/Prayer
- Acupuncture
- Chiropractic
- Colon hydrotherapy

Please see the appendix for details of the above therapies.

*Please see additional recommendations for all esophageal problems at the end of this chapter.

Barrett's Esophagus Facts:

- Approximately 1 in 10 GERD sufferers will also develop a condition called Barrett's esophagus. It can be serious and may lead to esophageal cancer.
- Approximately 700,000 adults GERD sufferers will develop Barrett's esophagus.

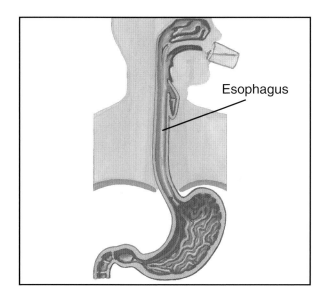

Esophagus

ESOPHAGITIS

What is it?
An "itis" anywhere in the body involves inflammation. Esophagitis, as its name implies, is inflammation of the lining of the esophagus.

What Causes it?
Esophagitis is most frequently caused by reflux of gastric contents into the esophagus, resulting in chemical esophageal burns. See the section on gastroesophageal reflux disease (GERD) for information on the cause of reflux.

Esophagitis may also be brought on by an infection. Infections can be fungal, viral or bacterial in origin. Candida (a yeast/fungus) and herpes (a virus) are the two most common forms of infectious esophagitis. Bacterial involvement is rarely a primary cause of esophagitis, though such infection may be secondary to a bacterial infection in the lungs.[1] Other fungi and viruses such as Human Immunodeficiency Virus (HIV) and Cytomegalovirus (CM) are possible but rare causes of esophagitis. In cases such as these, immunosuppression is the underlying cause. The weakening of the immune system may itself be caused by certain medications such as corticosteroids. Infectious esophagitis may also be caused by

parasitic infection with such organisms as Cryptosporidium, Pneumocystis and Leishmania donovani.[2]

Erosive esophagitis is caused by irritation. Such irritation may be of a physical, chemical or energetic nature. This latter type of irritation is brought on by radiation. For example, eighty percent of patients receiving radiation therapy for cancer will develop esophagitis if the esophagus is exposed to radiation.[3] The risk level is increased if chemotherapy is administered in conjunction with radiation therapy.[4]

There are a number of things that may cause physical injury to the esophagus. The most common of these are pills and capsules when swallowed just before bedtime with insufficient water. Should the pill or tablet become lodged in the esophagus, it may cause a superficial ulceration, which will typically heal within a few weeks. More rarely, a deep esophageal ulcer will form and cause perforation (piercing the entire wall, resulting in contamination of the adjacent pleural space and lung). Strictures (narrowing anywhere along the esophageal tube) may also result as a consequence of an esophageal ulcer. These types of complications are most likely to occur in patients with esophageal motility problems, characterized by the inability to quickly move food through the esophagus. Certain medications may wear away the lining of the esophagus as they pass through it because of their caustic nature. The antibiotic doxycycline and the anticholinergic emepronium bromide are two of the most common culprits. Nonsteroidal anti-inflammatory drugs [NSAIDs] and slow-release forms of potassium chloride are also frequently implicated.[5] Twenty percent of those who routinely take NSAIDs, such as aspirin or ibuprofen, will develop esophagitis.[6] Osteoporosis medications such as alendronate (Fosomax) and iron supplements may also be caustic to the esophagus, contributing to esophagitis.[7]

Esophagitis may result from the accidental or intentional ingestion of caustic chemicals, as in a

Chapter **2**

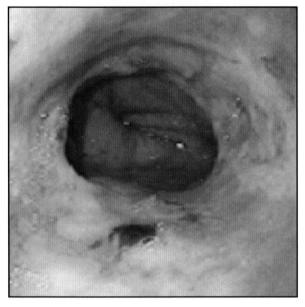

This is an internal scope of esophagitis.

suicide attempt. Strong acids and alkalis are both capable of causing significant injury by destroying tissue, but the alkaline agents are the more injurious to the esophageal mucosa, causing both tissue death and thermal burns. Additionally, healing may be complicated by extensive deposition of collagen (connective tissue), which may cause scarring and strictures.

Repeated vomiting, sometimes self-induced, as with some eating disorders, can cause an acid burn in the esophagus and may therefore be a cause of esophagitis. The disorder may also be the result of a hiatal hernia, where a portion of the stomach protrudes through the diaphragm muscle into the lower mediastinum (the lower portion of the chest). Finally, esophagitis may be caused by surgery.

Who Gets it?

Over 19 million Americans have chronic esophagitis.[8] People with weakened immune systems may be at risk for developing infectious esophagitis. This would include patients with Candida, CMV, herpes simplex and HIV, as well as those taking

immunosuppressive medications, undergoing chemotherapy or those who have had organ transplants. Heavy metal toxicity, often in the form of dental restorations, may be an unsuspected cause of immunosuppression. Patients with diabetes mellitus, adrenal dysfunction, alcoholism and those of advanced age can be predisposed to infectious esophagitis because of altered immune function.[9]

Other systemic disorders and conditions associated with esophagitis are listed below[10]:

- Behcet disease
- Chronic granulomatous disease
- Collagen vascular disease
- Inflammatory bowel disease
- Sarcoidosis
- Metastatic cancer
- Pemphigus vulgaris
- Cicatricial pemphigoid
- Epidermolysis bullosa
- Bullous pemphigoid
- Drug-induced skin disorders (i.e., Stevens-Johnson syndrome, toxic epidermal necrolysis, erythema multiforme)
- Lichen planus, psoriasis, acanthosis nigricans, leukoplakia
- Graf versus host disease (GVHD)

If you're not familiar with these disorders, don't worry about it. They'd sound familiar if you'd ever been diagnosed with any of them. The only one with which we'll deal directly will be inflammatory bowel disease, and that will be in Chapter 4.

People at risk for developing reflux esophagitis would be those exhibiting the risk factors described under GERD in this chapter of the book.

What Are the Signs and Symptoms?

Signs and symptoms of esophagitis may include:

- A burning sensation behind the sternum (breastbone)
- Difficult and/or painful swallowing

- Mouth sores or ulcerations (herpes lesions)
- The sensation of having something stuck in the throat
- Gagging
- Nausea
- Vomiting
- Thrush (white patches) in the mouth (may be present with Candida esophagitis)
- Rapid breathing/wheezing
- Mild to severe chest pain upon swallowing
- Loss of appetite
- Blood in stools
- Anemia
- Increased salivation or drooling

Not all of these symptoms will be present with every patient who has esophagitis. Some symptoms, such as stricture and bleeding, are only present in advanced forms of the disease. The type of esophagitis present will largely determine the nature of the symptoms experienced.

How is it Diagnosed?

In addition to taking a medical history and doing a physical examination, if your doctor suspects esophagitis, he or she will no doubt order special tests. Some of the medical tests that may be used to diagnose esophagitis include upper endoscopy with biopsy and upper GI series (described in the appendix of this book). Blood tests (including CBS and complete blood count) may also be performed to check for infection. Additionally, the acidity/alkalinity of the esophagus may be measured. Esophageal motility tests may be done as well to evaluate the movement of food through the esophagus.

Your medical doctor will not necessarily do all of these tests. S/he may do some and even order additional ones not listed here, depending on your symptoms.

What is the Standard Medical Treatment?

Treatment for esophagitis will depend on the type of esophagitis and the specific cause. To be fully effective, it must involve treatment of any underlying conditions such as diabetes, GERD, Candida, adrenal dysfunction, etc.

The traditional medical treatment for reflux esophagitis involves medications to suppress acid production. This is discussed more fully in the GERD section of this book, along with little known information about the benefits of stomach acid and risks involved in suppressing it. Lifestyle changes and dietary restrictions are often also recommended when reflux is found to be the cause of esophagitis. You will also find these discussed in the GERD section. For some difficult cases of reflux esophagitis where medications no longer control symptoms or where complications such as stricture or ulceration are present, surgery may be performed to repair the esophagus.

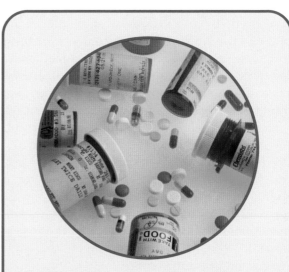

Antibiotics may create an unhealthy environment in your digestive system. Antibiotic usage requires a good probiotic to replenish good bacteria.

Did You Know?

- Probiotics produce important nutrients, eliminate toxins, destroy "bad" bacteria and enhance the body's immune system.

- Many modern day farming practices include antibiotics in the regular feed of animals to protect them from disease. When we eat the dietary products from these animals, we also eat the antibiotics they have ingested.

- The word antibiotic literally means "against life."

- The word probiotic literally means "for life."

- The over consumption of antibiotics is dangerous to our digestive health because we not only kill the problematic bad bacteria that make us ill, but we also kill the beneficial good bacteria essential to good health.

- Some of the most benefitial probiotics are Lactobacillus acidophilus and Bifidobacterium bifidum.

When infection is present, antibiotics are typically prescribed. Bearing in mind that antibiotics are only effective against bacterial infections, and most infectious esophagitis is not of a bacterial nature, the efficacy of such treatment is questionable. Even if the antibiotic is appropriately prescribed, we must be aware of adverse effects of such treatments – namely the killing off of all bacteria in the gut, the good and the bad. This opens the door to a condition of bacterial imbalance (dysbiosis) and the subsequent onset of more gastrointestinal stress and distress unless beneficial bacteria are replaced. If the cause is a viral infection, anti-viral medications will be prescribed. If the esophageal infection is found to be Candida, an antifungal medication will be prescribed

Where esophagitis is caused by medications, it may be necessary to discontinue the offending drug (always under the guidance of your physician) and find an alternative treatment. Whatever the case, it is very important to always swallow pills with large amounts of water, especially if medication is taken just before bedtime; this helps prevent esophageal irritation.

Where esophagitis is due to injury from a caustic

chemical, emergency medical treatment is required. Typically, the patient is given intravenous fluids and not permitted anything by mouth. Most often antibiotics and corticosteroids are used, although there is no good evidence documenting the efficacy of this approach.[11]

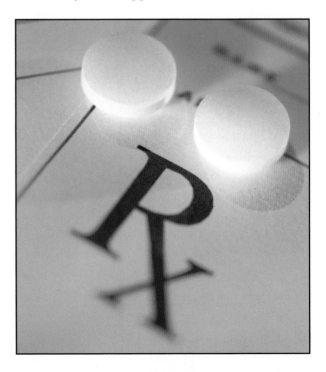

Optional Nutritional Approaches

It is of utmost importance to rule out any underlying Candida or herpes conditions (see Candida, Chapter 4 for details on Candida). If herpes is present, seek natural solutions for this condition.

DIET

- Follow the Digestive Care Diet in the appendix of this book.
- If you are in pain, a juicing diet for 2 to 3 days may be helpful. Follow the juicing recipes in the appendix of this book, and then start the Digestive Care Diet.
- Eat small meals slowly.
- Chew your foods to mush before swallowing.
- Do not drink cold liquids with meals; have no more than 1/2 glass of room temperature water with meals.

SUPPLEMENTS

- Take digestive enzymes before and after meals. This supplement should include protease (at least 20,000 H.U.T.), amylase and lipase, as well as papaya and bromelain. Other ingredients in this formula might include soothing herbs like marshmallow and slippery elm. Additionally, a good digestive enzyme formula would contain glutamine (an amino acid) and N-acetyl-glucosamine.
- Chew deglycyrrhizinated licorice (DGL) between meals.
- Drink aloe vera juice or syrup (about 5 ounces) between meals daily. Dilute 50% with water, and gradually increase concentration as tolerated (see appendix).
- Take 5,000 mg. to 10,000 mg. of glutamine powder with N-acetyl-glucosamine (NAG) and gamma oryzanol once to twice daily on an empty stomach (see appendix).
- Take a multivitamin/mineral supplement (see appendix).
- Take antioxidant supplements (vitamin C – 500 mg. to 3000 mg., vitamin A - 10,000 I.U. daily and zinc – 30 mg. to 60 mg. daily) after meals. Other antioxidants may also be taken with these (see appendix for specification on antioxidants).
- Take essential fatty acids (EFAs). A combination of fish and flax oils (Omega-3) with borage oil (Omega-6) is good to reduce inflammation in the gastrointestinal tract. Absorption of the oils may be enhanced with the addition of lipase (a fat-digesting enzyme). Take three to six 1000 mg. capsules twice daily with food.
- Take a multi-strain probiotic (good bacteria - Lactobaccilus and Bfidus) supplement daily. It should contain at least 2 to 6 billion cultures. A good prebiotic could be helpful (see appendix).

LIFESTYLE

- Sleep on your left side to avoid heartburn.
- Do not lie down for at least 3 hours after eating.
- Elevate head of bed 4 to 8 inches when sleeping.
- Make sure you have good bowel elimination daily.
- Exercise daily – even if it's just taking a walk.

COMPLEMENTARY MIND/BODY THERAPIES

- Yoga
- Massage
- Biofeedback
- Music therapy
- Meditation/Prayer
- Acupuncture
- Chiropractic
- Colon Hydrotherapy

Please see Appendix for details of the above therapies.

*Please see additional recommendations for all esophageal problems at the end of this chapter.

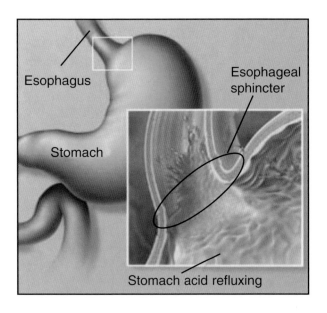

Esophagus

Esophageal
sphincter

Stomach

Stomach acid refluxing

GASTROESOPHAGEAL REFLUX DISORDER (GERD)

What is it?

You may know this condition by a variety of names. It is often referred to as acid reflux, chronic heartburn and acid indigestion. These terms are frequently used in advertisements to get you to buy the latest pill or tablet, guaranteed to ease your pain. But if you are experiencing discomfort on a regular basis, the recurring sensation of "heartburn" is likely a symptom of a larger problem.

GERD is a digestive disorder in which partially digested food from the stomach, along with hydrochloric acid (HCl) and enzymes, backs up into the esophagus. This process is known as "reflux." HCl has a very low pH, meaning that it is very acidic and can thus cause damage when it comes into contact with the delicate lining of the esophagus. This mucous lining or mucosa of the esophagus, unlike the lining of the stomach, was not designed to withstand the caustic effects of acid.

The term "GERD" came into use in the medical field in the 1980s to describe a group of conditions involving reflux. These conditions include acid indigestion (also known as heartburn), hiatal hernia and reflux esophagitis.

What Causes it?

Reflux occurs when the lower esophageal sphincter (LES), the muscle that connects the esophagus to the upper portion of the stomach, malfunctions, allowing the contents of the stomach to flow backwards into the esophagus. Normally, the LES opens to allow food from the esophagus into the stomach; then, it closes immediately to prevent that food and digestive secretions from the stomach from entering the esophagus. In GERD, the LES malfunctions, staying open after food has entered the stomach. So, LES weakness causes GERD. But what causes the LES to weaken?

A hiatal hernia may weaken the LES and cause reflux. This condition occurs when a portion of the stomach protrudes into the chest cavity through a small opening in the diaphragm, the muscle separating the abdomen from the chest wall. Hiatal hernia is discussed more fully later in this chapter of the book.

There are also a number of dietary and lifestyle factors that may contribute to GERD and esophageal irritation. These include:

- Overeating
- Overweight
- Stress (and eating when upset)
- Alcoholic beverages
- Chocolate, peppermint
- Eating too rapidly
- Spicy foods, including yellow onions
- Non-steroidal anti-inflammatory drugs (NSAIDs like aspirin, ibuprofen and naproxen), bronchodilating drugs used to treat asthma (like theophylline, albuterol, ephedrine), some blood pressure medications (calcium channel blockers, beta blockers), Valium, Demerol, nitroglycerine. These medications relax all muscles in the body, including the LES in the esophagus.[1]
- Drugs that irritate the GI lining – NSAIDs, the antibiotic tetracycline, the antiarrhythmic drug

quinidine, potassium chloride tablets and iron salts.[2]
- Fatty foods and fried foods
- Sugar
- Smoking
- Lying down after eating
- Bending from the waist, heavy lifting, straining at stool, pregnancy (all increase intra-abdominal pressure, which can give rise to a GERD by affecting gastric emptying)
- Inadequate chewing
- Swallowing large amounts of air when eating
- Coffee, tea and other caffeine-containing beverages
- Carbonated beverages
- Tight-fitting clothing (constricts abdomen)
- Insufficient water intake (dehydration)
- Tomato-based foods and citrus, raw onions, garlic, black pepper, vinegar

It is important to take your time while eating. When food is eaten too quickly, the stomach becomes distended, and the food is pushed against the top of the stomach, where it can force open the LES and wash into the esophagus, causing heartburn. This discomfort occurs from the partially digested food, gastric acid, enzymes and bacteria on the food, which can at times reach as high as the throat and windpipe and occasionally cause aspiration pneumonia. Also, swallowing air while eating – common if you are eating in an anxious state – results in heartburn when the air warms to body temperature, expands and is belched forcefully enough to push stomach acid into the esophagus.

Smoking inhibits production of saliva, salivary IgA (a protective antibody) and Salivary Epithelial Growth Factor (SEGF), which helps repair the intestinal lining. Both IgA and SEGF serve as a protective barrier against damage to the esophagus. Smoking also weakens the LES, as do the foods and beverages mentioned above.

Other factors that can contribute to GERD are:

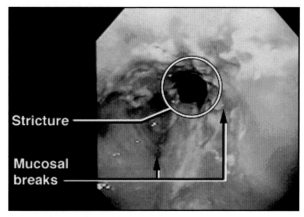

The squamous esophagus has a narrowed opening (lumen) due to chronic GERD with inflammation and scarring. This narrowed opening is called a stricture. The surrounding esophageal lining has ulcerations and erosions (mucosal breaks) from chronic acid injury to the esophagus.

- Ulcers
- Food allergies (especially milk and dairy products)
- Poor food combining (combining protein and carbohydrate at the same meal or eating fruit at the same time that other food is eaten)
- Gallbladder problems
- Enzyme deficiencies

It is commonly accepted by the medical profession that heartburn and GERD are caused by excess stomach acid. Virtually all drugs used to treat GERD neutralize, reduce, suppress or inhibit HCl production. This is very interesting in view of the fact that the 11th edition of the *Merck Manual*, published in 1966, states quite clearly that "[heartburn] is not due, as formerly believed, to excessive gastric acidity per se, as the same symptom often occurs in achlorhydria [absence of stomach acid]."[3] **The bottom line and shocking truth is that heartburn and GERD are more often caused by deficiency or lack of HCl than by too much of it.**[4] This is the basic premise of a fascinating book on the subject by Jonathan Wright, MD, and Lane Lenard, PhD, *Why Stomach Acid is Good for You*. Dr. Wright has found in his clinical practice that 90% of patients with GERD showed hypochlorhydria (too little HCl) when testing was done to measure exactly how much HCl they were producing.[5]

HCl deficiency has some far reaching consequences as far as overall health is concerned, for it results in electrolyte deficiency, which in turn inhibits enzyme production.[6] The net result is poor metabolism of other nutrients, disruption of homeostasis and development of degenerative disease conditions. Dr. Wright points out that people with serious diseases usually have low HCl. His clinical experience bears this out:

> As a physician practicing for more than thirty years, I've seen the harm that low stomach acid can do over a long period of time. I have worked with thousands of patients who arrived at the Tahoma Clinic with diseases as disparate as rheumatoid arthritis, childhood asthma, type I diabetes, osteoporosis, chronic fatigue, depression and many others only to find that they all had one thing in common: their stomachs were putting out a less-than-optimal amount of acid. In many cases, by restoring normal gastric function using safe, inexpensive acid supplements; pepsin and other digestive enzymes and amino acids, vitamins, minerals and botanicals, we have been able to help them improve or even eliminate their disease conditions. And we do this with almost no risk of dangerous side effects.[7]

Raphael Kellman, MD, has stated in his book *Gut Reactions* that he believes most cases of GERD to be related to poor motility. This, in turn, could be the result of an under-active thyroid gland, which would cause poor muscle tone that could disturb LES function.[8]

Who Gets it?

While chronic heartburn associated with GERD can strike anyone at any age, it is more common in older people than in younger people.[9] So is

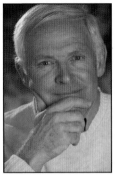

hypochlorhydria, or low HCl production. In fact, from the late nineteenth century to the mid-twentieth century, researchers regularly reported that the number of people with achlorhydria and hypochlorhydria increased with age from a low of about 4% at age 20 to as much as 75% after age 60.[10] If excessive HCl caused reflux, these findings should be reversed.

Although more common in older people, recent studies show that GERD in infants and children is more common than previously recognized.[11]

Because estrogens can weaken the LES, women who are pregnant, taking birth control pills or estrogen replacement therapy are more likely to suffer from heartburn than those who are not. Twenty-five percent of pregnant women experience daily heartburn, and more than 50% have occasional distress.[12] Obesity has been considered a possible risk factor for GERD; however, its causative role, as well as the benefits of weight loss, has not been proven.[13] Other people at risk for developing GERD would be those whose dietary and lifestyle factors match those listed under the causes section above.

What Are the Signs and Symptoms?

With GERD, there is, by definition, reflux, although the amount and frequency will differ from individual to individual; so does the degree of acidity of the stomach contents that are being regurgitated into the esophagus. Therefore, one person with GERD may have mild symptoms, while another could have severe ones. Along with the reflux quite often comes heartburn (70-85%). Other signs and symptoms of GERD may include:

- Regurgitation – 60%
- Angina-like chest pain – 33%
- Dsyphagia (difficulty swallowing) – 15-20%
- Bronchial spasms with asthma – 15-20%

- Laryngitis (voice problems – hoarseness)
- Shortness of breath
- Belching/bloating/gas
- A sense of fullness after eating (especially in conjunction with a chronic cough)
- Abdominal distention after eating
- Sore throat
- Nausea
- Vomiting of blood (may lead to anemia)

Not all people with GERD will experience all of these signs and symptoms. All GERD patients have reflux, but not all have burning, bloating and/or nausea.[14] Bloating and gas, when present, can be the result of swallowing air, undigested food being acted upon by bacteria, overeating and delayed gastric emptying. The stomach expands from gas, which travels up toward the esophagus, pushing HCl with it. The resulting heartburn is caused, not by too much HCl, but by HCl that is in the wrong place – the esophagus instead of the stomach. It is important to note that many of the symptoms listed above may be indicators of other problems. For this reason, and because GERD can lead to the more serious Barrett's esophagus (covered extensively at the beginning of this chapter) or even cancer for a small percentage of people, physicians will often perform tests to establish a definitive diagnosis.

How is it Diagnosed?

Medical tests help to:

1. Provide information on LES pressure
2. Confirm presence of acid or alkaline reflux in the esophagus
3. Evaluate the patient's ability to clear acid from the esophagus

Dr. Wright points out that, while x-rays and gastroscopes (fiber optic devices used to look inside the stomach) are routinely used for diagnosing GERD, actual measurements of stomach acid production are not routinely done. He goes on to say, "When we actually measure stomach acid output under careful, research-verified conditions, the overwhelming majority of heartburn sufferers are found to have too little stomach acid production."[15] **Once again, the problem we have in GERD is not that the stomach is producing too much acid; it is that the acid is in the wrong place: the esophagus.**

So what causes low HCl production? Low HCl production can result from a deficiency of vitamin A and B complex, as well as from a low intake of protein.[16] Chronic stress and zinc deficiency are other factors that may result in suppression of stomach acid.[17] Low salt diets may also contribute to HCl deficiency, as sodium and chloride are needed for HCl production.

Recognizing that low stomach acid may play an important role in GERD, the progressive physician may well do a gastric analysis to measure the stomach's acid-secreting capacity. This test involves swallowing a "Heidelberg capsule," which contains a tiny pH sensor and radio transmitter. Then a series of "bicarbonate challenges" is introduced to see how quickly the pH changes from alkaline to acid.

A less sophisticated but effective way to measure HCl output is described by Dr. Raphael Kellman in *Gut Reactions*. He describes an "HCl challenge test," which can be done at home. It is described in the appendix of this book.

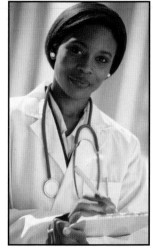

Another test that may be ordered by a holistic physician is a Complete Digestive Stool Analysis (see appendix). Elevated levels of vegetable and meat fibers (especially meat) present in this stool analysis may be yet another indicator of insufficient HCl production. The CDSA also gives information about the levels of digestive enzymes, the degree of fat digestion and the microbial population of the gut. This test can potentially identify problems not detected by standard GI tests, which are designed solely to identify structural not functional problems.

What is the Standard Medical Treatment?

The hallmark of standard medical treatment for GERD is the routine use of antacids to neutralize or suppress stomach acid production to reduce the symptoms of heartburn. The thinking with regard to use of such drugs is that by reducing acid production or neutralizing it, irritation to the esophagus will be minimized. Such thinking has given rise to widespread use of antacid drugs to treat GERD. Unfortunately, little press has been given to the long term adverse effects of continual use of such potent drugs.

These acid-blocking drugs may be divided into two categories, acid neutralizers and acid suppressors. Dr. Wright describes the effects of antacid drugs in detail in *Why Stomach Acid is Good for You*. A synopsis of his information is presented in the next four paragraphs.[18]

Acid-neutralizing drugs are alkalis, meaning they have an extremely alkaline (high) pH. Their active ingredients are mineral salts such as calcium, sodium, aluminum or magnesium. These minerals

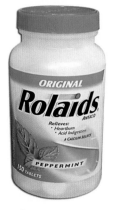

form a neutral salt upon contact with stomach acid, increasing the pH (reducing acidity). Their effects are temporary. They do not halt the production of HCl by the stomach. The acid-neutralizing products include such brand names as Rolaids, Tums, Alka Seltzer, Maalox and Mylanta These products are available over-the-counter without prescription. While their occasional use for isolated bouts of heartburn might not do much

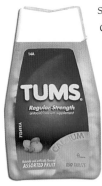

harm, habitual use can pose some serious problems. Most serious of the potential problems is a syndrome called milk-alkali syndrome, characterized by excess calcium in the blood, giving rise to a condition known as alkalosis (elevated blood pH) and kidney failure. This syndrome may result from over-consumption of milk (which is high in the alkaline mineral calcium) along

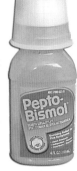

with an antacid over a long period of time, but it may also occur when no milk is consumed if calcium-based acid neutralizers are used habitually or excessively. Because some calcium-based acid-neutralizers are advertised as beneficial sources of supplemental calcium, some consumers – especially elderly women in an effort to stave off osteoporosis – overuse them. Ironically, the calcium contained in these products is calcium carbonate, an inorganic form of the mineral that is very poorly absorbed due to the fact that it neutralizes HCl needed for its utilization. Because calcium requires an acid environment in order to be properly absorbed by the body, the carbonates are a very poor dietary source of the mineral, as they have an alkalizing effect. Calcium-containing acid-neutralizers include Mi-Acid Gelcaps, Mylanta Gelcaps, Mylagen Gelcaps, Rolaids and Tums.

Some acid-neutralizing drugs contain aluminum, which poses an additional problem, as this metal has been shown to be a possible cause of such brain dementias as Alzheimer's disease. It would therefore be advisable to avoid long-term use of aluminum-containing antacids, which include Duracid, Tempo, Maalox, Mylanta, Gelusil, Gaviscon, Amphojel and Riopan.

There are two groups of acid-suppressing drugs: histamine H2-receptor blockers (H2-blockers) and proton pump inhibitors (PPIs). H2-blockers prevent acid secretion by blocking the action of histamine, which signals acid-producing cells to secrete HCl upon command of the hormone gastrin. These drugs were originally developed to treat peptic ulcers but came to be widely used to treat GERD instead, when it was found that the bacteria H. pylori, not excess HCl, causes ulcers. H2-blockers like Tagamet, Zantac, Pepcid and Axid can shut off acid flow for hours at a time and, like many other drugs, they have some serious side effects, including GI disturbances such as constipation, diarrhea, nausea, vomiting and heartburn (the very condition they're prescribed to treat).

Proton pump inhibitors are the strongest of the acid-suppressing drugs. They block the action of the proton pump, the HCl-producing and secreting mechanism inside some cells in the stomach lining. According to Dr. Wright, "Just one of these pills is capable of reducing stomach acid secretion by 90 to 95% for the better part of a day." Higher doses (recommended for "intractable" heartburn) totally eliminate HCl, producing a state of achlorhydria. Among the side effects that can be caused by PPIs are diarrhea, skin reactions, headaches, impotence, breast enlargement and gout. PPIs on the market today include Prilosec, Prevacid, AcipHex, Nexium and Protonix.

Because GERD is considered to be a motility problem (as well as an "acid problem"), motility enhancing drugs may also be prescribed. Their job is to help strengthen the LES and move food through the stomach more rapidly. This certainly makes more physiological sense than suppressing acid production. However, profound adverse side effects have limited the use of these drugs. For example, the FDA took Propulsid, one of the most potent motility enhancers, off the market when it was found to cause heart failure after a few years of clinical use.

When a person with low stomach acid is treated with antacids for heartburn, obviously the hypochlorhydria is exacerbated. And since in-

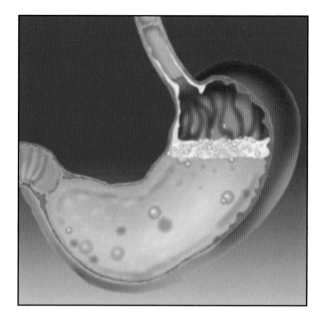

This is an illustration of the acid environment of the stomach.

adequate HCl production is more often the cause of GERD than is excessive acid production, it is apparent that we are making the problem worse in many cases with the treatment. Even if lack of stomach acid was not a problem before treatment with antacids, it can become one afterward. While they may provide short-term relief of heartburn, strong antacids, when used habitually, continually block the natural production of HCl. This knocks out one of the functions of stomach acid: to sterilize food before it enters the intestinal tract. Uncontrolled growth of every kind of microbe in the stomach can result, including yeast and Helicobacter pylori (H. pylori), the bacteria associated with gastric ulcers.[19]

Hydrochloric acid is one of nature's most essential antibiotics. Imagine a patient with virtually no stomach acid production eating a salad and being incapable of neutralizing the bacteria present on all the raw vegetables.[20] Obviously, we are inviting problems in such a scenario.

While acid-suppressing drugs may offer temporary relief of the symptoms of heartburn, antacids cre-

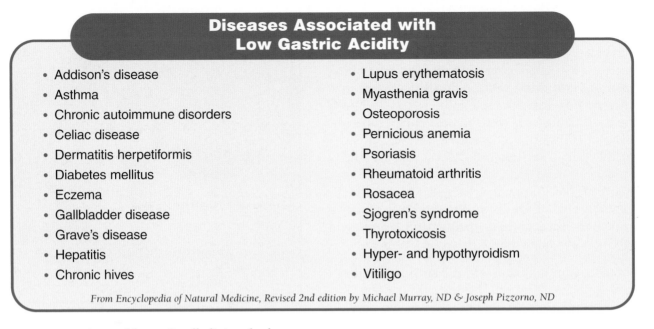

Diseases Associated with Low Gastric Acidity

- Addison's disease
- Asthma
- Chronic autoimmune disorders
- Celiac disease
- Dermatitis herpetiformis
- Diabetes mellitus
- Eczema
- Gallbladder disease
- Grave's disease
- Hepatitis
- Chronic hives

- Lupus erythematosis
- Myasthenia gravis
- Osteoporosis
- Pernicious anemia
- Psoriasis
- Rheumatoid arthritis
- Rosacea
- Sjogren's syndrome
- Thyrotoxicosis
- Hyper- and hypothyroidism
- Vitiligo

From Encyclopedia of Natural Medicine, Revised 2nd edition by Michael Murray, ND & Joseph Pizzorno, ND

ate many major problems. By alkalizing the lower stomach (antrum), the hormone gastrin is released, causing a huge rebound output of acid, thereby requiring more antacids to neutralize the increased acid output in response to the gastrin. Eventually the parietal cell mass that manufactures the acid ceases to function normally, resulting in low stomach acid (hypochlorhydria) or worse, no stomach acid (achlorhydria).

Dr. Wright observes that by promoting bacterial overgrowth and raising gastrin levels, habitual use of antacids produces hypochlorhydria or achlorhydria, which elevates the risk of stomach cancer.[21] While he emphasizes that there is no outright proof that use of acid-suppressing drugs causes cancer, he predicts that at least some of these drugs will be found to increase cancer risk, particularly when taken for a long time. He also makes the point that overuse of antacids "can inhibit the absorption of essential nutrients (vitamin B6, B12, folate, zinc, iron and calcium) and impair the digestion of protein, minerals and a few vitamins ... [and] the resulting malnutrition can, over many years, lead to depression, osteoporosis, arthritis, and other chronic degenerative diseases that reduce the quality of our lives and may ultimately shorten our life spans."[22]

Also, antacids create conditions conducive to yeast and fungus growth.[23] Additionally, they can also mask symptoms of an ulcer or even cancer of the stomach or esophagus. Ironically, they can actually cause stomach pain.

Should drugs and lifestyle/dietary adjustments fail to control symptoms of GERD, surgery may be suggested by a physician as a last resort. A procedure known as fundoplication involves wrapping part of the stomach around the lower esophagus to strengthen the LES.

GERD Fact:

- The medical term used for chronic heartburn is "GERD" (gastroesophageal reflux disease). GERD is defined as a digestive disorder in which partially digested food from the stomach, along with hydrochloric acid (HCl) and enzymes, backs up (or regurgitates) into the esophagus.

Optional Nutritional Approaches

According to Dr. Wright, the best way to treat heartburn/indigestion/GERD and other GI symptoms is almost always with more HCl, not less.[24] Use of supplemental HCl supports healthy digestion by assuring that the stomach has enough hydrochloric acid to begin the breakdown of protein and activate pepsin, a protein-digesting enzyme, in the stomach. Although it is difficult to comprehend taking acid to relieve heartburn, additional HCl helps the stomach to properly digest food, which ultimately helps to prevent putrefaction that leads to gas production, reflux and heartburn.

The condition of GERD can be difficult to address from any single approach since there can be many underlying factors contributing to the problem. Before using the suggestions that follow, it would be helpful to run tests to rule out underlying problems, as indicated below:

- Thyroid self test (see appendix)
- Adrenal dysfunction test (see appendix)
- Stool test for Candida or parasites (see appendix)
- HCl test (see Heidelburg test or self-test in appendix)

It is also advisable to take the following action:

- Rule out H-pylori infection
- If you are on medication (especially proton pump inhibitors) for GERD, please consult with your health care practitioner to help gradually decrease your medication as you implement the natural protocol. Share with your health care practioner that you understand this may only be a temporary trial, but if it works, you will decrease your risk of chronic high levels of gastrin and possible increased risk of cancer.

DIET

Follow the Digestive Care Diet in the appendix of this book indefinitely. After recovery, if you want to add other foods back into your diet, please do so slowly and with caution. Other dietary considerations are listed below:

- It would be helpful to do a juice fast 2 to 3 days before starting this diet. Please see the appendix for juice recipes appropriate for digestive conditions.
- Eat small meals frequently during the day.
- Chew food to mush or liquid, and eat slowly.
- Do not drink cold liquids with meals; have no more than 1/2 glass of room temperature water with meals.

Common Signs & Symtoms of Low Gastric Acidity

- A sense of fullness after eating
- Acne
- Bloating, belching, burning and flatulence immediately after meals
- Chronic Candida infections
- Chronic intestinal parasites or abnormal flora
- Dilated blood vessels in the cheeks and nose
- Indigestion, diarrhea or constipation
- Iron deficiency
- Itching around the rectum
- Multiple food allergies
- Nausea after taking supplements
- Undigested food in the stool
- Upper digestive tract gassiness
- Weak, peeling and cracked fingernails

From Encyclopedia of Natural Medicine, Revised 2nd edition by Michael Murray, ND & Joseph Pizzorno, ND

SUPPLEMENTS

- Take HCl/pepsin supplements before meals to make a rough determination if your stomach acid levels are low. Start with one capsule, and increase by one capsule daily with meals until symptoms of heartburn are gone. If you feel a burning sensation, back off to previous dose. The supplement may contain other soothing ingredients like quercitin, bromelain, gamma oryzanol, L-glutamine and N-acetyl-glucosamine.

- Plant enzymes can also be used with meals. These should include protease (20,000 H.U.T.) amylase, lipase and cellulase. This formula might also include ginger, marshmallow, papaya, bromelain and gamma oryzanol. Take one or two capsules before and after meals.
- Take 5,000 mg. to 10,000 mg. of L-glutamine powder with gamma oryzanol daily on an empty stomach (see appendix).
- Take a multi-strain probiotic (2 to 6 billion per cap), 2 to 4 caps daily. Take a pre-biotic, as well (see appendix).
- Take essential fatty acids (EFAs). A combination of fish and flax oils (Omega-3) with borage oil (Omega-6) is good to reduce inflammation in the gastrointestinal tract. Absorption of the oils may be enhanced with the addition of lipase (a fat-digesting enzyme). Take three to six 1000 mg. caplets twice a day with food (see appendix).
- Take a multivitamin/mineral supplement daily (see appendix).
- Take antioxidant supplements (vitamin C – 500 mg. to 3000 mg., vitamin A - 10,000 I.U. daily and zinc – 30 mg. to 60 mg. daily) after meals. Other antioxidants may also be taken with these (see appendix).

With irritation in the gut, you may want to do the following:

- Chew deglycyrrhizinated licorice (DGL) between meals.
- Drink aloe vera juice or syrup (about 5 ounces) between meals daily. Dilute 50% with water and gradually increase strength as tolerated (see appendix).

The formula given below could be very beneficial in relieving the symptoms of heartburn. This combination acts as a powerful antacid. It is natural and could be a better choice than taking an over-the-counter drugs or antacids. This formula, which is a combination of fava bean flour and ellagic acid, provides nutritional support for the upper GI tract while relieving the symptoms of heartburn, "sour stomach" and dyspepsia. This formula should be in chewable form and contain the following: (Refer to www.renewlife.com)

- Ellagic acid, a powerful antioxidant found in several fruits (especially raspberries and pomegranates) can counter the oxidative stress caused by H. pylori. It also has anti-inflammatory properties and can temporarily inhibit stomach acid.
- Fava Bean flour buffers stomach acid without producing side effects. Used in combination with ellagic acid, it provides nutritional support for upper digestive function, as well as long-lasting digestive support through extended acid section modification.

The formula should also contain additional antioxidant and anti-microbial nutrients, such as:

- Green tea (antioxidant)
- Tumeric (antioxidant)
- Mastic gum (antibacterial)

LIFESTYLE
- Sleep on your left side to avoid heartburn.
- Do not lie down for at least 3 or 4 hours after eating.
- Elevate head of bed 4 to 8 inches when sleeping.
- Make sure you have good bowel elimination daily.
- Exercise daily – even if it's just taking a walk.

COMPLEMENTARY MIND/BODY THERAPIES
- Acupuncture
- Colon Therapy
- Biofeedback
- Massage

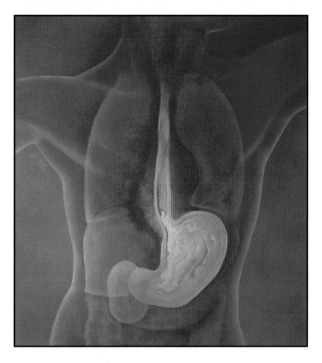

HEARTBURN
What is it?
Heartburn is basically reflux esophagitis, a condition wherein gastric juices back up into the esophagus, creating a burning sensation, which radiates upward. It is usually part of a larger symptom complex known as dyspepsia or indigestion. The medical term used for chronic (frequent) heartburn is gastroesophageal reflex syndrome (GERD).

What Causes it?
See GERD section.

Who Gets it?
Anyone can get heartburn. It is as common as the cold. According to the *Get Heartburn Smart* book-let published by the National Heartburn Alliance, "Twenty-five million adults experience heartburn on a daily basis."[1]

What are the Signs and Symptoms?
Apart from the burning sensation in the chest, the heartburn sufferer may experience:

• Nausea

• Upper abdominal pain (usually comes after meals)
• Flatulence and belching (gas)
• Abdominal distention after eating
• A sense of fullness after eating

Frequent and persistent heartburn, particularly if it is accompanied by any of the symptoms listed below, may be an indicator of GERD:

• Hoarseness or wheezing
• Painful or difficult swallowing
• Vomiting
• Dramatic weight loss
• Increased severity of symptoms over time

See the GERD section for more information if you have any of these symptoms.

How is it Diagnosed?
Simple heartburn may be diagnosed on the basis of symptoms alone. However, your doctor may want to perform tests – upper GI series or endoscopy (see appendix for description of these tests) to be sure and to rule out other conditions. To distinguish heartburn from angina (heart pain), a Bernstein test (acid perfusion) may be performed.[2] This test involves introducing first a saline solution, then a weak hydrochloric acid (HCl) solution into the esophagus through a tube inserted into the nasal cavity. Theoretically, if pain is felt with the HCl but not with the salt, it is indicative of reflux. An EKG and stress test, as well as a 24-hour pH probe, may also be used to distinguish heartburn from angina. See the GERD section of this book for other tests that may be performed.

What is the Standard Medical Treatment?
Standard medical treatment will involve use of antacids. See the GERD section for a discussion of these medications and the risks posed by using them on an ongoing basis.

Optional Nutritional Approaches

For diet, lifestyle and mind/body approaches, follow the guidelines at the end of the GERD section. The following are guidelines for symptom relief of heartburn:

- Drink a glass of room temperature water.
- Try ginger or slippery elm tea.
- Chew deglycyrrhizinated licorice (DGL) between meals.
- Take probiotics (2 to 6 billion cultures per cap). Open capsule and take with water.
- Drink aloe vera juice or syrup (about 5 ounces) between meals daily.

The formula given below could be very beneficial in relieving the symptoms of heartburn. This combination acts as a powerful antacid. It is totally natural and is a better choice than taking an over-the-counter drug or antacids such as Maalox, Mylanta, Tums Rolaids etc. and anti secretory drugs like Tagamet, Zantec, Pepcid, etc. This formula, which is a combination of fava bean flour and ellagic acid, provides nutritional support for the upper GI tract while relieving the symptoms of heartburn, "sour stomach" and dyspepsia. This formula should be in chewable form and contain the following: (Refer to www.renewlife.com)

- Ellagic acid, a powerful antioxidant found in several fruits (especially raspberries and pomegranates) can counter the oxidative stress caused by H. pylori. It also has anti-inflammatory properties and can temporarily inhibit stomach acid.
- Fava Bean flour buffers stomach acid without producing side effects. Used in combination with ellagic acid, it provides nutritional support for upper digestive function, as well as long-lasting digestive support through extended acid section modification.

The formula should also contain additional antioxidant and anti-microbial nutrients, such as:

- Green tea (antioxidant)
- Tumeric (antioxidant)
- Mastic gum (antibacterial)

****If you choose to take an over-the-counter antacid, don't make it a habit. A trial of baking soda with water, if it eliminates the heartburn, does suggest that acid reflux may be part of your problem. Try to get to the source of your problem with diet, lifestyle and stress reduction as outlined in this chapter.

Heartburn Facts:

- A recent survey from the National Heartburn Alliance reported that more than 50 million adults in the United States suffer from heartburn at least once a month.

- According to the National Heartburn Alliance, 25 million Americans experience heartburn on a daily basis.

- Half of frequent heartburn sufferers believe it is impossible to live heartburn-free, and more than 90% say that frequent heartburn negatively impacts their quality of life by severely limiting daily activities and productivity.

- Though multiple factors can contribute to heartburn, including alcohol consumption, pregnancy, hiatal hernia, smoking, overeating, overweight, stress, enzyme deficiencies, food allergies, insufficient water intake, inadequate chewing, eating when upset and some prescription medications, sufferers generally identity food as the primary cause of their symptoms.

- Heartburn, also called acid indigestion, is an irritation of the esophagus caused by acid that refluxes (comes up) from the stomach.

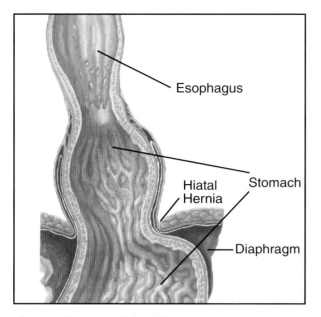

Esophagus

Hiatal
Hernia

Stomach

Diaphragm

This is an illustration of a hiatal hernia.

HIATAL HERNIA
What is it?

In order to understand what a hiatal hernia is, it is important to know that the esophagus passes through the diaphragm – the flat, dome-shaped muscle that separates the chest from abdominal contents – and into the stomach. The opening in the diaphragm through which this passage is made is known as a "hiatus," which gives this syndrome its name. With a hiatal hernia, a portion of the stomach rises up through the diaphragm due to weakness in the diaphragm muscles. The stomach is displaced to a position above the diaphragm, and the normal relation of the esophagus to diaphragm is altered, resulting in lower pressure at the junction of the stomach and the esophagus. This area, known as the lower esophageal sphincter high pressure zone (LES-HPZ), is not really a valve or sphincter but merely the site at which the diaphragm muscles attach to the junction of the esophagus and the stomach. This may give rise to gastroesophageal reflux, where the black-flow of stomach contents into the esophagus causes a burning sensation. When this happens, the patient is said to have gastroesophageal reflux disease (GERD).

What Causes it?

There are many contributing factors to hiatal hernia. Some include injury, trauma, obesity, thyroid dysfunction and age. By definition, the condition involves weakness in the diaphragm. It has also been theorized that, in some people, a congenital shortening of the GI tract[1] may be a causative variable. Here the person would be born with a predisposition to hiatal hernia, which would develop later in life as the result of some sort of stress, such as pregnancy or extreme physical exertion.[2]

Who Gets it?

Hiatal hernias affect women more frequently than men,[3] particularly pregnant women. They occur more often in people who are overweight than in people of normal weight[4] due to the increase in intra-abdominal pressure. These hernias also occur most often during middle age. In fact, the condition is so common that 25% of people aged fifty years and over are estimated to have a hiatal hernia,[5] although they may not know it if there is no discomfort. Though not as common, it has been found that hiatal hernias can be hereditary.[6]

What Are the Signs and Symptoms?

There are two types of hiatal hernias. The type present (and size of the hernia) will largely determine the degree of distress experienced, if any. Most common is the "sliding hiatal hernia." It occurs in 90% of all cases.[7] With this type of hernia, a portion of the stomach passes through the diaphragm. This condition may cause only mild, if any, symptoms. In fact, experts estimate that up to 40% of Americans have a sliding hiatal hernia and don't know it.[8]

The second type of hiatal hernia is the "para-esophageal hiatal hernia." Here a portion of the stomach outpouches through the diaphragm and actually positions itself next to the esophagus. This type of hiatal hernia may produce no symptoms because the LES is not displaced. However, should the stomach get pulled higher into the chest and

Chapter 2

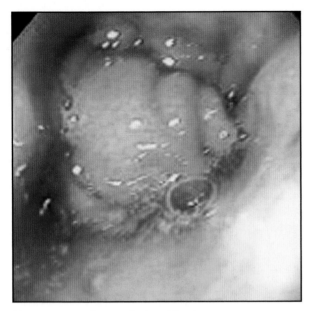

This is an internal scope of a hiatal hernia.

become pinched by the diaphragm, an emergency situation called "strangulation" may result, requiring immediate surgical intervention.[9]

A sliding hiatal hernia may cause heartburn and other symptoms associated with GERD (see GERD section) if the weakened LES permits reflux of stomach contents into the esophagus, causing a burning sensation. Both the sliding and the paraesophageal hiatal hernias may, on rare occasion, bleed (either a little or a lot) from their lining. A small amount of blood loss may lead to anemia, while massive blood loss can be life-threatening.[10]

How is it Diagnosed?
The hiatal hernia is typically diagnosed by use of an upper GI series, also known as the barium swallow (see the appendix for a description).

What is the Standard Medical Treatment?
Many hiatal hernias, particularly if they're small, cause no symptoms and require no treatment. When GERD symptoms arise, they are apt to be treated with antacids. See GERD section, under

"treatment" for information on the downside of habitual antacid use, as well as dietary and lifestyle modification recommendations. Also, see the GERD "alternatives" section for optional approaches to managing GERD symptoms.

If it is confirmed that reflux is caused by a hiatal hernia and symptoms cannot be controlled through diet, medications and lifestyle modification, your physician may recommend surgical repair of the hernia.

Unfortunately there are no known ways to reverse hiatal hernia without surgery. However, the following nutritional options can enhance digestion, minimize reflux, improve overall health and sense of well being.

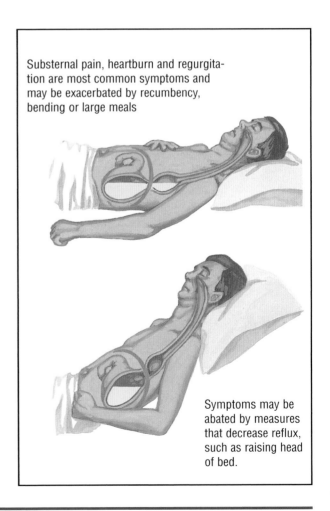

Substernal pain, heartburn and regurgitation are most common symptoms and may be exacerbated by recumbency, bending or large meals

Symptoms may be abated by measures that decrease reflux, such as raising head of bed.

Optional Nutritional Approaches

DIET

Follow the Digestive Care Diet in the appendix of this book indefinitely. After recovery, if you want to add other foods back into your diet, please do so slowly and with caution. Other dietary considerations are listed below:

- It would be helpful to do a juice fast 2 to 3 days before starting this diet. Please see the appendix for juice recipes appropriate for digestive conditions.
- Eat small meals frequently during the day.
- Chew food to mush or liquid, and eat slowly.
- Do not drink cold liquids with meals; have no more than 1/2 glass of room temperature water with meals.

SUPPLEMENTS

- Take HCl/pepsin supplements before meals to determine if your stomach acid levels are low. Start with one capsule, and increase by one capsule daily with meals until your heartburn symptoms are gone. (If you feel a burning sensation, back off to previous dose.) The supplement may contain other soothing ingredients like quercitin, bromelain, gamma oryzanol, L-glutamine and N-acetyl-glucosamine.
- Plant enzymes can also be used with meals. These should include protease (20,000 H.U.T.) amylase, lipase and cellulase. This formula might also include ginger, marshmallow, papaya, bromelain and gamma oryzanol. Take one before after meals.
- Take 5,000 mg. to 20,000 mg. of L-glutamine powder with gamma oryzanol daily on an empty stomach (see appendix).
- Take a multi-strain probiotic (good bacteria - Lactobaccilus and Bifidus) supplement daily. It should contain at least 2 to 6 billion cultures. A good prebiotic could be helpful (see appendix).
- Take essential fatty acids (EFAs). A combination of fish and flax oils (Omega-3) with borage oil (Omega-6) is good to reduce inflammation in the gastrointestinal tract. Absorption of the oils may be enhanced with the addition of lipase (a fat-digesting enzyme). Take three to six 1000 mg. caplets twice a day with food.

- Take a multivitamin/mineral supplement daily (see appendix).
- Take antioxidant supplements (vitamin C – 500 mg. to 3000 mg., vitamin A - 10,000 I.U. daily and zinc – 30 mg. to 60 mg. daily) after meals. Other antioxidants may also be taken with these (see appendix for specification on antioxidants).
- Follow a 30-day herbal detoxification program as described in the appendix,

30-Day Herbal Detox

With irritation in the gut, you may want to do the following:

- Chew deglycyrrhizinated licorice (DGL) between meals.
- Drink aloe vera juice or syrup (about 5 ounces) between meals daily.

LIFESTYLE
- Do not lie down for at least 3 hours after eating.
- Elevate head of bed 4 to 8 inches when sleeping.
- Make sure you have good bowel elimination daily (see constipation, Part 4).
- Exercise daily – even if it's just taking a walk.

COMPLEMENTARY MIND/BODY THERAPIES
- Yoga (see appendix)
- Massage (see appendix)
- Biofeedback (see appendix)
- Music therapy (see appendix)
- Meditation/Prayer (see appendix)
- Colon hydrotherapy (see appendix) – to cleanse the large intestine so as to relieve pressure in the digestive tract
- Chiropractic – Some chiropractors use a technique of soft tissue manipulation to help with hiatal hernia.

• Acupuncture – Acupuncture physicians can place needles or manipulate pressure points to help relieve hiatal hernia symptoms (see appendix).

*Please see additional recommendations for all esophageal problems at the end of this chapter.

Dr. Smith's Comments

I have seen many patients who, after occasional episodes of heartburn, have been put on acid-blocking medications for indefinite periods of time. Often, I have found that if they will lose a little weight, improve their bowel function, eliminate foods that lower their esophageal sphincter pressure, remove sensitive foods and change their eating habits as mentioned in this chapter, they can get off of their medications. Since these medications can have significant and potentially serious side effects, it is wise to minimize their use. Implementation of more natural and safer nutritional options should be undertaken whenever possible.

I would like to point out that all esophageal conditions mentioned in Chapter 2, namely Barrett's esophagus, esophagitis, GERD, heartburn and hiatal hernia, have features in common that could be addressed from a nutritional standpoint:

• *Material from the stomach periodically enters into the esophogus. This often causes an inflammatory reaction and can damage the esophageal lining. Researchers have recently observed that the damage to the lining may be more due to esophageal intra-cellular oxidative stress than to the direct contact of the acid and gastric contents. There are articles in the literature that support the fact that adequate antioxidant levels are protective against damage from reflux. (Gut 2001;49;364-371). In this article, it was shown that pretreatment with antioxidants minimized damage and decreased the inflammatory markers (malondialdehyde and NfkappaB). In addition, the antioxidants slowed down the loss of glutathione (a naturally produced beneficial antioxidant). It would be wise to supplement with vitamins A, C, E, and the minerals zinc and selenium.*
• *Mucus production has been shown to be variable,*

and people with lower levels tend to have more inflammatory problems in the esophagus and stomach. Normalizing cellular function with glutamine, glycine, and Omega-3 essential fatty acids can be helpful. Mucus-producing nutrients (N-acetyl-glucosamine, N-acetyl-galactosamine, fucose, galactose and sialic acid) and increased water intake are needed to make high quality and quantity of mucus. There is a good review article about probiotics and mucus and their role in intestinal health in the American Journal of Clinical Nutrition, 2003;78: 675-683.

Minimizing the possibility of inflammation is important. Checking for any type of infection especially H.pylori or Candida, can be helpful; if found, short courses of appropriate anti-microbials should be implemented. After removal of pathogens, restoration of the beneficial bacteria (Lactobacilli and Bifidobacteria) is very important and may help prevent future infections. Liquid aloe vera has potent anti-inflammatory benefits as well.

Hiatal Hernia Facts:

• A hernia occurs when one part of your body — usually the intestine — protrudes through a gap or opening into another part of your body.

• Hiatal hernias — also known as diaphragmatic hernias — form at the opening (hiatus) in your diaphragm where your food pipe (esophagus) joins your stomach. When the muscle tissue around the hiatus becomes weak, it can allow the upper part of your stomach to bulge through the diaphragm into your chest cavity.

General Recommendations For All Esophageal Problems

- Avoid foods and beverages that weaken the LES (such as chocolate, peppermint, fatty foods, caffeine-containing and alcoholic beverages).
- Decrease portion sizes at each meal.
- Don't lie down for at least two to three hours after eating.
- Don't wear clothing that constricts the abdomen.
- Reduce stress.
- Lose weight (if overweight).
- Quit smoking.
- Elevate the head 4" to 8" when sleeping.
- Eat in a relaxed environment.
- Minimize activities (such as bending and heavy lifting) that might increase intra-abdominal pressure.
- Exercise regularly.
- Identify, reduce and/or eliminate any medications that may be contributing to the problem (under a doctor's supervision).
- Chew food thoroughly (until liquid).
- Drink more water (1/2 oz. for every pound of body weight – i.e., 50 oz. for a 100 lb. person).
- Keep a food diary to identify any food that may trigger an episode of GERD.
- Identify and avoid food allergens. (See Resource section for testing information).
- Combine foods properly (Eat fruit alone; avoid eating starchy carbohydrates at the same time proteins are consumed).

- Treat constipation if present (see Chapter 4).
- At the first sign of heartburn, drink a large glass of water.
- Take supplemental digestive enzymes at the end of each meal.
- Take a small amount of "bitters" (an aqueous blend of bitter herbs such as gentian root, artemisia, yellow dock, dandelion and barberry) about 15 minutes before eating. These will help stimulate the secretion of gastric acid, bile and pancreatic enzymes and assist in control of reflux by increasing the tone of the LES.[1]
- Drink raw potato juice (prepare with skin intact, drink immediately), diluted 50% with water, three times per day.[2]
- Drink a glass of fresh cabbage or celery juice daily.
- In lieu of HCl supplementation, if you wish, sip 1 tablespoon of apple cider vinegar [or lemon juice] diluted in a glass of water with meals.[3] Do not drink any other fluids with meals.
- Eat fresh pineapple and/or papaya. These fruits are rich in enzymes, which will aid digestion.
- Drink chamomile tea to relieve esophageal irritation.[4] This herb has anti-inflammatory properties.
- Consider a trial series of vitamin B_{12} injections. ("In cases of achlorhydria, it is an established fact that vitamin B_{12} is neither well digested nor well absorbed."[5])

Stomach Problems

GASTRITIS

What is it?

An "itis" anywhere in the body involves inflammation. Gastritis is inflammation of the lining of the stomach that involves erosion of the uppermost mucosal layer. Erosion of this protective layer leaves the underlying stomach tissue vulnerable to damage from enzymes and hydrochloric acid (HCl), which may seriously affect gastric function.

Gastritis is inflammation of the stomach. It means that white blood cells infiltrate into the wall of the stomach as a response to some type of injury or disease.

What Causes it?

Gastritis can have many causes, but recent research has shown that the bacterium Helicobacter pylori (H. pylori), which grows exclusively in the mucus-secreting cells of the stomach lining, is responsible for the majority of chronic gastritis cases.[1] It is interesting to note, however, that many people who are infected with H. pylori do not develop gastritis or any other GI disorder. While 25% of the U.S. population is infected with H. pylori, only 10-15% of this 25% will develop gastritis or ulcers.[2] It is not clearly understood why some people with the H. pylori infection develop problems and others do not. However, the natural healing perspective holds the notion that it is not bacteria, but rather the context in which they're found, that leads to disease. With that in mind, other factors like diet and other elements of one's lifestyle can be viewed as important influences. While H. pylori is the bacterium most commonly associated with gastritis, E. coli can also play a role.[3]

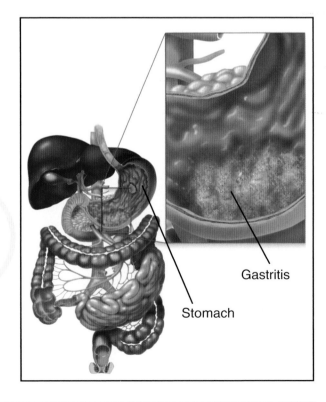

Gastritis

Stomach

Chronic erosive gastritis develops gradually as a result of the use of drugs that irritate the stomach lining (especially NSAIDs – see chart below), alcohol abuse, Crohn's disease (see Chapter 4) or from infections of a viral or bacterial nature.

Acute gastritis, characterized by severe symptoms of short duration, is caused by ingestion of mucosal irritants or high doses of radiation.[4] The irritants involved could be caustic chemicals or corrosive compounds that were accidentally swallowed, or they could be certain drugs used over a long period of time. Other irritants that may play a causative role in gastritis include heavy spices and tobacco.

Another type of acute gastritis is known as "acute stress gastritis." It is brought on by illness or injury, often an injury involving serious burns or profuse bleeding. Such conditions as high fever, heart attack and kidney failure may also give rise to acute stress gastritis.[5]

A type of gastritis known as "atrophic gastritis"

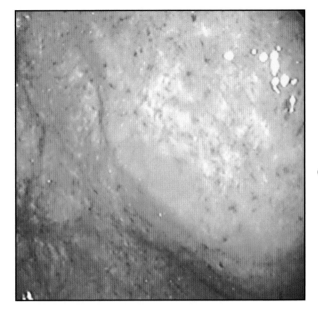
This is an internal scope of the stomach with gastritis.

occurs as a result of antibodies attacking the stomach lining, which causes a thinning of the lining and a loss of acid-producing and enzyme-producing cells.

A viral or fungal gastritis may develop in persons who have had or are having a prolonged illness, as well as those suffering from immune deficiency.

Two types of gastritis for which the cause is unknown are Mènètrier's disease and plasma cell gastritis. In the former, the walls of the stomach form thick folds, enlarged glands and cysts,[6] and there is an increased risk for stomach cancer. In plasma cell gastritis, white blood cells accumulate in various organs and in the stomach wall.[7]

Who Gets it?
Persons with H. pylori would be at greater risk for developing chronic gastritis than people without this bacterial infection, which is transmitted from person to person through contaminated food and water and through the use of diagnostic equipment, such as an endoscope, that has not been

Non-Steroidal Anti-Inflammatory Drugs (NSAIDs)

- Aleve/Anaprox
- Feldene
- Orudis
- Aspirin
- Indocin
- Relafen
- Ansaid
- Lodine
- Sodium salicylate
- Arthropan
- Mesalamine
- Tolectin
- Clinoril
- Motrin
- Toradol
- Daypro
- Nalfon
- Voltaren
- Dolobid
- Naprosyn

From Gastrointestinal Disorders and Nutrition by Tonia Reinhard, MS, RD

sterilized.[8] While the infection rate is only 25% in the U.S., it may be as high as 90% in underdeveloped countries where sanitation and hygiene are poor.[9] Those at greatest risk for developing the infection are the elderly, the impoverished, African Americans and Hispanics.[10]

Various types of gastritis would be:

- Acute gastritis – those receiving high-dose radiation therapy
- Acute stress gastritis – those who have experienced sudden onset of an illness or injury, especially one involving massive blood loss or extensive burns, or trauma
- Atrophic gastritis – elderly people and those who have had part of the stomach removed
- Chronic erosive gastritis – alcoholics, chronic users of NSAIDs, those with Crohn's disease, those with bacterial or viral infections
- Viral or fungal gastritis – those with an immunodeficiency (during or following a long illness)

What are the Signs and Symptoms?
Many cases of gastritis will cause no symptoms at all.[11] Where symptoms do exist, the type of gastritis will determine their nature. The most commonly experienced gastritis symptoms include:

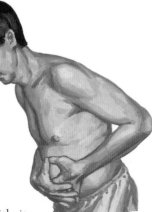

- heartburn
- pain in the upper abdomen
- bloating
- nausea/vomiting
- belching
- black, tarry stools (a sign of GI bleeding)
- loss of appetite
- weight loss

Acute stress gastritis, with its rapid onset, can lead to, ulceration and bleeding, which can be fatal.[12]

How is it Diagnosed?
As with all conditions, a thorough patient history is needed to assist in determining the cause of gastritis. A history of chronic NSAID use or alcohol abuse is particularly relevant.

Gastritis is typically diagnosed through endoscopic examination (see Upper Endoscopy in the appendix for description). A small piece of stomach tissue can be snipped off (biopsied) using the endoscope and later analyzed to help determine the type of inflammation. A biopsy can confirm the presence of H. pylori (as can special blood and breath tests). With the aid of the endoscope, the doctor is also able to cauterize any damaged tissue and thereby stop any bleeding that may be occurring.

In addition to gastroscopy, other tests may be performed. Your doctor may order a stool analysis to detect blood in the stool and/or a specialized stool test called the Comprehensive Digestive Stool Analysis (CDSA), described in the appendix. This test, as its name implies, yields comprehensive information about the patient's digestive capabilities. Raphael Kellman, MD, recommends the CDSA for patients with gastritis symptoms, as well as the adrenal saliva test,[13] which measures levels of the stress hormone cortisol (see appendix).

What is the Standard Medical Treatment?
If an irritant such as alcohol or a drug is found to be the cause of gastritis, the condition can be expected to resolve following removal of that irritant. If the culprit is H. pylori, standard treatment will involve a course of antibiotics and use of an acid-suppressing drug. Bismuth, an element that protects the stomach lining by protecting the mucous membranes from being dissolved by acid and pepsin,[14] may also be added to the regimen.

The use of acid-suppressing medications may well

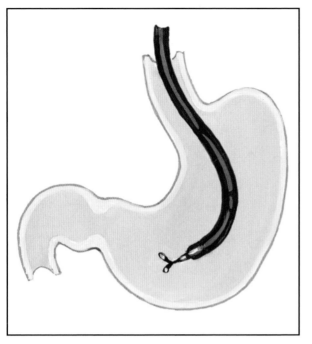

This is an illustration of an endoscope to the stomach.

gastritis, the patient, if hospitalized, is given no solid food for 24 to 48 hours, depending upon the severity of symptoms. Parenteral nutrition (placing nutrients directly into the bloodstream) may be administered if the patient is undernourished. As recovery occurs, the patient will progress to a soft or bland diet. The soft diet would be a low-fiber one that helps in the transition from a liquid to a solid diet. The bland diet eliminates foods that are irritating to the GI tract (see list below).

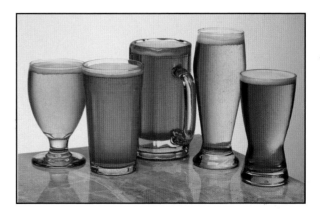

Fried foods may be eliminated as well, as these have been found to reduce gastric emptying.[17] Some patients may find dairy products cause problems and so will need to avoid these as well. The person with chronic gastritis would do well to eat small, frequent meals and avoid excessive fat intake.

eliminate heartburn symptoms, by protecting the damaged lining from acid. However, overuse of these drugs may be quite damaging to the body. According to holistic medical doctor Jonathan Wright, "Several studies have shown that gastritis … increases when people infected with H. pylori take Prilosec or other acid-suppressing drugs."[15] Dr. Wright further points out that H. pylori is the leading cause of atrophic gastritis, which is a major risk factor for stomach cancer. When a person with an H. pylori infection takes an acid-suppressing drug therefore, not only is the risk of developing atrophic gastritis increased but so is the risk of developing stomach cancer. In view of this information, Dr. Wright states quite bluntly, "…these drugs [acid-suppressors] should be classed as carcinogen-facilitators … Prescribing [them] without, at the very least, testing patients for H. pylori would appear to border on medical malpractice."[16]

In acute gastritis or in painful flare-ups of chronic

Vitamin B12 supplementation may be required for the gastritis patient since the chronic form of this disorder may reduce the ability to secrete acid and intrinsic factor.[18] Both of these are needed to absorb vitamin B12. In addition, low acid can cause malabsorption of most B vitamins, iron, zinc

Chapter 3

and amino acids. The supplementation of B12 may be best accomplished through injection since B12 may be reduced in the gastritis patient. Iron is best supplemented through whole food nutritional supplements or food sources.

Major iron-rich foods include:

- Eggs
- Fish
- Liver
- Meat
- Poultry
- Leafy green vegetables
- Whole grains

The type of iron used in "enriched" processed foods is synthetic and therefore not well utilized by the body. This form of iron can be constipating.

Reinhard also advises that in Ménétrier's disease (hypertrophic gastritis), "an important aspect of diet is to replace protein that is lost because of the disease.[19] We recommend emphasis on low-stress proteins (those that give more energy than they take), such as organic chicken, ocean fish, fermented soy products, eggs, seeds, sprouts and sea vegetables.

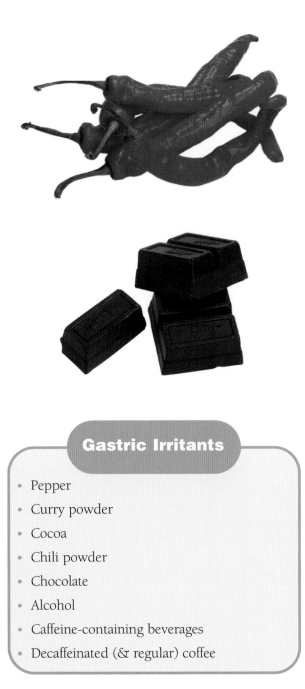

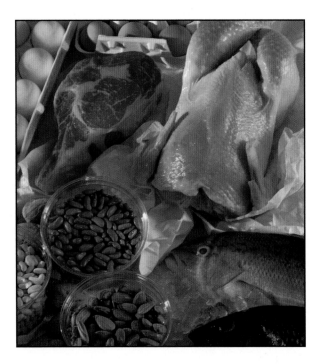

Gastric Irritants

- Pepper
- Curry powder
- Cocoa
- Chili powder
- Chocolate
- Alcohol
- Caffeine-containing beverages
- Decaffeinated (& regular) coffee

Optional Nutritional Approaches

Please follow general recommendations for all stomach problems at the end of this section. Since gastritis can have several contributing factors, further investigation will be needed to find the cause of the problem. The following factors can contribute and should be eliminated:

- Drugs, especially non-steroidal anti-inflammatory drugs, such as ibuprofen and aspirin (NSAIDS)
- Alcohol
- Smoking

Rule out the following:

- Any microbial infection
- Candida (see Chapter 4 on Candida)
- H. pylori infection
- Food sensitivity (see ELISA testing in appendix)

DIET

- Follow the Digestive Care Diet (see appendix).
- If there is pain, it may be helpful to do two to three days of juice fasting. Cabbage juice can be extremely helpful (see appendix for recipes).
- Eliminate foods known to cause a problem such as:
  - Pepper
  - Curry powder
  - Cocoa
  - Chili
  - Chocolate
  - Caffeine-containing beverages
  - Decaffeinated and regular coffee
  - Sugar-containing and processed foods in general

SUPPLEMENTS

If there are underlying conditions such as microbial infection (yeast or bacteria), a natural approach to this problem should be initiated immediately. The following are suggested to soothe and heal the stomach:

- Drink slippery elm tea or ginger to soothe.
- Take digestive enzymes (protease [at least 20,000 H.U.T.], amylase and lipase combination) before and after meals. This supplement could include marshmallow, ginger, papaya, bromelain, gamma oryzanol and N-acetyl-glucosamine.
- Chew deglycyrrhizinated licorice (DGL) between meals.
- Drink aloe vera juice or syrup between meals daily (see appendix).
- Take 5,000 mg. to 10,000 mg. of glutamine powder with N-acetyl-glucosamine (NAG) and gamma oryzanol once to twice daily on an empty stomach (see appendix).
- Take a multivitamin/mineral supplement (a liquid form could be helpful; find in health food store).
- Take antioxidant supplements (vitamin C - 500 mg. to 2000 mg., vitamin A - 10,000 I.U. daily and zinc – 30 mg. to 60 mg. daily) after meals. Other antioxidants may also be taken with these.
- Take essential fatty acids (EFAs). Use a combination of fish, flax oil and borage oil with lipase. A gel cap can help with better absorption of the oils. Take three to six 1000 mg. caplets twice daily with food.
- Take a probiotic (good bacteria) supplement with multiple strains as a daily supplement. It should contain a minimum of 2 to 6 billion cultures. A prebiotic could be helpful (see appendix).
- Take a B-12 supplement.
- Take supplemental folic acid.
- Take an iron supplement (liquid form – Floridex; see Resource Directory), only if your blood levels of iron or ferritin are low.

LIFESTYLE

- Sleep on your left side to avoid heartburn.
- Do not lie down for at least 3 or 4 hours after eating.
- Elevate head of bed 4 to 8 inches when sleeping.

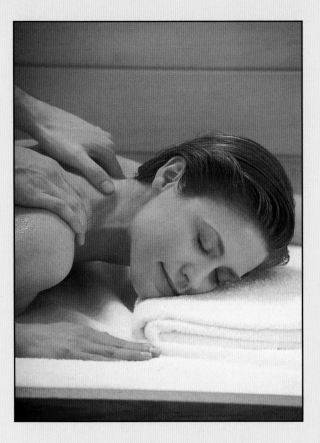

- Make sure you have good bowel elimination daily.
- Exercise daily (at the least, take a walk).

COMPLEMENTARY MIND/BODY THERAPIES

- Yoga
- Massage
- Biofeedback
- Music therapy
- Meditation/Prayer
- Acupuncture
- Colon hydrotherapy

See appendix for details.

Gastritis Facts:

- Gastritis means inflammation of the stomach. It usually involves only the mucosal lining not the entire stomach wall.

- Gastritis does not mean that there is an ulcer. It is simply inflammation — either acute or chronic.

- Helicobacter pylori is the name of a bacteria that has learned to live in the thick mucous lining of the stomach. It results in acute and chronic inflammation. It can occur early in childhood and remains throughout life. The infection can lead to ulcers and other gastric problems which are even more serious. Fortunately, there are now ways to treat this disorder.

- Currently in the United States, gastritis accounts for approximately 2 million visits to doctors' offices each year. Although gastritis can occur in people of all ages and backgrounds, it is especially common in:
  - People over age 60
  - People who drink alcohol excessively
  - Smokers
  - People who routinely use NSAIDs, especially at high doses

- Viral infections — Brief bouts of gastritis are common during short-term viral infections.

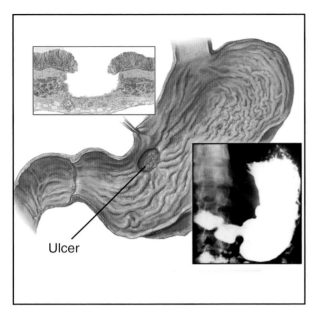

Ulcer

PEPTIC ULCERS

What is it?

"Peptic" means pertaining to pepsin or to digestion or to the action of gastric juices.[1] An ulcer is a sore or lesion. A peptic ulcer is a sore that develops in the mucous lining of the stomach (gastric ulcer), duodenum (duodenal ulcer) or the esophagus (esophageal ulcer) and underlying tissue as a result of exposure to stomach acid and pepsin (the protein-digesting enzyme produced in the stomach). Gastric, duodenal and esophageal ulcers then all fall under the category of "peptic ulcer." The duodenal ulcer is the most frequently occurring type, being four to five times more common than the gastric ulcer.[2] Esophageal ulcers are quite rare; they can develop as a consequence of gastroesophageal reflux disease (GERD), which involves regurgitation of stomach acid (and pepsin) into the esophagus where it burns delicate tissue (see GERD section in Chapter 2).

What Causes it?

Stress was once viewed as the major cause of peptic ulcers. The thinking was that stress caused an over-production of stomach acid, which irritated the mucosal lining, giving rise to an ulcer. While it is true that ulcers occur in the presence of stomach acid, it does not necessarily follow that excessive

quantities of hydrochloric acid (HCl) are the cause of the condition. In fact, given the fact that some people who have ulcers produce too little gastric acid and others without ulcers have too much acid,[3] it seems safe to conclude that the amount of acid produced is not a critical variable in determining who will get ulcers and who will not. More relevant seems to be the integrity of the protective mechanisms designed to shield tissues from the caustic effects of stomach acid. According to Steven Peikin, MD, it is a "distortion of the balance between acid and protective mucus"[4] that is the likely cause of ulcers. This being the case, "with inadequate mucosal defense, even a small amount of acid can cause an ulcer."[5]

There is, however, one very rare condition in which we can definitely say that excess stomach acid does play a major role in causing ulcers. That condition, known as Zollinger-Ellison syndrome, is characterized by elevated levels of gastrin in the blood caused by a tumor or tumors in the pancreas, duodenum or in the tissues around the stomach or spleen.[6] In ordinary peptic ulcers, gastrin levels are normal, and we do not see the massive production of gastric acid typical of Zollinger-Ellison syndrome.

For years, stress was considered the key factor in ulcer formation. Recently this supposition has been proved wrong. The stress-causes-ulcer model was largely abandoned in the earlier 1980s when Australian researchers discovered the presence of a bacterium, Helicobacter pylori (H. pylori), between the lining of the stomach and the protective mucous layer in ulcer patients. To prove the cause-effect relationship between H. pylori[7] and ulcers, they actually ingested the bacteria themselves and subsequently developed ulcers.[8]

It has been widely reported that the majority of patients with peptic ulcers have H. pylori, which is thought to weaken the mucosa over time, leaving the stomach vulnerable to the caustic effects of its own acid.[9] H. pylori has been identified in patients

Chapter 3

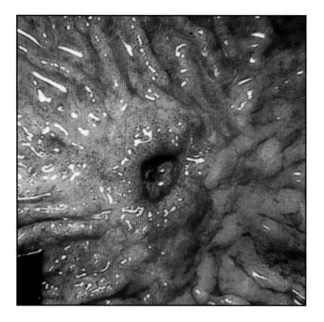

This is an internal view of an ulcer.

- Regular use of non-steroidal anti-inflammatory drugs (NSAIDs), such as aspirin (see gastritis section for full list)
- Use of steroid drugs like cortisone
- Alcohol consumption (moderate to excessive)
- Heavy smoking
- A family history of peptic ulcer disease
- Stress
- Nutrient deficiencies
- A low-fiber diet
- Food allergies
- Caffeine-containing beverages
- Dehydration
- Severe illness or trauma (causing a "stress ulcer")

with peptic ulcers but not all of them. Once H. pylori was estimated to be present in 65% to 100% of peptic ulcer sufferers. However, recent studies have suggested that the number is much lower, and could be below 50%.[10] If H. pylori were the sole cause of ulcers, we would expect to find it in all ulcer patients, and we would also expect it to be absent in those without ulcers. This is not the case, however. Many people in the U.S. have tested positive for H. pylori (about 20% under 40 years of age and more than 50% of those over 60) but most people with H. pylori will never develop ulcers.[11] It is estimated that 40 million people in the U.S. have H. pylori, but only 10-20% of them will develop an ulcer.[12]

While H. pylori does not appear to be the sole cause of peptic ulcers, it seems to be an important contributing variable, for the rate of recurrence of these ulcers is greatly diminished when H. pylori is successfully eradicated.[13] It would appear also that the cause of peptic ulcers is multi-faceted – that is to say, there is more than one cause. Other important causative variables appear to include:

It has been found that aspirin use at any level is a risk factor for developing peptic ulcers, although higher doses cause more gastrointestinal bleeding.[14] Those taking low-dose aspirin therapy in an effort to prevent heart disease may therefore be putting themselves at risk for developing peptic ulcers. Aspirin and other NSAIDs interfere with the stomach's ability to produce protective mucus and acid-neutralizing bicarbonate, and they affect blood flow to the stomach and interfere with cell repair.[15] Two to four percent of patients who take NSAIDs for a year develop serious gastrointestinal complications, including ulcers and bleeding from the stomach and small intestine.[16]

Stress is certainly not the major culprit in ulcer formation as it was once thought to be. In fact, several studies have shown that the number of stressful life events is not significantly different in peptic ulcer patients than in carefully selected, ulcer-free controls.[17] However, stress hormones do affect stomach acid secretions, and ulcer patients do tend to have flare-ups during stressful times. Stress would therefore appear to be a factor contributing to peptic ulcers.

We list dehydration as a cause of ulcers due primarily to the striking work of Dr. Batmanghelidj, an MD who found that the stomach needs plenty of water in order to

produce adequate mucus. Amazingly, while imprisoned in Iran, he was able to successfully treat ulcers in fellow inmates using nothing but water.[18]

Food allergies, especially to dairy products, have been found to be a primary factor in many cases of peptic ulcer.[19] The truth is, population studies show that the higher the milk consumption, the greater the likelihood of ulcer.[20] This is because food allergies can initiate histamine release, which in turn stimulates HCl-producing cells.

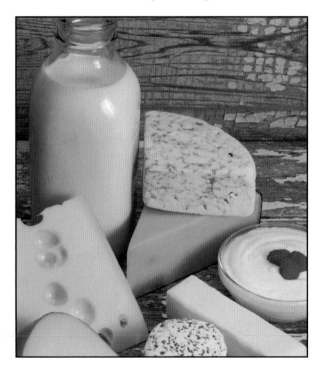

The antioxidant nutrients – vitamins A, C and E and the mineral zinc – protect the stomach lining from irritation by combating free radical damage. These renegade chemical fragments are injurious to cells. Inadequate levels of these nutrients, as well as a deficiency of vitamin B6 and the amino acid glutamine, may contribute to ulcers.[21] Where the antioxidant content of the GI tract lining is low, the likelihood of H. pylori infection is increased.

People who eat high-fiber diets have a lower rate of ulcers than those who consume low-fiber diets.[22]

Fiber is found in whole grains and in fruits and vegetables and is notoriously lacking in the processed standard American diet. Not only will a high-fiber diet help prevent ulcers, but it has been shown to reduce the recurrence of recently healed duodenal ulcers by half.[23]

Lifestyle and dietary choices play a key role in ulcer formation. For instance, smoking appears to play a major role in peptic ulcer disease. Those who smoke can expect to have a higher incidence of peptic ulcers, a higher rate of return of ulcers and a decreased response to treatment.[24] There are several reasons for this, the most significant of which is that smoking increases the reflux (backflow) of bile salts into the stomach, causing irritation to it and the duodenum.[25] Alcohol is also a problem. Alcohol irritates the stomach lining, and continued use of it interferes with healing of ulcers.

The rationale for the avoidance of coffee and other caffeine-containing beverages – and drugs like No-Doz, Anacin and Excedrin – is that caffeine seems to stimulate acid secretion in the stomach, increasing ulcer pain. Interestingly, decaffeinated coffee has the same effect as regular coffee, so clearly adverse effects are due to something more than just the caffeine.[26]

As with gastritis, trauma or severe illness can bring on an ulcer, which is identified as a "stress ulcer."

Who Gets it?

Over 25 million Americans will develop a peptic ulcer at some time in their lives.[27] Those at greatest risk are people with type "O" blood and those who have a family history of peptic ulcer disease.[28]

Although ulcers can affect people of all ages, it is rare for children to develop them. The risk of ulcer formation increases with age. Duodenal ulcers tend to occur more often in men than in women. Also, the age at onset of a duodenal ulcer is lower (30–50 years of age) than with the more rare stomach ulcers (over age 60). Interestingly, these rarer

Chapter 3

forms of ulcer affect more women than men.[29]

H. pylori infection, thought to be a major cause of ulcers, usually occurs during childhood and is more common in older adults, African Americans, Hispanics and lower socio-economic groups.[30] Interestingly, H. pylori infection rate is equal between men and women despite the fact that ulcers tend to affect men about twice as often as women.[31]

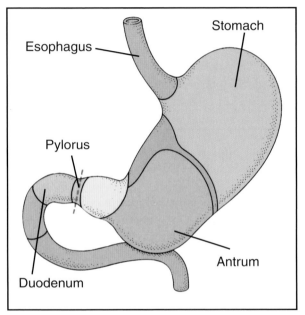

What Are the Signs and Symptoms?

Half of all people who have ulcers have no symptoms.[32] Those who do have symptoms will experience a pain in the upper abdomen underneath the breastbone. It may be a cramping, burning or gnawing sensation that feels like a "hunger pang." The pain may be constant or intermittent. Those with gastric ulcers will feel the pain just below the rib cage to the left, while the pain of duodenal ulcers is felt a little to the right of the mid-abdominal region. Quite often, this pain is worse at night and between meals – because gastric acid is more likely to cause irritation when the stomach is empty. Food acts as a buffer to neutralize acid and quickly relieves the pain of duodenal ulcers, although certain foods may irritate, causing more pain (see chart in Gastritis section). Food

may irritate gastric ulcers initially, but the burning generally subsides as acid is neutralized.[33] Other possible signs and symptoms of peptic ulcers include:

- Headache
- A choking sensation
- Nausea/vomiting
- Back pain
- Black tarry stools
- Paleness
- Weakness
- Loss of appetite
- Weight loss
- Dizziness

Incidents of black tarry stools and paleness are signs of internal bleeding. The symptoms are dizziness and weakness. Blood may also appear in vomit (looking like coffee grounds). These signs of bleeding should prompt one to seek immediate medical attention, as hemorrhage is an emergency situation. Perforation and obstruction also are considered acute and serious medical situations. All three are potential complications of peptic ulcers. With perforation, the ulcer literally eats a hole through the wall of the stomach or duodenum, and the stomach contents can spill into the abdominal cavity. With obstruction, the ulcer blocks the passage of food through the GI tract. These painful complications will likely require immediate surgical intervention, as they can be life-threatening.

Diarrhea is not typically a sign of ulcer, but is present in Zollinger-Ellison syndrome. If a patient has other ulcer symptoms along with diarrhea and has failed to respond to standard treatment, s/he may have this rare syndrome.

How is it Diagnosed?

Ulcers cannot be definitively diagnosed by symptoms alone for two reasons: Only half of those with ulcers have symptoms, and the symptoms typical of peptic ulcers are the same as those of stomach cancer.[34] Gastric ulcers may be malignant (cancerous), while duodenal ulcers are almost never malignant.[35] Also, symptoms of peptic ulcer may be similar to those of gastroesophageal reflux disorder (GERD).

Endoscopy (see appendix) is typically used to detect ulcers. H. pylori can be identified through biopsy taken with the endoscope. The bacterium also shows up in special blood and breath tests. All of these tests are about 90% effective in detecting H. pylori.[36] Endoscopic biopsy can also rule out malignancy in gastric ulcers.

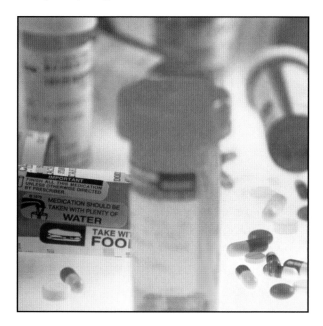

Another test for identifying gastric or duodenal ulcers (also described in the appendix) is the upper GI series, also known as a barium swallow. Additional tests may also be performed. Blood levels of gastrin will be measured if Zollinger-Ellison is suspected, as elevated gastrin is a sign of the disease. Special stool and/or blood tests may be done to check for hidden (occult) blood.

A test that is often performed by progressive physicians is the Comprehensive Digestive Stool Analysis (CDSA). In this test, stool samples are taken at home and submitted to a Diagnostic Laboratory (see appendix). The test helps identify problems with digestion and absorption, as well as microbial imbalances in the gut. This can be helpful in terms of getting to the cause of the problem, for H. pylori infection often results from an imbalance in the ecology of the gut.

Another test sometimes used by alternative practitioners is the adrenal hormone saliva test (see appendix).

What is the Standard Medical Treatment?

The standard medical treatment for ulcers, since it is viewed as an infectious disease aggravated by stomach acid, involves a combination of therapies, using all or some of the following:

- Antibiotics (usually two because H. pylori is believed to have a variety of strains)
- Acid-suppressing drugs called H2 blockers (like Tagamet and Pepsid) to block the action of histamine (which signals HCl production) or the more powerful proton pump inhibitors (like Nexium). See GERD treatment section in Chapter 2 for more information on these drugs.
- Drugs, such as sucralfate (sucrose plus polyaluminum hydroxide), to coat the lining of the stomach

Alternately, bismuth salts may be used along with antibiotics. These promote a protective layer in the stomach and halt the progress of H. pylori without reducing the amount of stomach acid.[37] Antacids are also used as needed to control heartburn or to block the pain of acute ulcer episodes. Care should be taken to avoid aluminum-containing antacids due to their toxicity (see GERD treatment section in Chapter 2).

Gastric and duodenal ulcers are treated in the same manner, but gastric ulcers are often treated more aggressively since they tend to heal more slowly than duodenal ulcers. Ulcers typically take 2 to 6 weeks to heal. Typically, antibiotics are administered for a period of 2 weeks, concurrently with antacids, which are often continued indefinitely.

If the use of NSAIDs is established as the cause of peptic ulcers, elimination of these drugs may in itself be sufficient to solve the problem. If not, standard treatment, as described, will be initiated.

A downside of the "combination treatment" approach is the manifestation of powerful side effects from the drugs typically used. Antibiotics can cause nausea, and their use can result in yeast infections when good bacteria are destroyed along with the bad. Acid-suppressing drugs have a number of undesirable side effects, many of them affecting the GI tract. This subject is covered at length in Chapter 2 in the GERD section. Interestingly, H. pylori secretes an enzyme called urease, which actually neutralizes HCl. And too little acid will allow H. pylori to reproduce more rapidly.[38] This being the case, the use of acid-suppressing drugs could actually make the H. pylori infection worse. Low gastric acid is considered by some to be an influential factor for development of H. pylori infection.[39]

While temporary initial use of antacids for symptomatic relief is relatively safe, taken regularly, these drugs can lead to malabsorption of nutrients, bowel irregularities, kidney stones and other side effects.[41]

Surgery is usually recommended for patients who don't respond to the therapies described above.

Ulcer Facts:

- It is an estimate that over 25 million Americans will develop a peptic ulcer at some time in their life.

- Helicobacter pylori (H. pylori), a type of bacteria that is believed to be a common cause of peptic ulcers, is very common in the United Sates, with 20% of people under 40 years of age and more than 50% of people over 60 years of age infected by it.

- Though H. pylori was first discovered in 1982, researchers still do not know how people contract it. They believe it may be contracted from food, water or mouth-to-mouth contact.

- Doctors, who orginally believed that peptic ulcers were solely caused by stress, spicy food or alcohol, simply recommended bed rest and a bland diet. Now, doctors focus on using antibiotics.

- Peptic ulcers are relatively common, affecting approximately 500,000 people in the United States each year.

- It has been estimated that about 10% of Americans will develop an ulcer at some time in their lives.

- Ulcers can develop in anyone at any age, but they are more common in older people.

- Duodenal ulcers tend to occur at an earlier age than gastric ulcers. While ulcers used to be more common in men, recent studies show that ulcers now occur at the same rate in men and women.

Optional Nutritional Approaches

Follow the General Recommendations for Stomach Problems at the end of this chapter.

Alternative approaches to ulcers can be two fold.

- Follow Step 1 if H. pylori is present, as a means to eradicate it.
- Follow Step 2 in order to soothe and heal the stomach.

Step 1

The following natural solutions could be effective in eradicating H. pylori infection:

- Mastic gum 250 mg. four times a day
- Vitamin C (see appendix to determine amount), but start with at least 3000 mg. per day.
- Bismuth subcitrate (different than Pepto-Bismol, which is bismuth salicylate), 240 mg. twice a day; available from compounding pharmacies.
- A natural anti-fungal and antibacterial with grapefruit seed extract, garlic, undecylenic acid, rosemary, thyme and bismuth could be helpful.
- Probiotics Lactobacillus and Bifidobacterium: A supplement that provides a combination of these bacteria, along with L. salivarius. L. salivarius has been shown to inhibit H. Pylori experimentally.

Step 2

Restoring and healing the stomach is the next approach and can be combined with the protocol from above.

DIET

If there is acute pain, you may want to do a juicing diet for a few days. An important factor would be cabbage juice. Follow the juicing recipes in the appendix.

Follow the Digestive Care Diet (see appendix). If symptoms are severe, you may want to ease from a juicing diet to a soft foods diet to include foods such as squash, potatoes, yams and avocados. See end of chapter for general recommendations.

SUPPLEMENTS

- Chew deglycyrrhizinated licorice (DGL) between meals.
- Aloe vera juice or syrup (see appendix)
- Glutamine powder with gamma oryzanol, ginger, calendula and cranesbill, 5000 mg. to 20,000 mg. daily on an empty stomach (see appendix).
- Take a probiotic (good bacteria) supplement with multiple strains as a daily supplement. It should contain a minimum of 2 to 6 billion cultures. A prebiotic could be helpful (see appendix).
- Antioxidant support – Vitamin C: at least 3000 mg. a day (or do the test for Vitamin C in appendix, and follow that recommendation), vitamin A: 10,000 I.U., vitamin E: 400-800 I.U. per day, zinc: 30 mg. to 60 mg. per day. A multiple antioxidant product that includes these would be fine.
- Take essential fatty acids (EFA's). A combination of fish and flax oils (Omega-3) with borage oil (Omega-6) is good to reduce inflammation in the gastrointestinal tract. Absorption of the oils may be enhanced with the addition of lipase (a fat-digesting enzyme). Take three to six 1000 mg. capsules twice daily with food.
- Take a fiber supplement that provides a balance of both soluble and insoluble fibers. A flax/borage seed combination is a good choice.
- Take an iron supplement (liquid form – Floridex; see Resource Directory). Take only if blood iron and ferritin levels are low.

LIFESTYLE

- Drink plenty of water and decaffeinated herbal teas daily.
- Make sure you have good bowel elimination daily.
- Exercise daily – even if it's just taking a walk.

Chapter 3

COMPLEMENTARY MIND/BODY THERAPIES

- Yoga can be extremely beneficial.
- Massage
- Biofeedback
- Music therapy
- Meditation/Prayer
- Acupuncture can be extremely beneficial.
- Chiropractic
- Colon hydrotherapy

For details, please see appendix.

Dr. Smith's Comments

Gastritis and ulcers are a spectrum of nutritional, inflammatory and infectious events that occur in the stomach and the first portion of the duodenum. During my lifetime as a surgeon, I have seen the treatment of ulcers change radically from surgery to medical therapy with antacids and antibiotics. The current medical therapy is so effective that surgery for ulcers has largely become a thing of the past. There are still some situations where surgery is urgently needed:

- *Ulcers can burrow through the stomach or duodenal wall (perforation) and spill acid, food and bile into the abdominal cavity; this is corrected by oversewing and patching the perforation and washing and cleaning the abdominal cavity.*
- *Ulcers can bleed uncontrollably and require lifesaving surgery.*
- *Ulcers can cause enough damage and swelling as to obstruct the outflow of the stomach and sometimes still require surgery.*
- *Ulcers are at times associated with cancer necessitating surgery.*

Nutrition is critical to protect the stomach. There must be adequate hydration, good mucus production and optimum cellular function. Research on vitamin C supplementation by Janoz, et. al. (European Journal Cancer Prevention 7:449-454) showed that 5 grams of vitamin C given daily to patients with chronic gastritis as the only therapy, resulted in eradication of H. pylori in 30% of the cases. Biopsies have shown significantly increased levels of vitamin C in the esophagus and stomach even after 1 gram of vitamin C per day. Other nutritional products of value include all B vitamins, particularly B12, sulforaphane from broccoli and various strains of lactobacillus bacteria.

Indiscriminate use of acid-blocking drugs can be a serious problem for some patients. A study in GUT (2003, 52:496-501) showed that patients with H. pylori gastritis had iron deficiency anemia, thought to be due to high gastric pH (7) and low vitamin C levels caused by the H. pylori, as compared to normal controls. Both an acid pH and vitamin C are needed for iron absorption. This study also pointed out that plasma vitamin C levels were uniformly lower in patients infected with H. pylori compared to controls. Stomach acid is our best natural antibiotic and is required for absorption of most B vitamins, zinc, as well as iron. This may well be why so many elderly people (who have low gastric acid) have problems with immunity (low tissue zinc levels), Candida infections, heart disease and Alzheimers (low B12, folate and B6, raising plasma homocysteine levels).

Acid-blocking drugs, when used briefly (10-14 days) with antibiotics to treat ulcers, constitute acceptable medical care. Unfortunately, I have seen patients left for years at a time on these acid-blockers. It is well known that the gastric hormone gastrin is markedly elevated when acid is blocked. Studies are now suggesting high gastrin levels increase cellular activity that could lead to cancer of the esophagus and stomach in genetically susceptible patients.

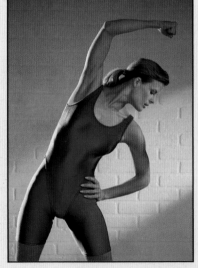

General Recommendations for all Stomach Problems

- For immediate relief of pain, try drinking a glass of room temperature filtered water; it can dilute acidity.

- No caffeine (or decaffeinated) coffee.

- No carbonated beverages.

- Teas are good: ginger, slippery elm or green tea.

- Cabbage juice is excellent (see appendix for recipes).

- Eat frequent small meals.

- Chew foods thoroughly.

- Millet and rice are usually the best tolerated grains.

- Eat soft foods after a 3-day juice fast if symptoms are severe (see appendix).

- Avoid fried foods, and follow the Digestive Care Diet for at least three months. Stay on it if you can.

- Avoid milk.

- Make sure you have good bowel elimination daily; if not, refer to constipation section.

- No smoking.

- No NSAIDS (aspirin, ibuprofen, etc.)

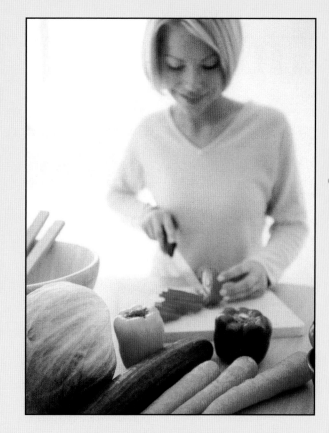

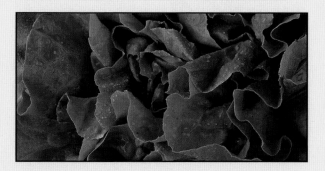

Ulcer Fact:

- Although it's still unclear what causes ulcers, current research suggests that the bacterium Helicobacter pylori plays a major role. In fact, this bacterium is believed to cause between 70% and 90% of all peptic ulcers. But infection is not the whole story, because only about 20% of people infected with H. pylori develop ulcers. In some people, H. pylori infection somehow upsets the delicate balance between the damaging effects of gastric acids and the body's natural protection.

Intestinal Problems

APPENDICITIS

What is it?

The appendix is a small tubular structure attached to the right side of the cecum, the lower right portion of the large intestine (colon). Appendicitis is an acute or chronic inflammation of the organ. Normally, the appendix resembles the little finger, being 3 to 4 inches long and one quarter of an inch in diameter. When inflamed, the appendix can swell, and the wall can fill with dead white blood cells (pus), and this local infection can rapidly spread to the rest of the body. The pathological definition of appendicitis is the microscopic presence of white blood cells in the wall of the appendix.

In the past, medicine has not been able to assign a particular function to the appendix. Today, however, it is becoming more apparent that the appendix and surrounding lymphatic tissue probably serve an important role in immunity. Bowel movements in a liquid or semi-solid state pass in and out of the appendix. Research now supports the concept that the microbes in the stool have a dynamic communication with the intestinal lining, including the lining of the appendix. Signals are sent from these microbes to the lymph tissue, which creates a memory bank of immune information. Future exposure will then cause the immune system to either accept or reject previously recognized microbial populations.

What Causes it?

The cause of appendicitis is not officially known, though there are several possible causes of the condition. Obstruction of the appendix can occur due to solid pieces of stool (faecaliths) or as a result of the stool becoming hard like stone (appendicoliths). Occasionally, impaction of the appendix can occur secondary to parasites, especially pinworms. Another cause of appendicitis can be swollen lymph nodes at the base of the appendix secondary to a viral or bacterial infection. This swollen tissue can impede lymphatic or venous drainage,

Sixty to 70 million people are affected by digestive disease.

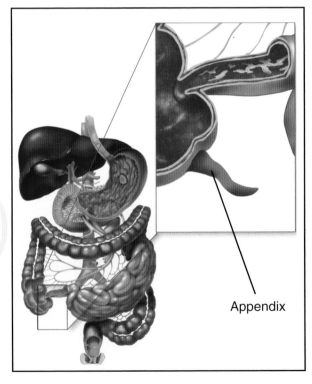

Appendix

causing the appendix to swell. The pressure from the swelling may hamper arterial inflow, resulting in decreased oxygen to the tissues, followed by inflammation, more swelling and finally gangrene and rupture of the appendix.

From the natural medicine perspective, chronic constipation, high concentrations of bad or pathogenic bacteria, absence of friendly bacteria and decreased fiber could play a role in appendicitis.

Who Gets it?

People of any age may develop appendicitis, but it most commonly occurs in pre-teens, teenagers and young adults. In fact, acute appendicitis is the most common cause for emergency surgery in children. Those with a family history of appendicitis are at greater risk for developing the disorder, and children under two years of age and adults over 70 are at higher risk for developing a rupture (described below).[1]

There is a 7% chance of developing appendicitis over the course of a lifetime, and one in 500 will be hospitalized because of it each year.[2]

Interestingly, women have about half the number of cases of appendicitis as men, and yet they have twice as many appendectomies.[3] This is due to the fact that appendicitis can mimic other disorders, such as inflammation and cysts of the ovaries and fallopian tubes. In these cases, a normal appendix may be removed to prevent further diagnostic dilemmas for the patient in the future.

The risk of developing appendicitis increases after a recent illness, especially a gastrointestinal infection or a roundworm infection.[4] It is also interesting to note who doesn't get appendicitis. Dr. Dennis Burkitt found that any colon infection, including appendicitis, was very rare in the African population he studied. It is suggested that diet may play a key factor in his findings, as his study group consumed an average of 60-80 grams of fiber every day!

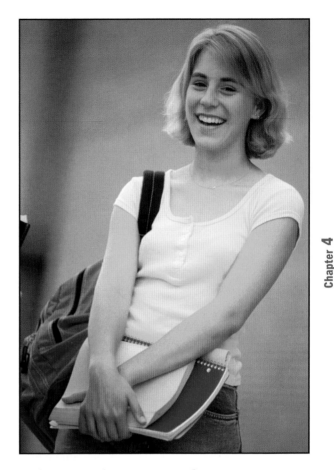

What are the Signs and Symptoms?

The hallmark symptom of appendicitis is a pain running from the navel toward the lower right portion of the abdomen. This pain may come in waves initially, but become progressively more constant and more pronounced. It is typically worse with movement, when coughing or when the area is touched. Other signs and symptoms may include:

- Nausea/vomiting
- Change in bowel habits (constipation or diarrhea, inability to pass gas)
- Fever
- Abdominal swelling
- Tenderness in right abdomen
- Loss of appetite
- Right-sided tenderness with walking, moving or coughing
- Elevated white blood count

It is important to know that many of these symptoms are typical of other diseases.[5] Among the diseases that may be mistaken for appendicitis are:

- Pelvic inflammatory disease
- Ovarian cysts
- Endometriosis
- Cervical inflammation
- Ectopic pregnancy (outside the uterus – usually in the fallopian tubes)
- Diverticulitis
- Kidney stones
- Bladder infection
- Inflammatory bowel disease

The first five disorders listed above occur only in females. This becomes important to note because the likelihood of misdiagnosis may be especially high in women. Misdiagnosis also occurs in men. In fact, surgeons find a normal appendix in 3 out of 10 appendectomies they perform.[6] This is considered acceptable because of the difficulty in obtaining an accurate preoperative diagnosis. At times, normal appendices are removed during the course of other abdominal surgeries for "prophylactic" reasons, to avoid future problems. However, this is less common now than in the past.

The rush to surgery may be due largely to the consequences of failure to promptly diagnose an inflamed appendix. Left untreated, complications may occur. These may include tissue death (gangrene) of the appendix, a collection of pus (abscess) in, or in the vicinity of the appendix, blood poisoning caused by infectious bacteria (sepsis) or rupture of the appendix. With rupture, the appendix bursts, spreading fecal liquid and material, as well as pus, throughout the abdominal cavity, causing an inflammation of the abdominal lining (peritonitis). This can be a life-threatening condition. The risk of these complications makes appendicitis an emergency condition. While the death rate for those whose appendix hasn't ruptured is quite low (less than 1%), it rises significantly (as high as 5%) if the appendix bursts.[7] These percentages increase for the very young and the very old. A ruptured appendix is found in approximately 1/5 of those patients who undergo appendectomies,[8] although the amount of contamination varies considerably from case to case.

How is it Diagnosed?

Appendicitis is generally diagnosed on the basis of medical history and physical exam. Blood and urine tests may be done to check for infection. Where there is uncertainty regarding diagnosis, an ultrasound or CT scan (computer-assisted tomography) may be performed. While these further diagnostics are not routinely performed, perhaps they should be, at least with women, as they could theoretically help doctors to make a more definitive diagnosis where gynecological problems are mistaken as appendicitis. A recent study with 500 patients who underwent appendectomy seems to

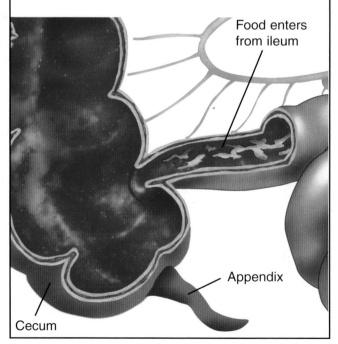

This illustration shows food from the small intestine going into the cecum. The appendix is located at the end of the cecum.

Food enters from ileum

Appendix

Cecum

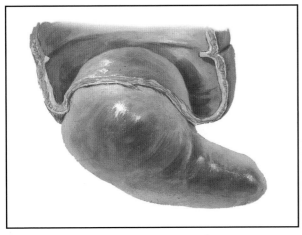

This is an illustration of an impacted appendix.

Appendicitis Facts:

- The risk of appendicitis increases with age and peaks between the ages of 15 and 30. However, appendicitis also is the main reason for abdominal surgery in children, with four of every 1,000 children requiring an appendectomy (surgical removal of the appendix) before age 14.

- Although the duration of symptoms varies, most patients will seek medical attention within 12 to 48 hours because of the abdominal pain. In some cases, a low level of inflammation exists for several weeks before a diagnosis is made.

confirm this; it was found that in women, if a CT scan or ultrasound was done before the surgery, a healthy appendix was removed 7% of the time compared to 28% of the time if a scan was not done. However, in some studies, this lowered rate did not hold up in men or children.[9] CT scan of the abdomen and pelvis is rapidly becoming a mainstay in the evaluation of the appendix.

When diagnostic tests are inconclusive, exploratory surgery may be performed.

What is the Standard Medical Treatment?

Because of the risks of rupture, appendicitis is treated as a medical emergency, with surgical removal of the appendix as the treatment of choice. An increasing number of surgeons are performing laparoscopic surgery in which a miniature camera and surgical instruments are inserted through tiny cuts in the abdomen. There are numerous claimed advantages to this procedure: less infection, fewer adhesions, less pain and scarring and more rapid recovery. There are instances, however, in which it is necessary to use traditional "open" surgical procedures to remove the appendix. Typically, antibiotics are administered, as well as intravenous fluids, and, if nauseated, the patient will be given medication to control vomiting.

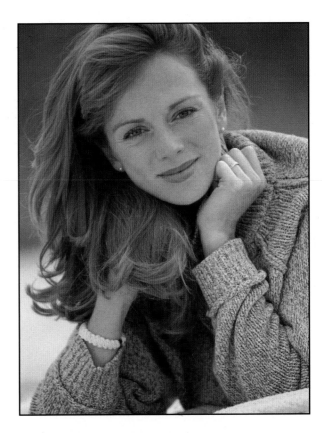

Optional Nutritional Approaches

Because appendicitis is a medical emergency, a patient needs to tread lightly where alternatives are concerned. On the other hand, because of the potential for misdiagnosis (particularly for women), people should insist upon a complete diagnostic work up before electing surgery – unless the appendix has ruptured, in which case, immediate surgery must be performed.

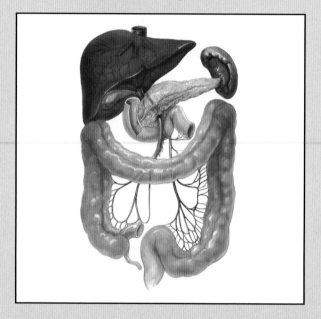

While accumulation of wastes in the colon is viewed as a causal factor, it is important to NOT take enemas or laxatives (even herbal ones) when appendicitis is suspected, for they could cause the appendix to burst (rupture), leading to a life-threatening situation. However, these measures, as well as colonic irrigation (a thorough colon cleansing therapy performed by certified colon therapists) can be very helpful in preventing appendicitis. They may also be used to advantage as an adjunct to herbal colon cleansing programs once the patient has thoroughly healed from appendectomy.

For prevention of appendicitis, follow the Digestive Care Diet (see appendix). If surgery has been performed, follow a soft diet of squashes, potatoes and freshly prepared juice for a few days, and then follow the Digestive Care Diet.

SUPPLEMENTS

The following is recommended for prevention of appendicitis, as well as following surgery should an appendectomy have been necessary:

- Take digestive enzymes (protease [at least 20,000 H.U.T.], amylase and lipase combination) before and after meals. This supplement could include marshmallow, ginger, papaya, bromelain, gamma oryzanol and N-acetyl-glucosamine.
- Take a probiotic (good bacteria) supplement with multiple strains as a daily supplement. It should contain a minimum of 2 to 6 billion cultures. A prebiotic could be helpful (see appendix).
- Take a multivitamin/mineral daily (see appendix).
- Take a fiber supplement that provides a balance of both soluble and insoluble fibers. A flax/borage seed combination is a good choice, particularly one that contains other beneficial ingredients such as a probiotic blend with fructooligosaccharides (FOS) and herbs like slippery elm bark, marshmallow and fennel seed. Another key ingredient would be L-glutamine, which the intestine uses as fuel to regenerate.

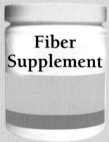

Fiber Supplement

- Take essential fatty acids (EFAs). A combination of fish and flax oils (Omega-3) with borage oil (Omega-6) is good to reduce inflammation in the gastrointestinal tract. Absorption of the oils may be enhanced with the addition of lipase (a fat-digesting enzyme). Take three to six 1000 mg. capsules twice daily with food.
- Take antioxidant supplements (vitamin C - 500 mg. to 3000 mg., vitamin A - 10,000 I.U. daily and zinc – 30 mg. to 60 mg. daily) after meals. Other antioxidants may also be taken

with these (see appendix for specification on antioxidants.)

If surgery has already been performed, the following may be added to the above supplements:

- Take 5,000 mg. to 10,000 mg. of glutamine powder with N-acetyl-glucosamine (NAG) and gamma oryzanol once to twice daily on an empty stomach (see appendix).
- Take aloe vera juice, 5 ounces twice a day, between meals. Dilute 50% with water, and increase concentration as tolerated (see appendix).

***PLEASE NOTE: Three to four months after surgery, it could be helpful to do a 30-day herbal cleansing program (see appendix under "30-day detox protocol").

LIFESTYLE

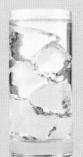

- Drink plenty of water daily. Ideally, you should consume half your body weight in ounces.
- Follow the 30-day herbal cleansing program twice a year for prevention (see appendix).
- Exercise daily – even if it's just taking a walk. Also, a mini-trampoline can be beneficial to stimulate lymph flow (see Resource Directory).
- Daily bowel elimination is important. Do not get constipated.

COMPLEMENTARY MIND/BODY THERAPIES

- Colon hydrotherapy can be very helpful in preventing many bowel problems. Incorporate it into your 30-day herbal detox program.
- Massage can be helpful, especially lymphatic massage, as the appendix is a lymphoid organ.
- Yoga
- Biofeedback
- Music therapy
- Meditation/prayer
- Acupuncture
- Chiropractic

See appendix for the above eight therapies.

Dr Smith's Comments

Appendicitis is a common surgical emergency requiring experience in making an accurate diagnosis. If the diagnosis is not clear, sometimes the judgment to proceed with operation is best. Still 10-20% of appendectomies are done when the diagnosis is for other conditions including diverticulitis, inflammation of the right fallopian tube or ovary and commonly lymphadenitis (swollen lymph nodes in the tissue surrounding the appendix). CT scan has decreased the incidence of non-therapeutic appendectomy from about 14% to 7%. Ultrasound is cheaper, and sometimes is very good in confirming the diagnosis. Either of these studies can be done when the diagnosis is not clear. This can often be the case with young children and older patients where the history, signs and symptoms may not be classical. Delay in surgery can result in ruptured appendix, which is still a very serious problem and can lead to recurrent intra-abdominal infection.

Nutrition may play a role in prevention. It has been shown that in societies with high fiber intake there is a much lower incidence of appendicitis. High-fiber, combined with probiotics, makes short-chained fatty acids that fuel and maintain the health of colonic and appendiceal cells. Many cases of appendicitis are due to either bacterial or viral infection. Dietary and supplemental antioxidants (especially vitamin C), as well as essential fatty acids, may help avoid the inflammatory changes that accompany the infection (a Th1 cellular type of inflammatory immune response) and thereby prevent the swelling that leads to full-blown appendicitis.

Chapter 4

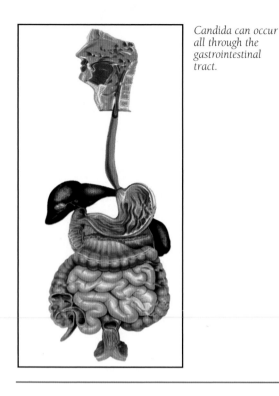

Candida can occur all through the gastrointestinal tract.

CANDIDIASIS
What is it?

The presence of Candida albicans, a benign sugar-fermenting yeast, in various parts of the body – the skin, genitals and especially the intestinal tract – is entirely normal. In small amounts, this yeast is an integral part of the intestinal ecology and, when kept in balance with other microorganisms, does no harm. Candidiasis, however, is a complex medical syndrome resulting from an overgrowth of Candida albicans. This yeast (or single-celled fungus) is one of 600 strains of Candida, and is among the minority that can become pathogenic (disease-causing).[1]

In candidiasis, normally harmless yeasts proliferate and change into a mycelial form (where they take root in tissues and colonize). This upsets the ecological balance in the gastrointestinal tract. When the friendly gut bacteria that normally control Candida die off, and Candida gains an upper hand, local problems can result – in the vagina ("yeast" infection), throat (thrush), nails (fungal infection), bladder (Candida cystitis), etc. When Candida colonizes in

the gut, it can cause problems throughout the body due to the fact that potent, immune-suppressing toxins are absorbed into the bloodstream. Candida is actually a form of parasite, an organism that feeds off of the human body and can pollute the system with its toxic waste products if it is present in disproportionate quantities.

What Causes it?

There are multiple factors that may trigger the form change and proliferation of Candida that result in candidiasis. This condition develops when the balance between yeast and bacteria is upset as a result of:

• Immune dysfunction
• Disruption in ratio of good to bad bacteria in the gastrointestinal tract
• Upset in intestinal pH

Immune dysfunction is caused by a number of factors: ingestion of certain drugs, like anti-inflammatories, cortisone, birth control pills, chemotherapy and antibiotics; exposure to toxic metals, such as mercury, lead, cadmium, nickel and aluminum, and other environmental toxins; generation of internal toxins as a result of poor digestion and focal infection (a walled off area of concentrated toxins and dead and/or infected tissue, often in the mouth); stress and over-consumption of refined carbohydrates. All of these factors create an imbalance of gut flora (with the bad bacteria outnumbering the good) called dysbiosis, which can result in reduced immunity.

An alteration of the ratio of good to bad bacteria in the GI tract is a very common cause of candidiasis. In fact, the prolonged – and sometimes inappropriate – use (and overuse) of antibiotics is perhaps the most widespread cause of chronic candidiasis today. These drugs suppress not only pathogenic or bad bacteria, but also the friendly bacteria whose job it is to prevent yeast overgrowth. The net result is proliferation of Candida. As Candida proliferates, the fungus releases toxins (waste products called mycotoxins) that further weaken

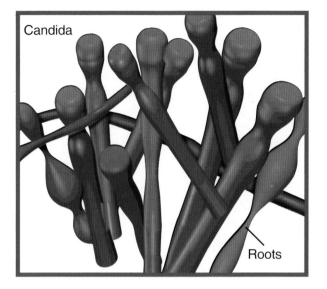

Candida

Roots

the immune system. Candida also secretes acids that can unfavorably alter pH (acid-alkaline balance). A by-product of Candida digestion of protein is Beta-alanine. Beta-alanine is absorbed through the intestinal lining and secreted by the kidneys. It competes for reabsorption with the amino acid taurine in the kidneys and thus lowers taurine levels. This is a significant problem because taurine enhances the intracellular uptake of magnesium and potassium. In addition, it helps to bind toxins and remove them from the liver. Thus, it has been clinically observed that patients with candidiasis of the intestinal tract may have problems absorbing magnesium and potassium, despite oral supplementation. (Personal communication with Dr. David Quigg, nutritional biochemist at Doctor's Data Laboratories.)

While the sources of heavy metals are many and varied, one of the most important with regard to candidiasis is the dental use of mercury. The "silver" amalgam dental filling routinely used by dentists is actually composed primarily (50-53%) of mercury.[2] It will be extremely difficult for the person with amalgam fillings to rid the body of Candida, for mercury has an antibiotic effect, killing off the friendly bacteria so they cannot control yeast overgrowth.[3]

Who Gets it?

Yeast-connected illness affects people of all ages, and although both sexes are affected, women are eight times more likely to experience the yeast syndrome.[4] Women may develop vaginal yeast infections following a course of antibiotics, during pregnancy or while using oral contraceptives. Progesterone from birth control pills changes the vaginal lining to make it more hospitable to yeasts [and] … also causes the release of yeast-feeding sugar into the bloodstream.[5] Candida may be transmitted sexually, and a mother may pass it on to her newborn.[6] Candidiasis in the form of oral "thrush" and/or diaper rash is common in babies.

Factors that might predispose one to candidiasis include:[7, 8]

- Use of antibiotics
- Use of corticosteroid drugs (which suppress the immune system and permit the overgrowth of yeast)
- A compromised immune system (evident in people with AIDS, cancer and autoimmune diseases, as well as those taking immunosuppressive drugs and people with a heavy body burden of toxins)
- A damp, moldy environment
- A diet high in refined carbohydrates and other yeast-promoting foods (see Optional Nutritional Approaches section for foods to exclude)
- Presence of mercury-containing "silver" amalgam fillings in the teeth
- Stress (which suppresses immune function)
- Decreased digestive secretions
- Nutrient deficiency
- Impaired liver function
- Altered bowel flora (bacteria)

Also at increased risk for developing yeast infections, according to Luc De Schepper, MD, PhD, CA, are patients who have undergone surgical interventions, catheterizations and dialysis, as well as burn victims and those with diabetes mellitus and hypothyroidism.[9]

Chapter 4

Autoimmune Diseases Resulting from Leaky Gut

- Lupus
- Alopecia areata
- Rheumatoid arthritis
- Polymyalgia rheumatica
- Multiple sclerosis
- Chronic fatigue syndrome
- Sjogren's syndrome
- Fibromyalgia
- Thyroiditis
- Crohn's disease
- Vitilego
- Vasculitis
- Ulcerative colitis
- Urticaria (hives)
- Diabetes
- Raynaud's disease

Chart 1

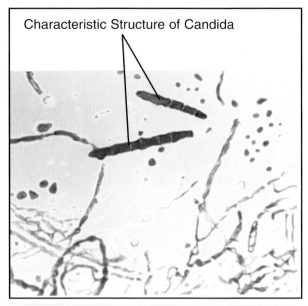

Characteristic Structure of Candida

This is a microscopic view of Candida.

What Are the Signs and Symptoms?

Candidiasis can affect many parts of the body and may be characterized by a wide variety of local and systemic signs and symptoms, including:[10,11]

- Chronic fatigue
- Food cravings (especially for sweets, fermented foods, alcoholic and carbonated beverages)
- Hyperactivity and learning disabilities in children
- Lack of libido
- Food and environmental sensitivities or allergies (adverse reaction to such items as perfume, dust, cut grass, tobacco smoke, chemicals, molds, pollen, etc.)
- Suppressed immune activity; autoimmune disorders (see chart I)

- Headaches
- Muscle aches
- Arthritis
- Change in bowel habits (or alternating diarrhea and constipation)
- Vaginitis
- Bladder and kidney infections
- Sunlight sensitivity
- Gas and bloating
- Abdominal pain
- Bad breath
- Rectal itching
- Impotence
- Prostatitis
- Sore throat
- Clogged sinuses/sinusitis
- Persistent heartburn
- Acne
- Night sweats
- Numbness in face or extremities
- PMS
- Burning tongue
- White spots on tongue and in mouth
- Nail infections
- Diaper rash

- Skin infection in groin, neck fold (in infants), under breasts (in heavy-breasted women) and under armpits
- Depression, irritability, poor concentration, brain fog

As mentioned, Candida releases waste products when it proliferates; these waste products are called mycotoxins. Among the mycotoxins produced by Candida is acetaldehyde – a poison that is transformed into ethanol and converted by the liver into alcohol. As alcohol builds up in the system, symptoms associated with drunkenness develop. This is how Candida can produce "brain fog" symptoms.

The development of allergies and other autoimmune disorders is viewed largely (by progressive physicians and alternative practitioners) as a consequence of mycotoxins entering the bloodstream. Normally, the semi-permeable lining of the intestinal tract will prevent contamination of blood with these and other toxins, microorganisms and undigested food particles. However, when the roots of Candida (known as rhizoids) burrow into the intestinal lining, they leave microscopic holes, through which these contaminants may pass. The

body sees undigested food particles as foreign bodies and therefore launches an immune reaction, giving rise to an allergic response or other manifestation of autoimmune disease.

Candida toxins are carried through the "leaky" gut via the bloodstream to the liver. From there, they proceed to other organs of the body – the brain, nervous system, joints, skin, etc. If the liver's detoxification ability is impaired due to inadequate nutrition and toxic overload, these toxins will be stored and can initiate states of chronic disease. In addition to suppressing the immune system, Candida also disrupts the endocrine (glandular) system, which has a regulating effect on the body. These effects make it possible for Candida to cause – or contribute to – virtually any disorder anywhere in the body.

Systemic Candida infection can follow an untreated local one, but it is important to know that systemic yeast infection can exist without any visible local symptoms. When present, symptoms can be varied, as the above list indicates.[12]

Yeast can harm the body in at least three ways:

1. Local infection, such as thrush, esophagitis, cystitis and vaginitis
2. Blood-borne infection resulting when the fungus burrows into the intestinal lining, causing inflammation and microvascular damage with the release of toxins directly into the blood and lymphatic systems. This causes further immune suppression in people with seriously depressed immunity as a result of conditions like AIDS or cancer.
3. Intestinal yeast infection, where direct damage to the intestinal lining increases intestinal permeability with subsequent absorption of Candida toxins and partially digested food, which can trigger food sensitivities

Additional local damage is done by the immune suppression caused by these toxins and possibly

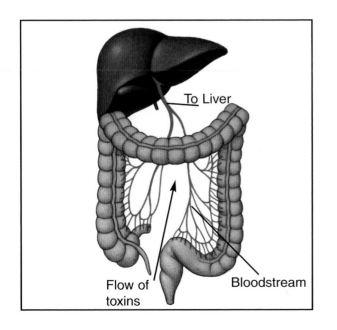

To Liver

Flow of toxins

Bloodstream

Chapter 4

by the body's allergic reaction to them. Traditional medical doctors do not generally recognize this last manifestation of candidiasis.[13]

How is it Diagnosed?

It is generally agreed that diagnosis of candidiasis is best made on the basis of a thorough patient history. A good questionnaire can be helpful toward this end. See end of this section (on candidiasis) for two versions of the self-scoring yeast questionnaire – adult and child – both developed by the late William G. Crook, MD, a pioneer in yeast-related illness.

Doctors may wish to confirm their diagnosis of candidiasis through use of specialized laboratory tests, such as stool cultures for Candida (Comprehensive Digestive Stool Analysis) and measurement of antibody levels to Candida or Candida antigens in the blood.[14] The Comprehensive Digestive Stool Analysis can also be useful in detecting parasites, which tend to co-exist with Candida. Since a certain amount of yeast is normally present in the GI tract, its detection in the laboratory tests does not necessarily mean that it has overgrown and is causing disease. For this reason, these tests alone may not offer a definitive diagnosis. That's why a thorough history should also be taken.

What is the Standard Medical Treatment?

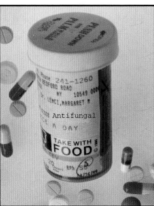

Traditional medicine employs fungicides (like Nystatin, Diflucan and Nizoral) to treat severe yeast infections. Fungistatic drugs that inhibit the growth of fungi, preventing it from getting worse, may also be employed. While these may effectively suppress fungal

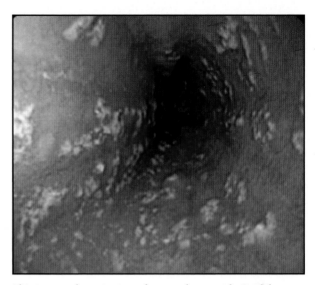

This is an endoscopic view of an esophagus with Candida overgrowth.

growth, it may resume once medication is discontinued unless the primary problem is handled and dybiosis corrected.

While many doctors of "complementary" medicine will rely upon herbal and nutritional remedies (as described on page 64-66) solely, some may opt to do a short course of drug (anti-fungal) therapy first in an effort to shorten treatment time. Diflucan, Sporanox and Nizarol are all absorbed in the upper GI tract and taken into circulation, so therapeutic doses do not reach the colon. Nystatin can be used in conjunction with the systemic drugs for a short period of time to help ensure elimination of Candida[15], but please understand that handling Candida is more than just taking a pill. It is a holistic approach, consisting of diet, supplementation, lifestyle modification, mental and emotional support.

Candidiasis Fact:

- In systemic candidiasis, Candida fungi contaminate the bloodstream and spread throughout the body, causing severe infection.

Optional Nutritional Approaches

The following should be ruled out for the effective elimination of Candida:

- Mercury toxicity, amalgam tooth fillings, over-consumption of fish and industrial exposure
- Oral focal infection, if you have been unresponsive to Candida programs in the past
- A holistic doctor or practitioner can test you for mercury toxicity through a stool analysis (see appendix).
- Consult a holistic dentist regarding testing for biocompatible materials and diagnosis and treatment of jawbone cavitations (hollow spaces in the jawbone not visible through x-ray or oral exam) if you have history of root canals, extractions or other trauma to the jawbone.
- Rule out hormone imbalance for women (see appendix).
- A questionnaire to determine if you have a potential problem with yeast overgrowth is located at the end of this section on Candida.
- A Complete Digestive Stool Analysis (CDSA; see appendix) is also available through a holistic practitioner. This could be helpful in detecting yeast overgrowth and determining the type of yeast overgrowth.

DIET

The diet below should be followed for at least one month. Many people suffer from hidden food sensitivities and are often addicted to the foods they are eating. When they begin to eliminate these foods from their diet, they can experience "withdrawal" symptoms. This can also cause one to feel angry due to a craving for foods that have been removed from the diet. This too shall pass! Try to start diet modifications at a time when you are able to take it easy and rest during the first few days. The first step is to remove certain foods from your diet:

- Clean out your kitchen, and get rid of sugar, corn syrup, white bread and white flour products, as well as all boxed sugar-laden cereals,

crackers and sodas (even diet soda).
- Eliminate fruit and fruit juices from your diet. Fresh green juices are excellent (see appendix under juicing).
- Eliminate sugar and artificial sweeteners. Have no sugar, honey, molasses or maple syrup during the first month.
- Eliminate cheese and commercial dairy products.
- Eliminate mushrooms, breads made with yeast, baked goods, (most packaged/processed foods in general) and peanuts. Find yeast-free breads in the health food store.
- Avoid caffeine-containing and alcoholic beverages.
- Eliminate vinegar (except raw apple cider vinegar from the health food store); also avoid vinegar-containing foods like mayonnaise, salad dressings and soy sauce.
- Avoid processed and smoked meats.

During the first month, you may eat:

- Plenty of vegetables, especially low carbohydrate - You may eat them raw, cooked or frozen. Organic is best. The vegetables to eat sparingly (1/2 cup serving) during this time include beans and potatoes (regular and sweet).
- Meat (organic is best), seafood, eggs and tofu. - Select chicken, lamb, turkey and lean cuts of beef, cod, salmon, mackerel, sardines, shrimp, lobster, tuna and wild game.
- Nuts, seeds, cashews, almonds, filberts, flaxseeds, pumpkin seeds - These need to be soaked overnight in distilled or purified water to ensure better digestion.
- Grains such as rice, spelt, teff, amaranth, buckwheat, millet, kamut, quinoa and oats - These need to be soaked overnight to ensure better digestion.
- Snacks may include raw pumpkin seeds, oil-free corn chips and nuts. Raw almond and cashew butter are excellent. Granny Smith apples are permitted.
- Oils (cold-pressed) - corn, olive, safflower and

walnut; butter in moderation.
- Plain organic yogurt, if you can tolerate it.
- Drink plenty of water, caffeine-free herbal teas; use sweeteners like lohan and stevia.
- Use fresh squeezed lemon juice to replace vinegar.

After the first month, begin to add in fruit, but limit yourself to one fruit at a time, and see how you feel that day. You can then start on the Digestive Care Diet in the appendix. Sugar and sugar-containing foods should be kept out of your diet indefinitely.

***Please note: If you are starting a Candida program (diet) and you have never cleansed (bowel or liver), it could be extremely helpful to do a 30-day herbal detox program (see appendix) before starting on the Candida supplement protocol below.

SUPPLEMENTS

A natural anti-fungal program would be essential during the first month. A product that combines a broad spectrum of natural anti-fungals can be effective since there are many different strains of yeast. Capsules and a liquid tincture in the morning and before bed can fit into anyone's schedule. Ideally, the following anti-fungal agents would be used:

- Uva ursi - shown in Germany to be effective in eliminating Candida
- Calcium undecylenate (from the castor bean) - shown to be six times more effective than caprylic acid in killing yeast
- Neem leaf - contains strong antibiotic alkaloids and tannins
- Olive leaf - a traditional anti-fungal
- Berberine sulphate - a concentrated anti-fungal, antibacterial compound found in barberry
- Oregon grape root - contains berberine, a strong anti-fungal/antibacterial
- Oregano leaf - contains the alkaloids carvacrol and thymol, both of which are strong anti-fungals

A 2-part system that contains the above should be combined with the following for best results:

- Enzyme supplements to support the anti-fungal program should be taken on an empty stomach to help break down the cell wall of the yeast, which is comprised of protein, fat and chitin. A good supplement would contain the following: 300,000 H.U.T. of protease, 112,500 C.U. of cellulase, 45,000 H.C.U. of hemicellulase, 22,500 mcg. lysozyme and 18,000 D.U. of amylase. It should also contain invertase, lactase, malt diatase and lipase. This should be taken before bed on an empty stomach.
- Plant enzymes can also be used with meals. These should include protease (20,000 H.U.T), amylase, lipase and cellulase. This formula might also include ginger, marshmallow, papaya, bromelain and gamma oryzanol. Take one before and after meals. HCl can be very helpful if the stomach acid level is low. Look for a product that combines both HCl and plant enzymes with soothing ingredients such as those above.
- Take essential fatty acids (EFAs). A combination of fish and flax oils (Omega-3) with borage oil (Omega-6) is good to reduce inflammation in the gastrointestinal tract. Absorption of the oils may be enhanced with the addition of lipase (a fat-digesting enzyme). Take three to six 1000 mg. capsules twice daily with food.
- Take a fiber supplement that provides a balance of both soluble and insoluble fibers. A flax/borage seed combination is a good choice, particularly one that contains other beneficial ingredients such as a probiotic blend with fructooligosaccharides (FOS) and herbs like slippery elm bark, marshmallow and fennel seed. Another key ingredient would be L-glutamine, which the intestine uses as fuel to regenerate.

To assist in rebuilding the intestinal lining and in reestablishing good bacteria:

- Take a probiotic (good bacteria) supplement

with multiple strains as a daily supplement. It should contain a minimum of 2 to 6 billion cultures. A prebiotic could be helpful (see appendix).

• Take 5,000 mg. to 10,000 mg. of L-glutamine powder with N-acetyl-glucosamine (NAG) and gamma oryzanol once to twice daily on an empty stomach (see appendix).

Enhancing the immune system is an important factor in eliminating Candida. For this:

• Take a multivitamin/mineral daily (see appendix).
• Take antioxidant supplements (vitamin C - 500 mg. to 3000 mg., vitamin A - 10,000 I.U. daily and zinc – 30 mg. to 60 mg. daily) after meals. Other antioxidants may also be taken with these (see appendix for specification on antioxidants).

***Please note: if you are constipated, add a colon cleanse before bed. Select an herbal blend that contains herbs such as cape aloe and rhubarb (which gently stimulate peristalsis) and magnesium hydroxide to help draw water to the bowel.

This protocol should be adhered to for at least 3 months. After that, drop the anti-fungal and L-glutamine powder, and stay on the rest of the protocol as good digestive maintenance.

COMPLEMENTARY MIND/BODY THERAPIES
• Colon hydrotherapy is excellent for removing waste from the colon.
• Massage - This stress-relieving therapy is also extremely beneficial for anyone with Candida.
• Yoga
• Meditation/Prayer
• Biofeedback
• Music therapy
• Chiropractic
• Acupuncture

See appendix for information on these therapies.

In conclusion, when dealing with Candida (and any problem in which the immune system plays an integral part), it is important to treat the whole person – mind, body, spirit and environment.

Dr Smith's Comments
Candida infections run a spectrum from minor oral thrush and vulvovaginal candidiasis to overwhelming Candida sepsis (usually in severely ill ICU patients or immunocompromised HIV patients). Hospital-based allopathic medicine does a great job with anti-fungals on the seriously ill. However, when patients have low-grade recurrent Candida infections, they are treated with appropriate anti-fungal agents, but then they are offered nothing else to prevent recurrences. This is another example of symptom-based medicine not focusing on the original nature of the problem. There are major considerations with regard to normal physiologic processes (such as normal HCl production and immune competence) and dietary and nutritional supplementation that help in prevention.

Many research findings support the concept that inadequate stomach acid is at least a double-edged sword: Higher pH promotes Candida growth and also blocks the absorption of iron, folate, vitamin B6 and zinc. It is well known that both zinc and vitamin A are critical for normal cellular immunity. So, it is easy to see that immune deficiency will further exacerbate the problem of chronic Candida overgrowth. It is also likely that the Candida may be consuming the deficient nutrients, oxidizing the essential fatty acids and leaving toxins in their place. Eradication of the problem does require dietary changes and anti-fungals (pharmaceutical, nutraceutical or both), depending on the clinical situation.

Chapter 4

Yeast Questionnaire – Adult

Section A – History

Circle the number next to the questions to which you answer 'yes,' then add all the circled numbers, and write the total in the box at the bottom.

1. Have you taken tetracycline (Sumycin®, Panmycin®, Vibramycin®, Minocin®, etc.) or other antibiotics for acne for 1 month or more? 50

2. Have you, at any time in your life, taken other "broad spectrum" antibiotics for respiratory, urinary or other infections for 2 months or more, or for shorter periods, 4 or more times in a 1-year span? . . .50

3. Have you taken a broad spectrum antibiotic drug – even a single dose? 6

4. Have you at any time in your life, been bothered by persistent prostatitis, vaginitis, or other problems affecting your reproductive organs? 25

5. Have you been pregnant...
    a) 2 or more times? 5
    b) 1 time? 3

6. Have you taken birth control pills for...
    a) more than 2 years? .15
    b) 6 months to 2 years? 8

7. Have you taken prednisone, Decadron® or other cortisone-type drugs by mouth or inhalation...
    a) for more than 2 weeks? 15
    b) for 2 weeks or less? 6

8. Does exposure to perfumes, insecticides, fabric shop odors, or other chemicals provoke...
    a) moderate to severe symptoms? 20
    b) mild symptoms? 5

9. Are your symptoms worse on damp, muggy days or in moldy places? 20

10. If you have ever had athlete's foot, ringworm, jock itch or other chronic fungus infections of the skin or nails, have such infections been...
    a) severe or persistent? 20
    b) mild or moderate? 10

11. Do you crave sugar? .10

12. Do you crave breads? .10

13. Do you crave alcoholic beverages? 10

14. Does tobacco smoke really bother you? 10

Section B – Major Symptoms

For each symptom that is present, enter the appropriate number on the adjacent line:

- If a symptom is occasional or mild,
  score 3 points
- If a symptom is frequent or moderately severe,
  score 6 points
- If a symptom is severe and/or disabling,
  score 9 points

Total the scores for this section, and record them in the box at the bottom of this section.

1. Fatigue or lethargy . . . . ____
2. Feeling of being 'drained' . . . . ____
3. Poor memory . . . . ____
4. Feeling 'spacey' or 'unreal' . . . . ____
5. Inability to make decisions . . . . ____
6. Numbness, burning or tingling . . . . ____
7. Insomnia . . . . ____
8. Muscle aches . . . . ____
9. Muscle weakness or paralysis . . . . ____
10. Pain and/or swelling in joints . . . . ____
11. Abdominal pain . . . . ____
12. Constipation . . . . ____
13. Diarrhea . . . . ____
14. Bloating, belching or intestinal gas . . . . ____
15. Troublesome vaginal burning, itching or discharge ____
16. Prostatitis . . . . ____
17. Impotence . . . . ____
18. Loss of sexual desire or feeling . . . . ____
19. Endometriosis or infertility . . . . ____
20. Cramps and/or other menstrual irregularities . . . . ____
21. Premenstrual tension . . . . ____
22. Attacks of anxiety or crying . . . . ____
23. Cold hands or feet and/or chilliness . . . . ____
23. Shaking or irritability when hungry . . . . ____

Total Score for Section A: _____

Total Score for Section B: _____

Section C – Minor Symptoms

For each symptom that is present, enter the appropriate number on the adjacent line:

- If a symptom is occasional or mild,
  score 3 points
- If a symptom is frequent or moderately severe,
  score 6 points
- If a symptom is severe and/or disabling,
  score 9 points

Total the scores for this section, and record them in the box at the bottom of this section.

1. Drowsy . . . . ._____
2. Irritable or jittery . . . . ._____
3. Lack of coordination . . . . ._____
4. Inability to concentrate . . . . ._____
5. Frequent mood swings . . . . ._____
6. Headaches . . . . ._____
7. Dizzy/loss of balance . . . . ._____
8. Pressure above ears...feeling of head swelling . . . . ._____
9. Tendency to bruise easily . . . . ._____
10. Chronic rashes or itching . . . . ._____
11. Psoriasis or recurrent hives . . . . ._____
12. Indigestion or heartburn . . . . ._____
13. Food sensitivity or intolerance . . . . ._____
14. Mucus in stools . . . . ._____
15. Rectal itching . . . . ._____
16. Dry mouth or throat . . . . ._____
17. Rash or blisters in mouth . . . . ._____
18. Bad breath . . . . ._____
19. Foot, hair or body odor not relieved by washing . ._____
20. Nasal congestion or post-nasal drip . . . . ._____
21. Nasal itching . . . . ._____
22. Sore throat . . . . ._____
23. Laryngitis, loss of voice . . . . ._____
24. Cough or recurrent bronchitis . . . . ._____
25. Pain or tightness in chest . . . . ._____
26. Wheezing or shortness of breath . . . . ._____
27. Urinary frequency, urgency or incontinence . . . . ._____
28. Burning on urination . . . . ._____
29. Spots in front of eyes or erratic vision . . . . ._____
30. Burning or tearing of eyes . . . . ._____
31. Recurrent infections or fluid in ears . . . . ._____
32. Ear pain or deafness . . . . ._____

Total Score for Section C: _____

Grand Total Score: _____

IF YOUR SCORE IS:	YOUR SYMPTOMS ARE:
180 (women) 140 (men)	Almost certainly yeast connected
120 (women) 90 (men)	Probably yeast connected
60 (women) 40 (men)	Possibly yeast connected
below 60 (women) below 40 (men)	Probably not yeast connected

The total score will help you and your physician decide if your health problems are yeast-connected. A comprehensive history and physical examination are also important. In addition, laboratory studies, x-rays, and other types of tests may also be appropriate.

Scores for women will be higher, as 7 items in this questionnaire apply exclusively to women, while only 2 apply exclusively to men.

If your total score for all three sections above was less than 60 for a woman or less than 40 for a man, then you are less likely to have a problem with Candida. However, if you scored higher than this, then you may wish to consider lifestyle and dietary changes, as well as a detoxification and cleansing program, all of which may help you feel healthy and more energetic.

Reprinted from *The Yeast Connection* by William G. Crook, MD with permission.

Chapter 4

Yeast Questionnaire – Child

Circle appropriate point score for questions you answer "yes." Total your score and record it at the end of the questionnaire.

Point Score

1. During the two years before your child was born, were you bothered by recurrent vaginitis, menstrual irregularities, premenstrual tension, fatigue, headache, depression, digestive disorders of 'feeling bad all over?' 30

2. Was your child bothered by thrush? (Score 10 if mild, score 20 if severe or persistent) 10/20

3. Was your child bothered by frequent diaper rashes in infancy?
    (Score 10 if mild, 20 if severe or persistent) 10/20

4. During infancy, was your child bothered by colic and irritability lasting over 3 months?
    (Score 10 if mild, 20 if moderate or severe) 10/20

5. Are his/her symptoms worse on damp days or in damp or moldy places? 20

6. Has your child been bothered by recurrent or persistent 'athlete's foot' or chronic fungus infections of his skin or nails? 30

7. Has your child been bothered by recurrent hives, eczema or other skin problems? 10

8. Has your child received:

    (a) 4 or more courses of antibiotic drugs during the past year? Or has he received continuous 'prophylactic' courses of antibiotic drugs? 80

    (b) 8 or more courses of 'broad-spectrum' antibiotics (such as amoxicillin, Keflex®, Septra®, Bactrim® or Ceclor®) during the past 3 years? 50

9. Has your child experienced recurrent ear problems? 10

10. Has your child had tubes inserted in his ears? 10

11. Has your child been labeled 'hyperactive?' (Score 10 if mild, 20 if moderate or severe) 10/20

12. Is your child bothered by learning problems (even though his early developmental history was normal)? 10

13. Does your child have a short attention span? 10

14. Is your child persistently irritable, unhappy and hard to please? 10

15. Has your child been bothered by persistent or recurrent digestive problems, including constipation, diarrhea, bloating or excessive gas? (Score 10 if mild, 20 if moderate, 30 if severe) 10/20/30

16. Has he/she been bothered by persistent nasal congestion, cough and/or wheezing? 10

17. Is your child unusually tired or unhappy or depressed? (Score 10 if mild, 20 if servere) 10/20

18. Has your child been bothered by recurrent headaches, abdominal pain or muscle aches?
    (Score 10 if mild, 20 if severe) 10/20

19. Does your child crave sweets? 10

20. Does exposure to perfume, insecticides, gas or other chemicals provoke moderate to
    severe symptoms? 30

21. Does tobacco smoke really bother him? 20

22. Do you feel that your child isn't well, yet diagnostic tests and studies haven't revealed the cause? 10

| **TOTAL SCORE:** | _____ |

Yeasts possibly play a role in causing health problems in children with
scores of 60 or more.

Yeasts probably play a role in causing health problems in children with
scores of 100 or more.

Yeasts almost certainly play a role in causing health problems in children with
scores of 140 or more.

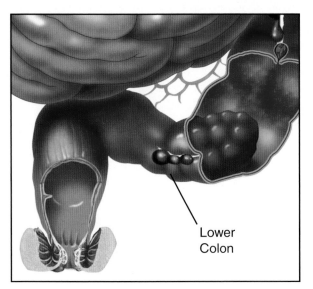

This illustration shows a commonly constipated area.

CONSTIPATION

What is it?

Constipation may be defined as infrequent or incomplete bowel movements often characterized by stools that are hard, dry and difficult to pass due to slow transit time through the gastrointestinal tract. Transit time is the amount of time that elapses between ingestion of food and excretion of it in the form of stool.

In conventional medical circles, it is considered "normal" to have a bowel movement as infrequently as three times a week.[1] In contrast, most holistic practitioners would consider the normal range of bowel movements to be one to three per day. The thinking here is that three movements would be ideal because we generally eat three meals daily. Ideally, when food enters the stomach, a nerve impulse is sent to the colon, prompting it to contract and release its contents. This gastrocolic reflex, when functioning properly, would cause us to empty our colons after each meal. Studies on Africans by Dr. Dennis Burkitt strongly support the concept that good hydration and 60 or more grams of fiber per day generally produce two or more bowel movements daily. These people were basically free from colon cancer and polyps, diverticular disease, hemorrhoids, constipation, varicose veins, gallstones and gastroesophageal reflux disease (GERD).

What Causes it?

There are many possible causes of constipation, ranging from simple to complex. Among them are:[2, 3, 4, 5]

- Insufficient fiber in the diet
- Too much fat in the diet and too many refined foods
- Side effects of some medications[6,7] (antidepressants; tranquilizers; painkillers that contain codeine, morphine or opium; some blood pressure and heart medications; diuretics; synthetic iron supplements; calcium-containing and aluminum-containing antacids; antispasmodic drugs; anesthetics; bismuth salts; anticholinergics; some antihistamines; cough syrups; calcium supplements; drugs for Parkinson's disease)
- Lack of exercise
- Travel (changing time zones especially)
- Pregnancy (hormonal and mechanical problems presented)
- Excessive use of laxatives or enemas (can damage nerve cells in the bowel, interfering with its ability to contract)
- Ignoring the urge to defecate
- Surgery (such as hysterectomy or back surgery that may result in severance of nerves in the bowel)
- Dehydration (water needed to provide bulk to stools)
- Extreme stress/depression
- Magnesium deficiency
- Deficiency of peristalsis-inducing nutrients: vitamin B5, vitamin C, choline and arginine[8]
- Prolonged bed rest
- Advanced age
- Spinal cord injury
- Growths, scarring or inflammation in colon or rectum
- Loss of body salts through vomiting or diarrhea (or from taking diuretics)

- Insufficient levels of digestive enzymes (hydrochloric acid, pancreatic enzymes, bile salts)[9]
- Insecticides[10]

Constipation is common in diseases such as:

- Parkinson's disease
- Autoimmune diseases such as Lupus and diabetes (see full list in candidiasis section)
- Glucose intolerance
- Hypercalcemia (too much calcium in the blood)
- Hirschsprung's disease (a rare congenital disease characterized by missing nerve cells in the rectum)
- Bowel diseases (such as irritable bowel syndrome, inflammatory bowel disorders and diverticulosis)
- Hemorrhoids and anal fissures (produce spasms of the anal sphincter muscle, delaying bowel movements)
- Scleroderma and other neuromuscular disorders
- Multiple sclerosis
- Kidney failure
- Stroke
- Colon cancer
- Dysbiosis (imbalance in bowel bacteria, where bad bacteria outnumber the good)
- Food allergies
- Parasites
- Hypothyroidism

If the body were a car, then the thyroid would be considered the spark plug. If it is sluggish, eliminations will also be sluggish. Many people today have what has been called "sub-clinical hypothyroidism." This means that their depressed thyroid activity does not show up on standardized tests. Alternative laboratory tests may be employed by progressive physicians to detect such thyroid problems. Some may test for and treat Wilson's thyroid syndrome, characterized by chronically low body temperature.[11]

Identifying and treating a sluggish thyroid is

important, but something as simple as common dental work may complicate the treatment. For example, it is possible that treatment for a sluggish thyroid may fail in the presence of silver amalgam dental fillings. These fillings are over 50% mercury, a toxic heavy metal that has the effect of binding to selenium and thereby interfering with the 5'deiodinase enzyme that is necessary for thyroid hormone production.[12] The thyroid hormone T4 cannot convert to T3 if this enzyme is not working properly. Thyroid hormone T3 is responsible for prompting cells to continue making and replacing damaged mitochondria (the principal energy generators of the cell). Without good mitochondrial

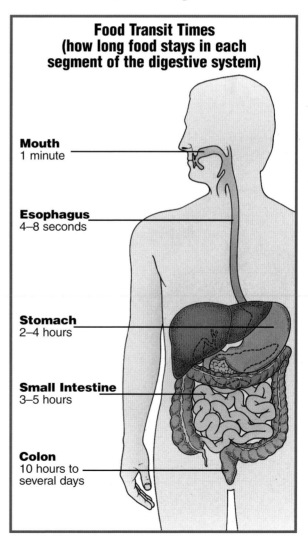

Food Transit Times
(how long food stays in each
segment of the digestive system)

Mouth
1 minute

Esophagus
4–8 seconds

Stomach
2–4 hours

Small Intestine
3–5 hours

Colon
10 hours to
several days

Chapter 4

function, there will not be enough ATP (adenosine triphosphate, the cell's primary high energy molecule) to allow for normal intestinal function. In view of this information, replacement of amalgam fillings with a biocompatible material may be considered followed by a good mercury detoxification program.

A slow intestinal transit time (the time it takes for food to pass through the gastrointestinal tract – from mouth through rectum) is an underlying factor in many cases of constipation. The optimal transit time is 24 to 30 hours; however, in the U.S., the normal transit time is 48 or more hours.[13]

Another possible cause of constipation has to do with the position we assume when having a bowel movement. In Western "civilized" cultures, we sit on a toilet, whereas the squatting posture is used in more "primitive" cultures. Actually, the squatting posture makes a good deal more physiological sense in terms of bowel stimulation and support that's achieved when the thighs come in contact with the abdominal wall.

Who Gets it?

Chronic constipation is the top gastrointestinal complaint in the United States. It affects people of all ages, but older adults are five times more likely than younger people to have the problem.[14] Low-fiber, highly processed diet of soft, easy-to-chew foods, inadequate water intake and use of constipating medications typical of many elderly people, sets the stage for chronic constipation problems.

Constipation is much more common in Western cultures than elsewhere due to our sedentary lifestyles and consumption of processed foods. Fiber (indigestible complex plant carbohydrates found in fruits, vegetables and whole grains) is removed from most processed foods because it decreases shelf life.[15] A high intake of dietary fiber:

• Decreases transit time of stools

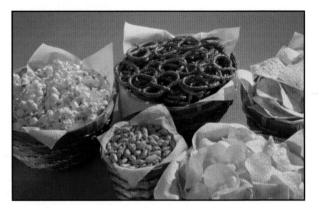

• Decreases absorption of toxins from stools
• Bulks and softens stools, increasing frequency and quantity of bowel movements

Indigenous cultures that have a high intake of dietary fiber invariably enjoy superior intestinal health and are virtually free of the diseases of modern civilization.

What Are the Signs and Symptoms?

With constipation, a wide range of symptoms may be experienced. These could include:

• Abdominal discomfort/fullness
• Rectal discomfort
• Bloating
• Nausea
• Loss of appetite
• Headache
• Lower back pain
• General feeling of malaise

When bowel transit time is slow, waste is not promptly eliminated from the body. It will consequently decay or ferment, producing poisonous chemicals. As toxins are reabsorbed into the body, the risk of developing colon diseases and other health problems increases.[16]

In addition to the symptoms listed above, constipation can give rise to:[17]

• Appendicitis
• Bad breath

- Body odor
- Bowel cancer
- Coated tongue
- Depression
- Diverticulitis
- Fatigue
- Gas
- Hemorrhoids
- Hernia
- Indigestion
- Insomnia
- Malabsorption syndrome
- Obesity
- Varicose veins

James F. Balch, MD, and his nutritionist ex-wife, Phyllis, tell us that antigens and toxins from bowel bacteria and undigested food particles may play a role in a host of symptoms and conditions in addition to those listed above. These include diabetes mellitus, meningitis, myasthenia gravis, thyroid disease, candidiasis, migraines and ulcerative colitis.[18] To this list, we may add predisposition to skin conditions, allergies, anxiety, depression and female disorders, as well as slower healing time, based on the observations of D. Lindsey Berkson.[19] The generation of toxins in the colon puts a strain on the entire body, particularly the liver, the body's major organ of detoxification.

Toxins created in the constipated bowel damage digestive enzymes in the intestinal wall and cause digestive problems and nutrient deficiencies. The walls of the colon can weaken and herniate, giving rise to diverticulosis (detailed later in this chapter).[20]

Besides diverticulosis, the excessive bowel transit time associated with constipation can contribute to such bowel disorders as irritable bowel syndrome and colitis. It also creates conditions favorable to the overgrowth of bad or putrefactive bacteria that can have health-damaging effects on the body.

Studies suggest that constipation may indirectly cause estrogen to be reabsorbed.[21] With slow tran-

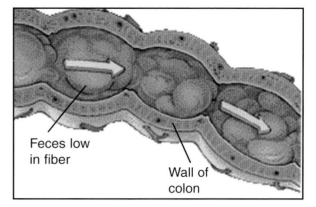

Pressure inside colon: *Feces high in fiber are able to pass easily along the colon. If feces are low in fiber, the force of contractions must increase, putting pressure on the wall of the colon.*

sit times, a low-fiber diet and low concentrations of Lactobacilli and Bifidobacteria, there will be resorption of estrogen. Elevated estrogen can give rise to many female problems, including breast, ovarian and uterine cancer.

Excessive bowel transit time means increased exposure to waste and toxins. These toxins stress the gallbladder, pancreas and liver (giving rise to fatigue and headaches) and may give rise to an increase in gas formation and a change in gas pressure, which can lead to esophageal damage from reflux. It also creates vulnerability to varicose veins, arthritis and low back pain, as well as putting an extra load on the immune system.[22]

How is it Diagnosed?

After taking a detailed medical history, your doctor may perform a rectal exam and order a stool analysis to look for hidden (occult) blood. Blood and urine tests may also be performed.

Where constipation is long-standing (chronic), your doctor may want to have special tests done to rule out bowel obstruction. Such tests may include sigmoidoscopy, colonoscopy, barium enema or virtual colonoscopy (see appendix for details). Motility tests to measure movement within the colon and a test to measure transit time may also be performed. Testing transit time involves x-rays of the colon on successive days after barium is swallowed.

Berkson describes a self-test for determining bowel transit time.[23] In it, 20 grains (5 to 12 tablets) of charcoal are swallowed all at once with water, and a note is made of the time. The time is again recorded when the black color of the charcoal is first seen in the stools. Ideally, this would be within 16 to 30 hours. Any longer indicates an excessive bowel transit time. If the black is not seen for 78 hours or never appears, this is indicative of a toxic bowel. If you continue to see the black in your stools for several more days, this is also a sign of a sluggish bowel.

What is the Standard Medical Treatment?

Because lack of dietary fiber in the diet is thought to be the most common cause of constipation, many doctors recommend the use of fiber supplements, as well as the addition of more high-fiber foods (fruits, vegetables, whole grains) to the diet. Bran, prunes, figs and apricots are particularly high in fiber. If you follow this protocol, add bran to your diet slowly, because adding bran to the diet too rapidly can cause gas and bloating.

Additional fiber may also be obtained through the use of "bulk" laxatives. Of the many different types of laxatives on the market, these most closely approximate the body's natural process of elimination. See chart 2 for a description of these and other commonly used laxatives.

It is important to note that laxative abuse is actually a cause of constipation. Habitual use interferes with the normal defecation reflex. Also, it can lead to the loss of potassium and calcium, causing muscle cramps, insomnia, anxiety and fatigue.[26] Other adverse effects can include nausea, malabsorption and diarrhea. The stimulant class of laxatives produces most of the adverse effects.

In addition to recommending the addition of more dietary fiber (in the form of food or dietary supplement) and possibly another form of laxative, many doctors will recommend lifestyle changes to help combat constipation. These may include increased water intake, exercise and establishment of regular bowel habits. This later suggestion involves heeding the defecation urge, taking time out each day (preferably after meals) to allow nature to take her course. If medications are suspected as the cause of constipation, these may be discontinued or switched by your doctor. If a disease process, such as hypothyroidism, diverticulitis, malignant tumor, polyps or inflammatory bowel condition, is identified, appropriate treatment of that condition will be initiated.

Drugs and surgery are the major tools of the medical doctor, so some form of these will likely be employed regardless of the cause of the constipation when and if it is established. If your constipation problem is due to parasites, candidiasis or food sensitivities, the traditional medical doctor is

Fiber Content of Foods

Apple	1 medium	= 4 grams
Peach	1 medium	= 2 grams
Pear	1 medium	= 4 grams
Acorn squash, fresh, cooked	3/4 cup	= 7 grams
Broccoli, fresh, cooked	1/2 cup	= 2 grams
Zucchini, fresh, cooked	1 cup	= 2.5 grams
Brown rice, cooked	1 cup	= 3.5 grams
Cereal, bran flakes	3/4 cup	= 5 grams
Oatmeal, plain, cooked	3/4 cup	= 3 grams

Source: www.nal.usda.gov/fnic/cgi/nut_search.pl

Chart 1

Types of Laxatives

Bulk-forming – These increase the bulk and water content of the stools. Some commonly used bulk-formers are psyllium (Metamucil), methylcellulose (Citrucel), calcium polycarbophil (FiberCon) and bran (used as a food and in supplement form). The only downside of the regular use of these products is that they can interfere with absorption of some drugs.

Osmotic Agents – These contain salts or carbohydrates that draw water to the colon to facilitate the passage of stools. While safe for occasional use, dependency can result if used habitually, and minerals can be washed out of the body. Examples of osmotic agents are lactulose, sorbitol, milk of magnesia and Epsom salts.

Stool Softeners – These wetting agents moisten and soften the stool so that it passes through the intestines more easily. Examples of this type of laxative are Colace, Dialose, Surfak and mineral oil. These products should not be used on a regular basis, as mineral oil reduces absorption of fat-soluble vitamins, and docusate sodium (in Colace and Dialose) may increase the toxicity of other drugs taken at the same time, causing liver damage to occur.[24]

Stimulant Laxatives – These irritate the intestinal wall, causing muscular contractions (peristalsis). Prolonged use can lead to dependency and damage the bowel. Examples are bisacodyl (found in Dulcolax), castor oil (Purge, Neoloid), casanthranol (Peri-Colace), senna (Senokot, Perdiem, Fletcher's Castoria) and phenolphthalein (once found in Correctol, Ex-Lax, Dialose Plus). It should be noted that phenolphthalein, the active ingredient in prune juice, was recently removed from the market. Overuse of this substance causes depletion of potassium in the blood and reduced absorption of vitamin D, calcium and other minerals.[25]

Chart 2

Chapter 4

unlikely to discover this, as these conditions generally lie outside their area of interest.

While lack of dietary fiber is generally agreed upon as the major cause of constipation in Western cultures, the fact of the matter is that published studies show that a significant number of chronically constipated people do not find relief from fiber supplements.[27] One study showed that the majority of patients with slow transit times and defecation disorders did not benefit from fiber therapy.[28] For patients like this, the issue of insufficient peristalsis must be addressed. Medically, this is done with prescription drugs used to enhance bowel motility (movement). Unfortunately, one such drug, used effectively for this purpose, Propulsid, was taken off the market when it was found to be causing an unacceptable number of potentially fatal heart failures.[29]

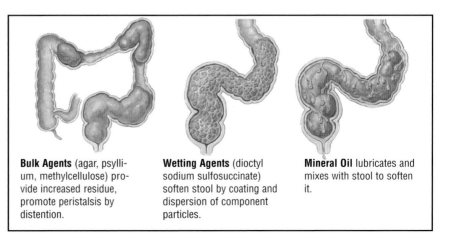

Bulk Agents (agar, psyllium, methylcellulose) provide increased residue, promote peristalsis by distention.

Wetting Agents (dioctyl sodium sulfosuccinate) soften stool by coating and dispersion of component particles.

Mineral Oil lubricates and mixes with stool to soften it.

Optional Nutritional Approaches

If you suffer from persistent constipation, and your standard medical doctor has ruled out other causes, you may wish to consult a progressive practitioner who might order testing to rule out the following:

- Food allergies - ELISA test (see appendix)
- Parasites, Candida or dysbiosis test - Comprehensive Digestive Stool Analysis (CDSA: see appendix)
- Thyroid test - self-monitoring or blood test (see appendix).

***Please note: The following is suggested in cases of extreme constipation when a person has not had a bowel elimination for 3 to 7 days or more: Do not take any fiber! Try one of the following to encourage elimination before starting the constipation program:

- Try a colon cleanse product. Look for one containing herbs, like cape aloe and rhubarb (that will gently stimulate peristalsis), as well as magnesium oxide to bring water to the bowel. Start with one capsule before bed, and increase by one capsule each night until bowel elimination occurs. Drink plenty of water during the day (see general recommendations at end of chapter).
- Do a vitamin C "flush" (see appendix).
- Colon hydrotherapy can be used alone or in conjunction with the above to help clean out the colon before starting on the constipation program.

The following is an ongoing, alternative therapy program for constipation:

Diet
- A 3 to 4 day juice diet prior to initiation of the Digestive Care Diet could be helpful (see appendix).
- Follow the Digestive Care Diet (see appendix). Make sure at least 80% of your diet is composed of fruits and vegetables.

- Drink water (see recommendations at end of chapter).

Supplements
Take a 30-day herbal detox formula, which addresses the whole body. Customized formulas to cleanse the channels of elimination (colon, liver, lymphatics, kidneys, skin and lungs) are available. These formulas come in two bottles and contain the following in Part I:

- Milk thistle stimulates bile secretion in the liver, acts as an antioxidant and strengthens the cells of the liver to protect them.
- Dandelion stimulates bile and acts as a gentle laxative.
- Beet helps reduce damaging fats in the liver.
- Artichoke leaf stimulates secretion of bile and protects cells of the liver.
- Mullein is an expectorant for the lungs
- Burdock is good for the skin.
- Corn silk helps flush the kidneys.
- Red clover purifies the blood.
- Larch gum helps the immune system.
- Hawthorne supports the heart.
- Ashwaganda supports the adrenals.
- Bupleurum is an anti-viral.
- Celandine supports the liver.
- Chlorella is a blood purifier.
- Turmeric is an antioxidant. It stimulates bile flow and protects the liver.

Part II would be a colon cleanse taken before bed. It would contain:

- Magnesium hydroxide to hydrate the colon
- Colon cleansing herbs like aloe and rhubarb to stimulate, as well as triphala to help strengthen the colon

This 30-day detox helps strengthen the channels of elimination: colon, skin, lungs, kidneys, lymph and liver. It should be combined with the following for best results:

- Take digestive enzymes before and after meals.

This supplement should include protease (at least 20,000 H.U.T.), amylase and lipase, as well as papaya and bromelain. Other ingredients in this formula might include soothing herbs like marshmallow and slippery elm. Additionally, a good digestive enzyme formula would contain glutamine (an amino acid) and N-acetyl-glucosamine.

- Take a fiber supplement that provides a balance of both soluble and insoluble fibers. A flax/borage seed combination is a good choice, particularly one that contains other beneficial ingredients such as a probiotic blend with fructooligosaccharides (FOS) and herbs like slippery elm bark, marshmallow and fennel seed. Another key ingredient would be L-glutamine, which the intestine uses as fuel to regenerate. This fiber supplement may be added to juices and taken any time of day.
- Take essential fatty acids (EFAs) to lubricate the digestive tract. A combination of fish and flax oils (Omega-3) with borage oil (Omega-6) is good to reduce inflammation in the gastrointestinal tract. Absorption of the oils may be enhanced with the addition of a fat-digesting enzyme (lipase). Take three to six 1000 mg. capsules twice daily with food.
- Take a probiotic (good bacteria) supplement with multiple strains as a daily supplement. It should contain a minimum of 2 to 6 billion cultures. A prebiotic might also be helpful (see appendix).

The above basic program for constipation should be followed for at least 30 days. After the 30-day period, this type of cleansing should be done bi-annually. Stay on fiber, oils, probiotics and enzymes indefinitely, as they are the basics for good digestive health. If you get constipated periodically, use a colon cleanse (described on previous page) as needed before bed.

LIFESTYLE
- Make time to go to the bathroom in the morning, even if it means getting up earlier.

- Make sure when you are on the toilet that your feet are elevated (assume a squatting position). This puts the colon in the proper position for elimination. Try the Lifestep™ (see Resource Directory), which will help you simulate a squatting position. It is made of plastic and fits around the toilet.
- Skin brushing – The skin is a major organ of elimination, and should be considered in all detoxification programs. Skin brushing should be done in the morning before showering. Use a natural bristle brush (found in health food stores). Start with the legs, and brush up towards the heart. Do the arms and torso (avoid the face and breast). Skin brushing will help stimulate the lymph and remove dead skin cells.
- Exercise helps to stimulate your body. Do at least 30 minutes of cardiovascular exercise daily. A mini-trampoline can also be helpful to stimulate the lymph (see Resource Directory).
- Sauna, steam or a hot tub bath can be helpful in detoxification (see appendix).
- Castor oil packs (see appendix)

COMPLEMENTARY MIND/BODY THERAPIES
- Colon hydrotherapy can be extremely beneficial in constipation conditions. It cleanses the large intestine and can help initiate peristalsis.
- Massage – Benefits include invigoration of skin tissue, promotion of suppleness of muscle tissue, stimulation of body fluid circulation, balancing of nerve impulse distribution and improved relaxation.
- Yoga/deep breathing - helps to stimulate the body overall and oxygenate the cell for better elimination.
- Acupuncture could also be beneficial in the management of constipation by stimulating the energy meridians of the colon and digestive tract.
- Chiropractic – Spinal adjustment can help resolve constipation.
- Meditation/Prayer
- Music therapy

• Biofeedback

See appendix for more information on these therapies.

Dr. Smith's Comments

This is one of the most common and expensive problems for Western society. A recent review article from the <u>New England Journal of Medicine</u> (349: 1360-1368, Oct. 2, 2003), describes this problem in detail. Constipation is a problem for up to 27% of the population of Western countries. There are 2.5 million visits to physicians and 92,000 hospitalizations per year for this problem. Laxative sales exceed several hundred million dollars per year for constipation.

The article goes on to divide constipation into three groups: normal transit time, disorders of rectal musculature (defectory disorders) and slow transit time constipation.

- *Normal Transit Time – most common; responds well to hydration, fiber and osmotic laxatives to keep stool soft. Severe cases may require prescription drugs like Tegoserod (5-hydroxytrptamine receptor agonist).*
- *Defectory Disorders – Often structural abnormalities like rectocoele, rectal intussusception or excessive perineal descent; these are often due to lack of coordination of abdominal, rectoanal and pelvic floor muscles during defecation. The condition is often helped by biofeedback training (see appendix for biofeedback).*
- *Slow Transit Time – usually occurs in young females with one or less bowel movements per week; often starts at puberty with symptoms of bloating, abdominal pain and no urge to defecate. Fiber, water and osmotics help in mild cases, but severe cases are made worse with fiber. The worst of the slow transit patients have histological changes with decreased Cajal cells (regulate motility) and in myenteric nerve plexus cells as well. Often these patients require total or subtotal colectomy to solve the problem. Thirty-two studies showed a patient satisfaction rate of 39-100% with this surgery.*

In my own experience, constipation is certainly one of the most common complaints of hospital patients. I believe that it has directly or indirectly led to hospitalization and surgery and kept patients in the hospital longer than necessary. I have had patients who were slow to recover and, by treating their constipation, their problems rapidly resolved.

I have lectured for and worked with the International Association of Colon Hydrotherapists for the last four years. In addition, I have personally experienced colon hydrotherapy. I believe it is an important therapy for anyone who cares about his/her health. It is interesting how often patients who try this therapy are amazed by the gentle and effective results they achieve. It is my opinion that all detoxification and chelation centers will be enhanced by adding colon hydrotherapy to their program.

I look forward to the day that colon hydrotherapy becomes a standard of care for the medical profession, both in the hospital and outpatient setting. In fact, I believe that colon hydrotherapy should be the standard of care for prepping seniors and children for colonoscopy. In addition, it could become the mainstay treatment for constipation in childhood. Recent research has shown that childhood constipation is largely the result of fear of painful bowel movements, which occurs when children are forced to evacuate by giving them laxatives.

In summary, most everyone can enhance their colonic eliminative process with a balance of soluble and insoluble fiber, probiotics, oils, good hydration and exercise.

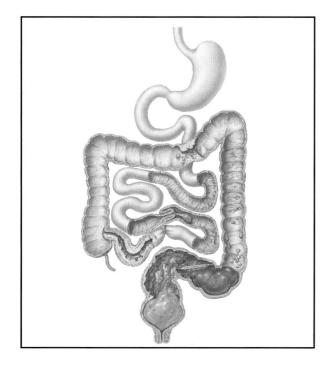

DIARRHEA

What is it?

Diarrhea, the frequent passage of watery stools, is a symptom, not a disease. It can occur for many reasons. A common one is increased bowel motility, which causes a rapid transit time (the time elapsed from ingestion to elimination of food). Put simply, with an increase in motility, there is insufficient time for water in the intestinal tract to be reabsorbed into the body. The result is that the stool retains water and becomes liquified.

Diarrhea may be either acute or chronic. Acute diarrhea takes the form of an isolated incident caused by a temporary problem, usually an infection that lasts 3 to 7 days. Chronic diarrhea is much more complex, with a multitude of causes and can last for months.

What Causes it?

The causes of diarrhea are many and varied. Basically, the condition stems from intestinal irritation or increased motility (muscular action) in the intestinal tract. These can be brought about by a variety of causes, including:

- Incomplete digestion of food
- Use of certain drugs (especially antibiotics like tetracycline, clindamycin and ampicillin and NSAIDs, like aspirin – see complete list in "Gastritis" section, Chapter 3 – that damage the gut lining)
- Food poisoning
- Food allergies (especially milk, eggs, wheat)
- Excessive consumption of alcohol
- Regular or excessive use of caffeine-containing beverages (coffee, tea, sodas), foods (chocolate) and drugs (No-Doz, Excedrin)
- Laxative use/abuse
- Sugar intolerances/overuse of sweeteners such as sorbitol, xylitol, mannitol, fructose and lactose
- Infections: bacterial, viral, fungal (including Candida) and parasitic
- Pancreatic insufficiency or pancreatic tumor
- Emotional stress
- Bowel diseases: Crohn's disease, irritable bowel syndrome, diverticulitis, ulcerative colitis, cancer
- Consumption of contaminated water
- Radiation or chemotherapy
- Nutrient deficiencies (vitamin A, B complex vitamins, glutamine, zinc)[1]
- Deficiency of hydrochloric acid (HCl – stomach acid)[2]
- Celiac disease (gluten intolerance)
- Surgical resection of the small intestine
- Short bowel syndrome
- Inadequate bile secretion (hepatitis or bile duct obstruction), causing malabsorption of fat
- Use of magnesium-containing antacids
- Bacterial toxins
- Malnutrition (deficiency of calories, protein)
- Heavy metal poisoning[3]
- Neurological disease (diabetic neuropathy)
- Metabolic disease (hyperthyroidism)
- Fecal impaction

Acute diarrhea is often caused by infection

(usually viral) or food poisoning. Such food-borne illnesses include:

- Salmonella – from raw eggs, undercooked chicken or ham
- E. coli – from undercooked red meat
- Botulism – found in canned high-protein foods
- Staphylococcus – from infected food handlers

Bacteria like salmonella and E. coli give off toxins that can stick to the intestinal lining, causing a profuse secretion of fluid, which gives rise to diarrhea. Parasites may be passed on from those who handle food and through the water supply. Parasites like Giardia lamblia, Entamoeba histolytica and Cryptosporidium interfere with digestion and/or damage the intestinal lining, often causing diarrhea. People who have insufficient stomach acid (HCl) will be more susceptible to parasitic and other infections. Food and water-borne diarrhea is frequently associated with travel to underdeveloped countries but occurs in developed ones as well, though to a lesser degree.

Antibiotic use can result in a type of diarrhea (pseudomembranous colitis) caused by overgrowth of the bacterium Clostridium difficele. This bacterium, common in hospitals, gives off a toxin that damages the lining of the colon and causes severe diarrhea, as well as lower abdominal cramps and fever. If untreated, it can lead to intestinal perforation.[4]

When a food allergen is ingested, histamine and other allergic compounds from white blood cells (known as mast cells) in the intestinal lining are released. These can have a strong laxative effect.

Chronic diarrhea is often due to a bowel disease. With chronic diarrhea, the body is not absorbing all the nutrients from food, and malnourishment results.

People with gallbladder disease or who have had their gallbladders removed may experience diarrhea after eating a fatty meal.

Who Gets it?

People of any age who can relate to any of the causes listed above can develop diarrhea. It is a particularly serious condition when it occurs in the very old or very young. Diarrhea has long been the leading cause of death among infants and children worldwide. For most people in the U.S., it is an acute, self-limiting condition brought on by a pathogen. The average American will have a bout of diarrhea about four times a year.[5] Interestingly, younger adults seem to develop traveler's diarrhea slightly more often than older ones.[6]

What are the Signs and Symptoms?

Diarrhea, which consists of the frequent passage of loose, watery stools, is often accompanied by:

- Abdominal cramps/pain
- Bloating/gas
- Malaise (generalized feeling of illness)
- Blood and mucus in the stools
- Rectal soreness
- Fever
- Weakness
- Loss of appetite/weight loss
- Intestinal rumbling sounds
- Increased thirst

The last symptom above, increased thirst, can be a sign of dehydration. Other signs may include a dry mouth, anxiety or restlessness, strong body odor, little or no urination, severe weakness and dizziness or lightheadedness. If any of these signs of dehydration occur, a doctor should be contacted immediately. Medical help should also be sought if diarrhea persists for more than a few days, if severe abdominal or rectal pain is experienced, if other family members are affected with the same symptoms, if fever exceeds 101 degrees F. or there is blood in the stool (which will have a black, tarry appearance).

Diarrhea can lead to extremely serious problems including dehydration, malabsorption of nutrients (leading to malnutrition), electrolyte (mineral) imbalances (upsetting homeostasis) and even death. Death from diarrhea is not just a third world problem; even in the U.S., diarrheal diseases are the third major cause of sickness and death.[7]

How is it Diagnosed?

While diarrhea is obviously not difficult to recognize from symptoms, zeroing in on the cause can be more difficult. As with other disorders, a thorough patient history can help point to possible causes. Knowing what medications the patient is taking, if s/he has recently traveled outside the country, is taking magnesium-containing supplements or products (like antacids or laxatives) or large doses of vitamin C, can all be very helpful. So can knowledge of dietary habits, for ruling out food allergy, as well as gluten and lactose intolerance, can be important.

Because most cases of diarrhea in the U.S. are self-limiting and relatively mild, specific laboratory tests are not always done. With more severe cases, a stool test for pus cells (stool leukocyte count) will help identify such pathogens as Shigella, Salmonella, Campylobacter and Yersinia.[8] If symptoms are severe, the stool will be cultured for abnormal bacteria to help determine the appropriate antibiotic to use.[9] In the case of traveler's diarrhea, a test for parasites will probably be ordered if diarrhea persists once the traveler has returned home. Unfortunately, many doctors will not order a parasite test unless the patient has traveled outside of the country. Holistic physicians are more likely than traditional ones to test for parasites (and digestive disorders) in those with no history of travel, recognizing the widespread nature of the problem. See the "parasite" section of this chapter for more detailed information on parasites and testing for them.

In the case of "secretory diarrheas," caused by a disease process that results in fluid secretion in the intestine, your doctor may choose to run tests to rule out hidden tumors, especially in the pancreas.

These tumors release chemical messengers (hormones) that stimulate the bowel to pour out large volumes of liquid.[10] Special blood and urine tests for these hormones, along with other screening techniques, can help to locate these rare tumors. It is important to bear in mind that the effects of laxatives and diuretic medications can mimic secretory diarrhea. It is therefore necessary to let your doctor know if you are taking either of these.

A stool test for the presence of fat will help detect malabsorption problems, which may be due to a disease of the small intestine. A hydrogen breath test may be performed to detect small bowel overgrowth, or a small bowel biopsy may be ordered. If the biopsy is negative, then a sigmoidoscopy or colonoscopy (described in the appendix) may be performed. Another option is the upper GI series (see appendix). These tests will help rule out inflammatory bowel disorders like Crohn's disease and ulcerative colitis.

A lactose breath test may be ordered to rule out lactose intolerance and/or an ELISA blood test (see appendix) performed to screen for food sensitivities.

What is the Standard Medical Treatment?

Treatment of diarrhea depends upon the cause: If it is lactose intolerance, dairy foods will need to be eliminated from the diet; if it is Celiac disease, gluten-containing grains must be avoided; if it is medication-related, it will be necessary to adjust, switch or discontinue medications; if it is food allergy, the food allergen must be avoided or eaten infrequently on a rotating basis; if the diarrhea is caused by over-consumption of alcohol, sweeteners, vitamin C, magnesium (in supplement or other form) or caffeine, it will be necessary to reduce, or in some cases discontinue, intake of these items. Where nutrient deficiency – of HCl, digestive enzymes, zinc, glutamine, vitamins A and B complex – is established to be a factor, supplementation of the deficient nutrients becomes part of the treatment plan if the deficiency is recognized. This is not apt to be the case in traditional medical circles, where nutritional awareness is limited. Where infection is present, medicine will treat with the appropriate drug – usually an antibiotic, anti-fungal or anti-parasitic agent. Natural health care practitioners will gravitate more toward the use of herbal remedies, as described below, for this purpose. Some may combine antibiotic and herbal treatments.

There is some disagreement in medical circles with regard to the treatment of acute diarrhea. Some doctors will prefer to let a mild case run its course, while others will offer symptomatic relief through the use of such drugs as bismuth subsalicylate (Pepto Bismol), which reduces the secretions of the intestines, and loperamide (Imodium) or diphenoxylale (Lomotil). These last two medica-

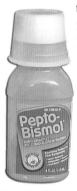

tions slow down the movement of the intestines and their secretions. However, they may worsen the diarrhea by retarding the elimination of organisms responsible for it.[11] While Lomotil and Imodium may offer temporary symptomatic relief, they should not be used if symptoms last more than a few days.[12] Non-absorbable earth mixtures of kaolin (clay) and pectin (dietary fiber), in the form of Kaopectate, have also been used to bulk up the stool. It is important to note that antidiarrheal drugs are not recommended for people suffering from food poisoning.[13] Keep foods refrigerated to help prevent food poisoning – Never allow them to sit out without refrigeration for more than three hours.[14]

Traditional medical doctors have often recommended the BRAT diet, consisting of bananas, rice, apples and toast. This diet, however, has its drawbacks: the sugar from the fruit can aid bacterial growth, and the gluten content of the bread (toast) can aggravate any underlying gluten sensitivity.

It is hugely important to bear in mind that over-

the-counter medications for diarrhea may slow the elimination of the infectious agent and so actually prolong the diarrhea.[15] Michael D. Gershon, MD, offers these words of wisdom in this regard: "Stopping the motility of the colon by taking an opiate, such as paregoric (camphorated tincture of opium), loperamide or Lomotil, is effective in putting an end to diarrhea, but cleansing is brought to a halt as well. What might have been a disturbing but relatively short-lived episode can be prolonged by these drugs and made worse."[16] Most cases of diarrhea are just the body's self-cleansing mechanism in action – a way of eliminating an irritant. A short-lived case of diarrhea can actually be therapeutic, as it will facilitate the removal of an undesirable substance from the body. In such a case, it's easy to see how we can make the situation worse through the use of symptom-suppressing medications. And yet, some medical doctors actually prescribe medication on a "preventive" basis for patients who will be traveling to developing countries. The use of some "preventive" antibiotics (like doxycycline) can cause unpleasant side effects like photosensitivity, preventing the traveler from sunbathing while on vacation, and ringing in the ears.[17] Worse yet, they will destroy the beneficial bacteria in the intestine, the body's first line of defense against pathogens. Bear in mind also that antibiotics can cause the intestines to become inflamed, resulting in diarrhea, abdominal cramps and fever.[18] Onset of these symptoms is usually 4 to 10 days after starting the medication, though symptoms may not surface until after the drug has been discontinued.[19]

Perhaps a better preventive measure than antibiotics where traveler's diarrhea is concerned would be to avoid the following when traveling to developing countries:

• Drinking the local water
• Using ice cubes made from local water
• Eating raw vegetables
• Eating dairy products
• Eating unpeeled fruit

Optional Nutritional Approaches

Acute diarrhea - In this condition, it is best to let the diarrhea run its course for the first two days. It is the body's way of eliminating bacteria, toxins and other foreign invaders.

DIET (FOR A FEW DAYS)
- Stop eating solid foods. Go on a liquid diet. Drink plenty of fluids.
- Include broth, bouillon, herbal teas and green drinks (freshly juiced green vegetables or a pre-mixed food powder of same).
- Sports drinks can help with electrolyte replacement.
- Drink rice water. Boil brown rice (1 cup) with 5 cups of water for 40 to 45 minutes. Strain and add salt to taste. Drink periodically through the day.
- Avoid dairy products, sugar, greasy fatty foods and highly seasoned foods.

After symptoms begin to subside:

- Start with a soft diet for a day: potatoes, soups, squashes, steamed vegetables. Go very slowly. Drink plenty of water.

SUPPLEMENTS
- Charcoal tablets, four every hour, until the diarrhea subsides; this helps absorb toxins from the digestive tract. Don't take charcoal with medication and/or supplements.
- Probiotics - Lactobacillus acidophilus should be taken to re-establish good bacteria (see appendix).
- Saccharomyces boulardii, a harmless yeast, has been found to be useful in treating diarrhea (see appendix).
- Take a fiber supplement that provides a balance of both soluble and insoluble fibers. A flax/borage seed combination is a good choice, particularly one that contains other beneficial ingredients such as a probiotic blend with fructooligosaccharides (FOS) and herbs like slippery elm bark, marshmallow and fennel

seed. Another key ingredient would be L-glutamine, which the intestine uses as fuel to regenerate. This fiber supplement may be added to juices and taken any time of day.
- Insoluble rice fiber supplement with herbs and nutrients (see appendix)
- Take 5,000 mg. to 10,000 mg. of L-glutamine powder with N-acetyl-glucosamine (NAG) and gamma oryzanol once to twice daily on an empty stomach (see appendix).

Chronic diarrhea – In this case, rule out the following with testing:

- Check for lactose intolerance (see appendix).
- Food sensitivities - ELISA test (see appendix)
- Parasitic infection - Parasite test (see appendix)
- Low stomach acid (see appendix)

If you have one of the above problems, see the section on that problem in this book, and follow the suggested guidelines.

DIET
Try the diet in the Candida section for one month. This diet excludes many foods to which you could be sensitive, thus creating a diarrhea condition. Upon completion of the Candida diet, go on the Digestive Care Diet (see appendix).

SUPPLEMENTS
- Take digestive enzymes before and after meals. This supplement should include protease (at least 20,000 H.U.T.), amylase and lipase, as well as papaya and bromelain. Other ingredients in this formula might include soothing herbs like marshmallow and slippery elm. Additionally, a good digestive enzyme formula would contain glutamine (an amino acid) and N-acetyl-glucosamine, which helps soothe an irritated mucosal lining.
- Take a fiber supplement that provides a balance of both soluble and insoluble fibers. A flax/borage seed combination is a good choice, articularly one that contains other beneficial ingredients such as a probiotic blend with

Chapter 4

fructooligosaccharides (FOS) and herbs like slippery elm bark, marshmallow and fennel seed. Another key ingredient would be L-glutamine, which the intestine uses as fuel to regenerate. This fiber supplement may be added to juices and taken any time of day.
- Use insoluble rice fiber with herbs and nutrients.
- Take a probiotic (good bacteria) supplement with multiple strains as a daily supplement. It should contain a minimum of 2 to 6 billion cultures. A prebiotic could be helpful (see appendix).

To help with inflammation, try the following:

- Take essential fatty acids (EFAs) to lubricate the digestive tract. A combination of fish and flax oils (Omega-3) with borage oil (Omega-6) is good to reduce inflammation in the gastrointestinal tract. Absorption of the oils may be enhanced with the addition of lipase (a fat-digesting enzyme). Take three 1000 mg. capsules twice daily with food.
- Take 5,000 mg. to 10,000 mg. of L-glutamine powder with N-acetyl-glucosamine (NAG) and gamma oryzanol once to twice daily on an empty stomach (see appendix).

It could also be helpful to add the following to the protocol:

- Multivitamin/mineral (see appendix)
- Take antioxidant supplements (vitamin C - 500 mg. to 3000 mg., vitamin A - 10,000 I.U. daily and zinc – 30 mg. to 60 mg. daily) after meals. Other antioxidants may also be taken with these (see appendix).

LIFESTYLE
Try to determine if there have been any changes in your lifestyle recently that might have brought about the diarrhea condition. You can then refer to the causes listed earlier in this section and take the appropriate steps.

COMPLEMENTARY MIND/BODY THERAPIES
- Colon hydrotherapy can be helpful in ridding the colon of bacteria and toxins. It is contraindicated in cases of anemia.
- Acupuncture could be helpful in balancing the meridians (energy channels) and therefore relieving diarrhea.
- Massage
- Yoga
- Meditation/Prayer
- Biofeedback
- Music therapy
- Chiropractic

See appendix for information on the above therapies.

Dr. Smith's Comments
Diarrhea can cause inflammation and damage the intestinal lining. In viral diarrhea, there are changes in small intestine cells, such as flattening and shortening of the villi, an increase in crypt cells and generally an increase in cellularity in the intestinal wall. The mucous barrier and brush border enzymes are damaged or destroyed, and there is a likelihood of increased intestinal permeability. It follows that partially digested food could pass through and, in the presence of an already activated immune system, cause an autoimmune type of reaction. This sets up a potential for the development of food sensitivities if foods with a higher allergic potential are eaten during, or even a few days after, an episode of diarrhea. Unfortunately, this would include many 'comfort' foods, such as wheat, dairy, tomatoes, eggs, sugary foods, etc. I recommend starting with water, then rice water and progressing to vegetable juices, vegetable soup and then cooked vegetables. For convenience, a hypoallergenic, nutritionally balanced powdered drink, such as Living Fuel (see Resource Directory), could be very helpful. I suspect that many childhood allergies, especially to wheat and dairy, could develop as the result of introducing these foods back into the diet while the child is in a hyper-immune and hyper-permeable state, which could last 3 to 7 days after the diarrhea has subsided.

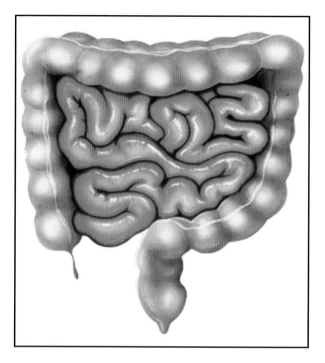

DIVERTICULAR DISEASE (DIVERTICULOSIS AND DIVERTICULITIS)

What is it?

Diverticula (the plural form of diverticulum) are herniations or protrusions that out-pouch from the inner lining of the colon. These outpouchings occur between the outer muscular coat and the arteries and veins, which penetrate the outer wall of the colon. Colonic diverticula generally are pea-sized, but vary in diameter from a few millimeters to several centimeters. The number of diverticula in a patient varies from one to several dozen. Diverticula usually form in the lower left (sigmoid) portion of the colon, though they may also be present in the transverse colon (which runs horizontally from right to left side). These sacs may form in the right side (ascending) of the colon, as well, although this is not common. When diverticula are present, the condition is known as diverticulosis. When a diverticulum becomes inflamed, the condition is referred to as diverticulitis. These types of diverticula are more usually an incidental finding on

x-rays or in surgery, but occasionally can be the source of bleeding.

What Causes it?

The cause of diverticular disease is not known with certainty, but it is believed that lack of dietary fiber may play a key role, for it has long been noted that diverticular disease is practically non-existent in groups of people who eat high-fiber diets. Fiber is abundant in fruits, vegetables and whole grains, which are largely lacking in the standard American diet. Such a low-fiber diet disrupts normal motility (movement of food waste through the colon), setting the stage for development of diverticula.[1] Dietary fiber increases the bulk of the stool, softens it and maintains normal colonic diameter.

Dietary fiber gives the colon something to push against; in a sense, it exercises the colon. In the words of Dr. Michael Gershon, "What running does for our bodies, dietary fiber does for our colons."[2] When stool stays in the colon too long, it becomes dry, small and hard, which creates higher pressure inside the undistended colon. The colonic muscles have to contract harder, working against the greater pressures in the colon. Eventually, the muscle layer hypertrophies (thickens) and can become rigid. It is thought to be the combination of the abnormally strong muscle contractions and increased intraluminal pressure that creates the diverticula. In addition, straining to pass stool may further increase intracolonic pressure and also promote diverticular formation.

Some patients with extensive diverticulosis may have other conditions that actually weaken the colonic wall. Connective tissue disorders, such as scleroderma, Marfan's syndrome and Ehler-Danlos syndrome, would be included in this category.

It has also been proposed that diverticula form as a result of spasms of the muscles in the intestinal wall. The thinking here is that such spasms cause the lining of the intestine to bulge through the weakest area of the muscular wall.[3] Here again, lack of dietary fiber would play a role, for by giving the muscles bulk to work against, the likelihood of spasm is decreased. Emotional stress is another factor that can adversely affect musculature and increase intestinal pressure.[4]

It is thought that diverticulitis may result from the entrapment of a piece of hard, dry stool in a diverticular pouch. The diverticulum impacted with stool is subject to inflammation. This is due to pressure, bacteria and free radicals in the stool, which can damage the adjacent blood supply and lead to perforation, infection and abscess formation. In more severe cases, there can be significant leakage of stool into the abdominal cavity, leading to sepsis (blood poisoning).

Who Gets it?

While diverticular disease can affect people of any age, it most commonly makes its first appearance in people between the ages of 50 and 90.[5] The incidence and severity of diverticular disease tends to increase with age, with an estimated 30 to 40% of Americans over 50 years of age having diverticulosis.[6] It is estimated that three-fifths of people over 70 years of age have the disease.[7] Those who live to age 90 stand very little chance of not developing diverticulosis.[8] Only 20% of those with diverticulosis will go on to develop diverticulitis (infected or inflamed diverticuli), and of those, only a small number will have serious or life-threatening complications.[9]

Diverticula tend to occur more commonly in men than in women,[10] and those with a family history of the disease are more apt to develop it. Also at increased risk are those who eat a poor diet, as well as those who have gallbladder or coronary artery disease.[11] It has also been established that smoking and stress make the condition worse.[12]

Diverticular disease is a disease of modern civilization, with its industrial "advances." Interestingly, diverticulosis was not reported in the U.S. until the beginning of the 20th century, when it became routine to remove fiber from grain products ...[13] Also of interest is the fact that diverticulosis is seldom seen in vegetarians and is almost unknown in India and parts of Africa where high-fiber diets are the standard.[14]

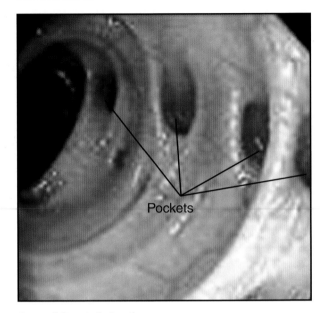

Scope of diverticula in colon

What Are the Signs and Symptoms?

As stated, the majority of people who develop diverticulosis are asymptomatic (without symptoms). They may not even know they have the condition unless it shows up on a diagnostic test done for another purpose. Where symptoms are present, they may include localized tenderness or pain, usually over the left side of the abdomen. The pain may be intermittent and vary in intensity. Often it increases when pressure is applied to the abdomen. There may be muscle spasms in the abdomen and, in some cases, blood in the stool when feces get trapped inside a pouch and cause an adjacent blood vessel to rupture. Bleeding is often not present and usually not severe when it does occur. Abdominal distress may increase after eating. The mere presence of diverticlar pouches is not a problem requiring treatment; only when the pouches become inflamed is action needed.

While diverticulosis may be asymptomatic, a person with diverticulitis will definitely know that something is amiss. The symptoms, in fact, will probably move a sufferer to seek immediate medical attention, which is a correct course of action, since this disease can lead to potentially life-threatening consequences. A person who has developed diverticulitis may experience any of the following symptoms:

- Abdominal pain, cramping, tenderness (usually left-sided)
- Fever
- Chills
- Bloating
- A change in bowel habits (constipation or diarrhea)
- An almost continual need to eliminate
- Blood in the stool
- Elevated white blood cell count (an indication of infection)
- Nausea
- Vomiting

Serious complications, including intestinal obstruction and perforation, may develop. With obstruction, there is blockage of the flow of fecal material out of the body. In perforation, a tear or hole in the wall of the colon develops, allowing colon bacteria to spill over into other areas of the body. If the person is lucky, the body will seal off the infection in the form of an abscess (boil). If the inflammation does not seal this perforation, the colon bacteria can infect the peritoneal (chest) cavity in a very serious condition called peritonitis. If the infection gains systemic access through the bloodstream, septicemia, infection of the bloodstream, results. Such infections are very serious and can lead to death if not promptly treated.

Infection can spread to other areas of the body in the form of a fistula, which is an abnormal passage between two organs or between an organ and the skin. Most commonly this occurs between the colon and the bladder when colonic bacteria invade the bladder, causing infection there.[15] Formation of a fistula is a serious medical problem usually requiring surgical intervention.

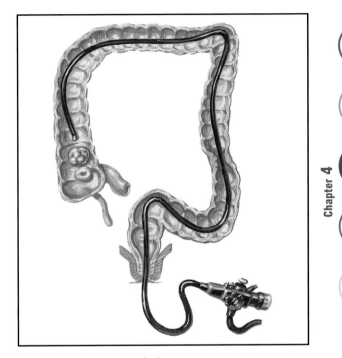

Colonoscope examination of colon

How is it Diagnosed?

Many times, diverticular pockets are found in the course of routine diagnostic procedures (x-rays or endoscopy, visual inspection of the colon) done for other purposes. Since many people with diverticulosis have no symptoms, they are surprised to learn of the presence of the condition.

Abdominal palpation will give the examining physician a clue regarding the correct diagnosis, for even with mild diverticulitis, discomfort tends to increase as pressure is applied. Routine blood tests can be helpful in that an elevated white cell count will indicate infection, a common sign of diverticulitis. An x-ray of the colon can show the outline of diverticular pouches and rule out perforation. A sonogram (sound wave examination) or CT (computerized tomography) scan can provide more information if a mass is felt or suspected. A

Chapter 4

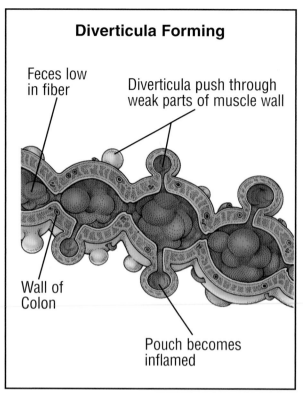

Diverticula Forming

Feces low in fiber

Diverticula push through weak parts of muscle wall

Wall of Colon

Pouch becomes inflamed

The illustration shows how increased pressure pushes the intestinal lining through weak points in the muscle of the intestinal wall. The pouches (diverticula) that form trap feces in which bacteria multiply, resulting in inflammation.

barium enema (see appendix) may be used to confirm the diagnosis, but some doctors caution against using this procedure during acute episodes since it involves filling the colon (or a portion of it) with liquid barium.[16,17] The reason for concern is that if the bowel has already perforated, there will be spillage of barium, which is quite irritating, into the abdominal cavity.

A sigmoidoscopy or a colonoscopy (see appendix) may also be performed. In these procedures, the doctor is also able to take tissue samples for later analysis. As with the barium enema, some doctors feel that "even the sigmoidoscope (or endoscope) may be a dangerous instrument to pass into the inflamed colon."[18] It may be prudent to hold off on any invasive diagnostic procedures until inflammation has subsided.

Where bleeding is present, a special x-ray (angiography) is done. In this procedure, a dye is injected into an artery that goes into the colon, so that the site of the bleeding can be located. Bleeding scans are also commonly employed as an initial screen, since they are non-invasive and cheaper. An isotope (a mildly radioactive material) is injected into an arm vein and allowed to circulate in the body. If it is positive, there will be blush on the monitor scanning to let the physician know the approximate location of the bleeding. This is very helpful in the event that emergent surgery is needed to locate the general problem area, which is usually then removed. In some cases, bleeding has been stopped with Barium enema, or colonoscopic couterization

In the rare instance where inflamed diverticular pouches occur in the ascending colon (right side of abdomen), distinguishing diverticulitis from appendicitis can be problematic for the physician. It is also significant that soft tissue abdominal muscular or ovarian problems can mimic diverticular disease.[19] Additionally, the inflammation of diverticulitis can resemble the segmental inflammation characteristic of Crohn's disease, and the symptoms of diverticulitis may mimic those of colon cancer. Differential diagnosis in these situations becomes extremely important.

What is the Standard Medical Treatment?

Where diverticula are found but no symptoms or inflammation are present, treatment is not recommended, though the patient may be counseled to increase the amount of fiber in the diet as a preventive measure. One very large study has found that insoluble fiber, especially cellulose, is of particular importance.[20] Fruits, vegetables and legumes are higher than cereal grains in cellulose, though all of these foods have a mix of both soluble and insoluble fibers. The insoluble fiber seems to have the greatest effect in terms of bulking up the stool. That is why it is particularly helpful in diverticular disease. A good diet, one that is free of processed foods and high in fiber, can help keep existing diverticula free of infection. There is no known way to get rid of diverticula once they have formed, but we can take steps to prevent more of them from forming and to avoid their development into diverticulitis.

In the acute stages of an episode of diverticulitis, whether it is a mild or severe case, there are two critically important steps that must be taken to successfully treat the condition: rest the bowel, and control the infection.[21] Bowel rest is accomplished through elimination of solid foods by adhering to a clear liquid diet during the initial phases of the episode. If the condition is severe, the patient may be strictly on intravenous fluids and, with improvement, be permitted to drink sips of water or chew on ice chips, then progress to clear liquids. As symptoms subside, a soft, low-fiber diet is initiated. Keeping fat intake low may also help in reducing pressure inside the colon.[22] Infection control is traditionally accomplished through the use of antibiotics. These will be administered intravenously to the patient whose condition is severe enough for him/her to be hospitalized. S/he will also receive intravenous fluids and pain medication. Total bed rest will be required. In milder cases, bed rest is still advised, though the patient need not be hospitalized. The patient will be given oral antibiotics and put on a clear liquid diet initially (then a soft, low-fiber one). A high-fiber diet can be initiated within a month of recovery from the acute episode of diverticulitis.

The majority of diverticulitis patients recover without surgery. However, in severe cases and in the case of repeated attacks, surgery may be needed to drain an abscess that has resulted from a ruptured diverticulum. In addition, it may be necessary to remove the affected portion of the colon and rejoin the bowel. In some cases, before the rejoining of the bowel, a temporary colostomy, which diverts the intestinal contents to the outside of the abdomen, may have to be performed and reversed

several weeks later when healing has progressed to the point that the patient can resume natural bowel movements. Surgery is also required in the case of perforations or fistulas. Potential post-surgical complications, which occur 30% of the time, include bleeding, obstruction and fistula.[23]

Once a normal diet is resumed, in addition to emphasizing high-fiber foods, the patient is often counseled to avoid tiny seeds such as poppy seeds or strawberry seeds, as it is believed that these may get trapped in diverticula, causing inflammation.

Although diverticulitis is a serious condition, it's encouraging that diverticula do not predispose a person to colon cancer or even to precancerous polyps.[24]

Chapter 4

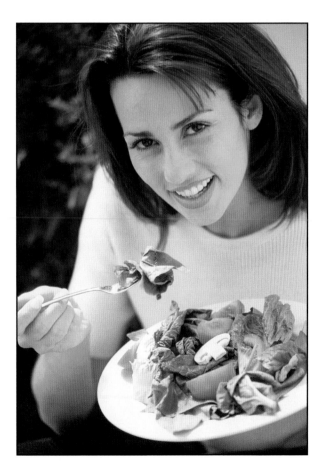

Optional Nutritional Approaches

A medical doctor should be consulted in the case of diverticulitis. If you have been treated by a doctor, are coming out of an attack of diverticulitis and are allowed to eat food, the following may be helpful:

DIET

- Put all foods through a blender.
- When using whole seeds and nuts, soak overnight and then grind with high-speed blender or coffee grinder.
- Cook whole grains with twice as much water as usual, and cook twice as long.
- Take garlic or garlic capsules with meals.
- Use freshly prepared juices (see appendix).

SUPPLEMENTS

- Chew deglycyrrhizinated licorice (DGL) on an empty stomach.
- Drink 5 ounces aloe vera juice twice a day (see appendix).
- Take 5,000 mg. to 10,000 mg. of L-glutamine powder with N-acetyl-glucosamine (NAG) and gamma oryzanol once to twice daily on an empty stomach.
- Take a multivitamin/mineral supplement – A liquid form could be helpful; it can be found in health food stores.
- Take antioxidant supplements (vitamin C - 500 mg. to 3000 mg., vitamin A - 10,000 I.U. daily and zinc – 30 mg. to 60 mg. daily) after meals. Other antioxidants may also be taken with these (see appendix).

If the condition of diverticula has developed (diverticulosis without inflammation), the following are suggestions for maintenance:

DIET

Follow the Digestive Care Diet in the appendix. A 2 to 3 day juice fast (see appendix for recipes) could be helpful a few times a year.

***Please note: A 30-day herbal detox program (see appendix) twice a year is very important for addressing the common cause of diverticula, namely chronic constipation. It is also important to keep the colon clean and make sure constipation does not reoccur. If there is a tendency for constipation, see section on constipation in this chapter and follow directions.

Follow-up on the 30-day herbal detoxification program would include taking L-glutamine powder for 30 days twice a year, as follows:

- Take 5,000 mg. to 10,000 mg. of L-glutamine powder with N-acetyl-glucosamine (NAG) and gamma oryzanol once to twice daily on an empty stomach (see appendix).

The following supplements should also be taken daily as maintenance:

- Take digestive enzymes before and after meals. This supplement should include protease (at least 20,000 H.U.T.), amylase and lipase, as well as papaya and bromelain. Other ingredients in this formula might include soothing herbs like marshmallow and slippery elm. Additionally, a good digestive enzyme formula would contain glutamine (an amino acid) and N-acetyl-glucosamine, which help soothe an irritated mucosal lining.
- Fiber is extremely important in the maintenance of this condition. Take at least 30 grams per day minimum. Take a fiber supplement that provides a balance of both soluble and insoluble fibers. A flax/borage seed combination is a good choice, particularly one that contains other beneficial ingredients such as a probiotic blend with fructooligosaccharides (FOS) 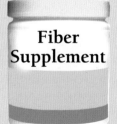 and herbs like slippery elm bark, marshmallow and fennel seed. Insoluble rice fiber with herbs and nutrients is another option. With increased

fiber, a proportional increase in water is essential to prevent constipation. Another key ingredient would be L-glutamine, which the intestine uses as fuel to regenerate. This fiber supplement may be added to juices and taken any time of day.

- Take essential fatty acids (EFAs) to lubricate the digestive tract. A combination of fish and flax oils (Omega-3) with borage oil (Omega-6) is good to reduce inflammation in the gastrointestinal tract. Absorption of the oils may be enhanced with the addition of lipase (a fat-digesting enzyme). Take three to six 1000 mg. capsules twice daily with food.

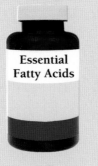

Essential Fatty Acids

- Take a probiotic (good bacteria) supplement with multiple strains as a daily supplement. It should contain a minimum of two to six billion cultures. A prebiotic could be helpful (see appendix).

Probiotic

- Take a multivitamin/mineral supplement (see appendix).
- Take antioxidant supplements (vitamin C - 500 mg. to 3000 mg., vitamin A - 10,000 I.U. daily and zinc – 30 mg. to 60 mg. daily) after meals. Other antioxidants may also be taken with these (see appendix).

LIFESTYLE

- Chew your foods to mush. To prevent diverticulitis, keep food (especially seeds) out of the pockets of the colon.
- Eat slowly.
- Drink plenty of water (see general recommendations at end of chapter).
- Do not get constipated!
- Use a squatting position when having a bowel elimination. Use the LifeStep™ (see Resource Directory).

COMPLEMENTARY MIND/BODY THERAPIES

- Colon hydrotherapy - Because it cleans out the

colon, colon hydrotherapy can be extremely helpful with diverticulosis. During your twice-yearly herbal detox program, do colon irrigation. It could also be done during the year periodically. Colon hydrotherapy should not be used in a diverticulitis attack.

- Yoga could be beneficial in diverticular conditions, as there are exercises to strengthen the abdominal area.
- Acupuncture
- Massage
- Biofeedback
- Meditation/Prayer
- Music Therapy
- Chiropractic

See appendix for information on these therapies.

Diverticular Facts:

- The condition is more prevalent as people age. For example, it is estimated that half of people in the United States ages 60 to 80 have diverticulosis, but only one person in 10 develops it by age 40. It is equally common in women and men.

- About 10 percent to 25 percent of people with this condition develop diverticulitis. This occurs when the diverticula become inflamed or infected.

- People whose diets contain large amounts of fiber are less likely to develop diverticular disease. The American Dietetic Association recommends 20 to 35 grams of fiber a day, preferably from fruits, vegetables and grains.

- Physical activity also may lower the risk of diverticulosis.

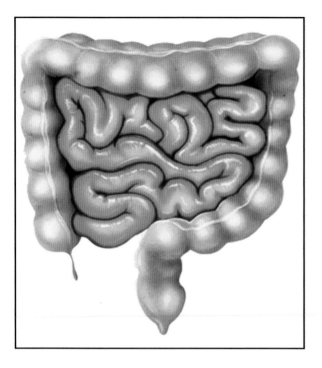

GAS
What is it?

The presence of excessive gas in the stomach and intestines is known as flatulence. Flatulence, when paired with other gastrointestinal symptoms, can be a sign of a serious GI disorder such as malabsorption, bacterial imbalance in the intestines (dysbiosis), parasites, irritable bowel syndrome, colitis, gallbladder disease, Candida, gastroesophageal reflux disease (GERD) or even a pancreatic tumor. At the very least, excessive gas production is a signal of incomplete digestion and a risk factor for intestinal problems. In and of itself, the passing of gas is not considered a medical problem unless it is excessive, or the person passing it is hypersensitive to it. Trapped gas that we're unable to pass can cause us a great deal more distress than that which is passed either through the rectum or by belching.

Certain gases are normally present in the GI tract and have no odor. These include nitrogen, oxygen, carbon dioxide and hydrogen. It is other gases like hydrogen sulfide, indole, butyric acid, cadaverine, putrescine and skatole that give off the foul-smelling odor with which we're all familiar. It is the sulfur content of methane and hydrogen sulfide that give these gases a rotten egg smell. People who pass excess gas have more sulfate-reducing bacteria in their feces. These bacteria cause high levels of sulfides in the feces, which is associated with disease of the colon.[1]

What Causes it?

There are three major sources of intestinal gas:

- Gas that is swallowed from the air, which contains nitrogen and oxygen
- Carbon dioxide gas, which is formed in the duodenum by a chemical reaction of hydrochloric acid from the stomach with the bicarbonate of the pancreatic secretions[2]
- Gases – primarily methane and hydrogen sulfide – that are formed through bacterial fermentation in the colon

This last group of gases is formed when bacteria in the colon or distal small bowel act on undigested food (food that was not absorbed in the small intestine), primarily carbohydrates, sugars and some fat. Some common sugars, which can be fermented to gas include fructose, lactose, sorbitol, trehalose (mushrooms), raffinose and stachyose (legumes and cruciferous vegetables). The more sulfide gases that are generated by intestinal bacteria, the more unpleasant the odor.

Swallowed air mostly causes belching. Much of it is absorbed in the small intestine, with the remainder being passed on to the colon and out the rectum. When rectal gas is high in nitrogen and oxygen, it is a sign that the cause is swallowed air (aerophagia).[3] Air is normally swallowed unconsciously in small amounts when we eat and drink. Some people repeatedly swallow it when eating and at other times, especially when they are anxious. We may swallow air by talking too much while eating, eating too rapidly, drinking carbonated beverages, chewing gum, smoking or sucking on hard candies. Any activity that causes excessive salivation may cause aerophagia. Also, excessive salivation may be associated with certain medications or nausea of any cause. Postnasal drip and ill-fitting dentures can also cause us to swallow air due to excessive salivation.

People who are lactose intolerant lack the enzyme lactase needed to break down the lactose (milk sugar) present in milk. The milk therefore is not properly digested and undergoes fermentation in the large intestine, causing gas. Some people are intolerant to other sugars (and sugar substitutes), as well, due to a deficiency in the enzymes that digest those sugars. Other foods that may give rise to gas production include:

- Cauliflower
- Brussels sprouts
- Legumes (peas, beans, lentils)
- Broccoli
- Cabbage
- Dried and sulfured fruits
- Cucumbers
- Celery
- Apples
- Carrots
- Onions
- Garlic
- Rutabaga
- Cantaloupe
- Kohlrabi
- Radishes
- Grapes
- Raisins
- Prune juice
- Bananas

Not all of these foods will cause excess gas in all people, but any can be a potential problem. The cruciferous vegetables – kale, collard greens, broccoli, cauliflower, cabbage, Brussels sprouts and turnips – contain a special type of carbohydrate (stachyose) that is poorly absorbed by the body but is quickly digested by bacteria in the intestines.[4]

Starches like wheat, oats, corn and bran and products made with the flours of these grains may pose

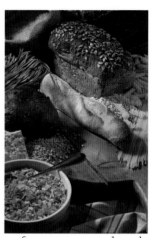

a problem too since bacterial fermentation occurs when carbohydrates are not being digested and absorbed in the small intestine as they should be. These carbohydrates then pass intact into the colon where they are acted upon by bacteria. The result is gas production. Bacterial fermentation is the cause of most gas produced. Much of that gas is methane, which may deplete specific short-chain fatty acids that are needed for the health of the colon lining.[5] People who eat a steady diet of processed foods are more apt to experience bacterial fermentation than those who eat whole foods because many of the nutrients needed for carbohydrate combustion are removed from grains when they are milled in the refining process.[6] Fiber is also removed in the refining process.

Even though fiber is needed to prevent constipation, some people find that when they add extra amounts to their diet, they experience excess gas production. This is most likely to happen if too much fiber is added too quickly. Making the transition gradually can reduce the likelihood of having this problem. It is not just the introduction of high-fiber food that may cause excessive gas; the introduction of any new dietary or supplement regime can have the same effect. For that reason, it is always wise to make changes slowly.

Overeating can result in excess gas production because when we gulp our food, it isn't digested properly. Over-consumption of caffeine, alcohol, salt, refined sugar and processed oils can be particularly problematic, as they serve as irritants.

Nutritional deficiencies – of digestive enzymes, hydrochloric acid and B vitamins (needed for carbohydrate combustion) – and food allergies or

Chapter 4

sensitivities may also result in excessive gas production. Too much vitamin C can also cause gas.

Poor food combining may result in excess gas production for some people. Improper food combining results primarily from mixing starchy foods, like grains and potatoes or fruits, with protein foods, like meat, eggs or cheese. Starchy foods and fruits are relatively low in protein and fat, and are more quickly absorbed and digested when eaten alone (especially raw fruit with its high enzyme content). It is believed that when protein and fat are combined with starch and fruit, the slower overall absorption allows for more bacterial fermentation of the starch and sugars, thereby creating more gas. Alternatively, it may be that with a large meal containing complex food combinations of protein, fat, starch and fruit, the total digestive need for more enzymes becomes a factor (particularly with aging), resulting in an increased load of undigested food, which promotes fermentation and gas. In any case, eating small meals slowly and chewing thoroughly are a health habits that may be more important than food combining. The food combining becomes more critical in people with digestive health challenges.

Gas may be associated with a variety of gastrointestinal disorders including constipation, diarrhea, malabsorption syndrome, parasites, candidiasis, gastroesophageal reflux disease, gastritis, dysbiosis (bacterial imbalance in the colon), colitis, gallbladder dysfunction or inadequate bile production, irritable bowel syndrome or, in rare cases, pancreatic tumor.

Who Gets it?
Everyone passes gas. The average person passes it approximately thirteen times a day[7] in amounts varying between a pint and a half-gallon.[8] About 30% of the U.S. population has bacteria in the colon or small intestine that produce excessive amounts of methane and hydrogen.[9] These are the people who are likely to be the most disease-prone. Overgrowth of bacteria in the colon or

small bowel can cause serious problems due to increased intestinal permeability, with absorption of bacterial toxins and partially digested food, and a decrease in short-chain fatty acid production, which feed the colonic cells and prevent cancer. Those who would fall in this 30% are those who have digestive problems stemming from the causes previously listed.

What Are the Signs and Symptoms?
Excess intestinal gas is thought to produce belching, bloating, abdominal distention and discomfort, bad breath, a feeling of fullness and release of malodorous gas through the anus. It appears that some people who suffer from these symptoms (especially those with irritable bowel syndrome) produce normal amounts of gas and yet are hypersensitive to it. Heartburn and nausea may also be experienced, and the tongue may be coated.[10]

How is it Diagnosed?
Unless the passage of gas is chronic and accompanied by other symptoms, no special diagnostics are indicated. Taking a thorough and detailed medical history can help give the attending physician an idea of the cause of the problem. Author D. Lindsey Berkson suggests the following guidelines for determining the cause of gas production in *Healthy Digestion the Natural Way:*[11]

- Gas and belching that occur during, immediately after, or within a half hour of eating suggests a hydrochloric acid deficiency or food allergy.
- Gas within 1 to 1.5 hours after eating may suggest overgrowth of bad bacteria in the small intestine. This can be more accurately documented by collecting expired air from the lungs and sending it for methane and hydrogen testing. Great Smokies Diagnostic Laboratories (see appendix) is one laboratory that does this type of testing.
- Belching that worsens after eating fatty foods – possibly associated with sharp pain in upper right shoulder and/or abdomen and spreading to the back – may signify gallbladder disease.

- Flatulence with foul smelling stools and possibly unexplained weight loss may be associated with malabsorption syndrome, parasites, dysbiosis or pancreatic dysfunction.
- Belching of gas that increases on bending over and lying down may signify reflux of stomach contents from the stomach to the esophagus.
- Gas associated with diarrhea and/or constipation, lower abdominal pain that lessens or goes away once gas is passed and excessive gas accompanying most bowel movements may indicate intestinal problems such as colitis, diverticular disease, irritable bowel syndrome, dysbiosis, parasites or candidiasis.

Consultation with a physician is recommended for anyone experiencing any of the above. Further tests will then be done to rule out or confirm the suspected diagnosis. The Comprehensive Digestive Stool Analysis, often used by holistic physicians, can be used to detect candidiasis and other dysbiotic imbalances. Special ELISA testing can identify food allergies, which can also be spotted by keeping a food diary. See the appendix for information on these tests.

What is the Standard Medical Treatment?

The Merck Manual (used by medical doctors for diagnosis) flatly states that "…most complaints [of excess gas] are caused by unconscious aerophagia or by exaggerated sensitivity to normal amounts of gas."[12] Therefore, recommended treatment is aimed primarily at: (1) altering lifestyle elements so that air swallowing is reduced and (2) suppressing symptoms through use of drugs.

The following measures may help to reduce air swallowing:

- Eat slowly; chew thoroughly (and with the mouth closed).
- Avoid chewing gum.
- Quit smoking.
- Eliminate carbonated beverages.
- Make sure dentures fit properly.

- Seek treatment for any disorder (such as peptic ulcer) that may cause reflex hypersalivation.
- Don't talk excessively while eating.
- Drink iced cold beverages in moderation, if at all.
- Eliminate or reduce sorbitol and xylitol, undigestible sugars that may cause gas.
- Exclude dairy products if lactose intolerant.
- Reduce or eliminate medications (under doctor's supervision) that may cause excessive salivation.
- Try biofeedback and relaxation therapy.
- Eliminate antacids if associated with belching.

Most of the above recommendations are included in the Merck Manual, which also offers the following observation: "Few well-controlled studies have demonstrated clear-cut benefit from any drug."[13]

Several drugs incorporating simethicone, an agent that breaks up small gas bubbles, have been used (with variable results) to treat gas. Anti-cholinergic drugs have been used with similar results. These affect the nervous system.

The Merck Manual also suggests that roughage (fiber), in such forms as bran or psyllium seed, may be added to the diet to correct constipation, but adds that it may have the effect of actually increasing gas production. Activated charcoal is also mentioned for its ability to reduce gas and the unpleasant odors sometimes associated with it.

Chapter 4

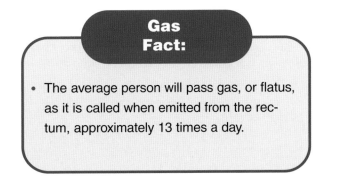

Gas Fact:

- The average person will pass gas, or flatus, as it is called when emitted from the rectum, approximately 13 times a day.

Optional Nutritional Approaches

It is important to rule out the following if you have excessive gas:

• Candida (see Chapter 4 on Candida)
• Parasites (see Chapter 4 on parasites)
• Food sensitivities (the Candida diet in the Candida section could be helpful to follow for one month. This diet excludes most common foods to which people are sensitive.)

The following food combining guide could be helpful in controlling excess gas:

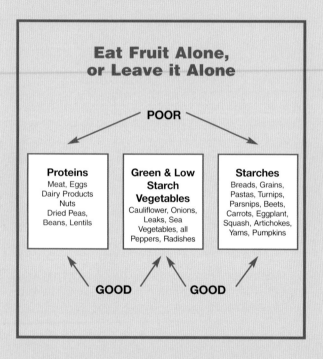

Eat Fruit Alone, or Leave it Alone

POOR

Proteins
Meat, Eggs
Dairy Products
Nuts
Dried Peas,
Beans, Lentils

Green & Low Starch Vegetables
Cauliflower, Onions,
Leaks, Sea
Vegetables, all
Peppers, Radishes

Starches
Breads, Grains,
Pastas, Turnips,
Parsnips, Beets,
Carrots, Eggplant,
Squash, Artichokes,
Yams, Pumpkins

GOOD   GOOD

Diet

• Juicing can be beneficial in healing the digestive tract. Try from one to three days of a juice diet to start (see appendix for recipes). You can also work some of these juices into you daily diet. Green juices are excellent for the digestive tract and immune system.
• Follow the Digestive Care Diet in the appendix. It is very important to follow food combining rules for this condition.

• As indicated in the Digestive Care Diet, two very important considerations for food combining are:
  – Eat fruit alone or thirty minutes before a meal.
  – Avoid eating protein and starch at the same meal.

Supplements

If gas occurs after starting a new supplement or detox program, it could be the result of starting too fast. The intake of supplemental dietary fiber can also cause gas. Slow the program down. Go to 1/2 strength with everything you are taking, and see if this helps.

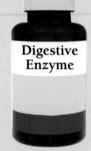

Digestive Enzyme

A plant enzyme should be specially designed for gas and bloating. This supplement should include (at least) 20,000 D.U. of amylase; galactosidase, 1,000 G.A.L.; cellulase, 3,000 C.U. and 40 U. of phytase. This enzyme blend is specific for poor carbohydrate digestion, which can be the cause of gas and bloating.

Digestive enzymes are important with meals. There are two kinds that could be helpful. One contains HCl (take this when acid levels are low in the stomach); the other contains a plant enzyme blend. The following are descriptions of each supplement:

• The plant enzyme blend: This supplement should include protease (at least 20,000 H.U.T), amylase and lipase, as well as papaya and bromelain. Other ingredients in this formula might include soothing herbs like marshmallow and slippery elm. Additionally, a good digestive enzyme formula would contain glutamine (an amino acid) and N-acetyl-glucosamine.
• Take HCl/pepsin supplements before meals if stomach acid levels are low. Start with one capsule, and increase by one capsule daily

with meals until symptoms are gone. (If y ou feel a burning sensation, back off to previous dose.) The supplement may contain other soothing ingredients like quercitin, bromelain, gamma oryzanol, L-glutamine and N-acetyl-glucosamine.

Additional supplements that may be helpful include:

- Take a probiotic (good bacteria) supplement with multiple strains as a daily supplement. It should contain a minimum of two to six billion cultures. A prebiotic could be helpful (see appendix).

- B complex vitamin supplement (see appendix) - Add extra pantothenic acid: 1,000 mg. to 2,000 mg. per day for the first week; then go to 500 mg. once to twice per day.[14]
- Aloe vera juice, five ounces, one to two times a day.
- Take 1,000 mg. to 5,000 mg. of L-glutamine powder with N-acetyl-glucosamine (NAG) and gamma oryzanol, once to twice daily on an empty stomach.

- Try fennel or peppermint tea (hot). This helps eliminate gas.

LIFESTYLE
- Check with you doctor, and see if any medication (including over-the-counter) could be causing gas.
- Do not eat late at night. Stop eating between 6:00 pm and 7:00 pm.
- Exercise to help stimulate the passage of gas through the GI tract.
- Sweeteners can cause excessive gas. Eliminate or reduce sorbitol, sucralose and xylitol. Artificial sweeteners like Nutrasweet and Equal should be eliminated.

COMPLEMENTARY MIND/BODY THERAPIES
- Colon hydrotherapy is indicated for removing excess gas from the colon. Try it along with the protocol above.
- Massage (abdominal massage) can be helpful in moving out trapped gas. Benefits include invigoration of skin tissue, promotion of suppleness of muscle tissue, stimulation of body fluid circulation, balancing of nerve impulse distribution and improved relaxation.
- Acupuncture
- Chiropractic
- Meditation/Prayer
- Biofeedback
- Music therapy
- Yoga

See appendix for information on the above therapies.

Gas Facts:

- Almost half of Americans (46%) claim to have been embarrassed by intestinal gas in public.
- According to the Canadian Society of Intestinal Research, careful analysis of intestinal gas has shown that about 90% is ingested air, and only 10% is actually formed in the intestine.
- Gas within one to one & one-half hours after eating may suggest overgrowth of bad bacteria in the small intestine.
- There are some people who lack the enzyme that is needed to digest lactose, the sugar in milk, resulting in the production of gas in the large intestine.

Chapter 4

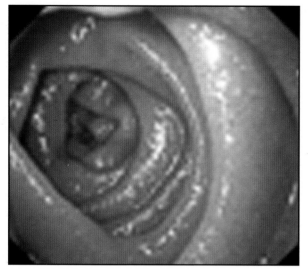

Internal view of the digestive tract.

GLUTEN SENSITIVITY
What is it?

Gluten is the insoluble protein constituent of wheat and other grains, a mixture of gliadin, glutenin and other proteins.[1] It is the gluten in grains that makes the rising of flour possible. Gluten sensitivity is an inflammatory reaction to eating foods containing gluten. It occurs mainly in the lining of the small intestine where an immune response is triggered. The degree of gluten sensitivity can be minor to life-threatening. Thus, there are numerous terms, encompassing several different conditions, that involve some degree or form of gluten sensitivity. This can be very confusing for those not acquainted with this subject. Primary emphasis here will be on what is known as celiac disease, a condition that can go by six different names: sprue, non-tropical sprue, celiac sprue, gluten-induced sprue, gluten-induced enteropathy and gluten-sensitive enteropathy. The dictionary definition of sprue (American Heritage, 4th edition) is "a chronic disease characterized by diarrhea, emaciation and anemia, caused by defective absorption of nutrients from the GI tract." We can use this same definition for celiac disease.

What Causes it?

Although the prime cause of gluten sensitivity is not completely understood, there is a great deal that can be asserted regarding cause. Infection or toxicity is thought to be the cause of tropical sprue, while leaky gut syndrome is believed to be responsible for the allergic form of gluten sensitivity. Celiac disease is a chronic disorder caused by an inability to properly digest foods that contain gluten. These foods include wheat, rye, barley, triticale, spelt, amaranth, buckwheat, spelt, kamut, millet and possibly oats.[2] This failure to properly digest these foods results in damage to the cells lining the small intestine, which in turn causes malabsorption of nutrients from food. Gliadin is the main protein component in wheat that causes difficulty for those suffering from celiac disease. However, similar proteins in other grains may cause the same reaction: hordein in barley, secalin in rye and avidin in oats. Current research suggests that the gliadin is absorbed between cells, and certain fragments of gliadin induce intense immune inflammatory reactions that injure the bowel lining, further exacerbating the injury. In addition, these antibodies produced in the immune reaction can cross react with other tissues and produce a wide array of autoimmune diseases, as mentioned below. Interestingly, gliadin that has been completely broken down by digestion does not activate celiac disease in susceptible individuals. This suggests that celiac disease may arise from a deficiency of enzymes that break down gliadin or other factors involved with protein digestion.[3]

The immune inflammatory response typical of celiac disease will eventually destroy the small hair-like villi in the intestine through which nutrients are absorbed into the bloodstream. This can lead to leaky gut syndrome.[4] However, it is important to realize that not everyone with gluten intolerance has full blown celiac disease. Some people who don't test positive for it nonetheless feel better avoiding grains. They just don't have the enzymes to properly break them down, which can cause leaky gut and inflammation.[5]

The stage may be set for development of celiac disease in infancy. The early introduction of cow's milk is believed to be a major causative factor in celiac disease.[6] Early introduction of cereals appears to be another factor. In fact, research has indicated that "delayed administration of [both]

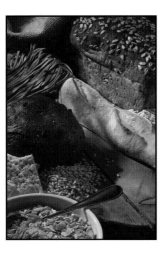

cow's milk and cereal grains are the primary preventive steps that can greatly reduce the risk of developing celiac disease.[7]

Who Gets it?

Celiac disease, in some cases, has an hereditary component. Therefore, many family members may be affected. The disease is usually identified in early childhood, but may disappear in adolescence and reappear later in adulthood.[8] It may also make its first appearance in adult years. Celiac disease occurs twice as often in females as in males[9] and primarily affects Caucasians and people of European descent.[10] It rarely occurs in people of African, Jewish, Mediterranean or Asian descent.[11] The highest incidences of the disease occur in Northern and central Europe, the northwestern Indian subcontinent and any other areas where wheat cultivation is a relatively recent development.[12] Celiac disease is especially common in Ireland, where it is estimated to affect one in every 300 people.[13] Estimates of the frequency of the disease in the United States vary widely from source to source, often ranging from one in 1,000 to one in 5,000 people. However, recent studies show that celiac disease is a great deal more prevalent than previously thought. According to Dr. Joseph Mercola:

> …Traditional diagnostic methods in recent studies show as many as 1 in 33

in the US have this disease. This is a far cry from 1 in 5000! Due to the fact that celiac disease was considered rare in this country, it often went undiagnosed or misdiagnosed as irritable bowel syndrome or lactose intolerance. My experience is that the true incidence is probably much higher still, perhaps on the order of 1 in 10 people.[14]

Celiac disease can be triggered by many factors, including viral infection, surgery, extreme stress and childbirth.[15] Others who have an elevated risk of developing celiac disease are those who have Down's syndrome, type 1 diabetes or chronic arthritis in childhood.[16] It may be difficult to always know, with certainty, which came first, the celiac disease or the autoimmune disorder (like diabetes or arthritis).

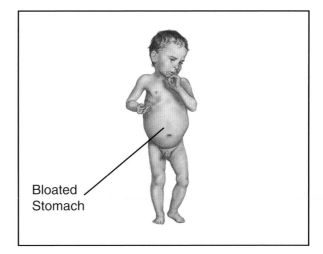

Bloated Stomach

What are the Signs and Symptoms?

Some people with celiac disease have no symptoms, while others become quite ill with:

- Weight loss
- Gas and bloating
- Diarrhea (which is typical of malabsorption)
- Abdominal pain
- Nutritional deficiencies
- Anemia (due to iron deficiency)

Chapter 4

- Edema (fluid accumulation in the extremities due to a decrease in blood protein)
- Steatorrhea (gray or tan, fatty, greasy, foul-smelling stools that float)
- Dermatitis herpetiformis (a chronic skin condition)
- Weakness
- Lack of appetite
- Early satiety (feeling full after eating a small amount of food)
- Nausea/vomiting
- Depression
- Fatigue
- Irritability
- Muscle cramps and wasting
- Joint and/or bone pain

The first five listed on the previous page are usually the first to develop.

Celiac disease may cause slow growth in children and suppress the onset of menses in adolescent girls. Also, children may exhibit behavior changes, develop blisters and sores or a red rash all over their bodies; they may also develop mouth ulcers.[17] On the other hand, symptoms in children may be mild and are apt to be dismissed as a simple stomachache.

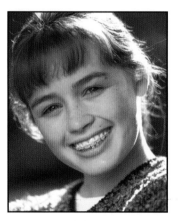

Celiac disease can be quite serious, even life-threatening, if not treated. Among the serious impairments that may result from it are:[18]

- Bone disease (due to malabsorption of all nutrients involved in bone health)
- Central and peripheral nervous system impairment

- Seizures (due to folic acid deficiency)
- Internal hemorrhaging
- Pancreatic disease
- Infertility
- Miscarriages
- Birth defects
- Gynecological disorders
- High risk of developing intestinal malignancies (possible result of decreased vitamin and mineral absorption, ongoing inflammation and low antioxidant levels)
- Hypothrombinemia (lack of clotting factors in the blood, a result of vitamin K deficiency)

The celiac disease patient is also at increased risk of developing other autoimmune disorders, including:[19]

- Kidney failure
- Sarcoidosis (the formation of lesions in lungs, bones, skin and elsewhere)
- Insulin-dependent diabetes
- Systemic lupus erythematosus
- Thyroid disease
- Chronic active hepatitis
- Scleroderma
- Myasthenia gravis
- Addison's disease
- Rheumatoid arthritis
- Sjögrens's syndrome

These last six diseases are more rarely developed than the others. Hives and psychiatric disorders, including schizophrenia, have also been linked to celiac disease.[20] Partially digested wheat gluten produces opiate-like activity. This activity is believed to be the factor responsible for the association between wheat consumption and schizophrenia established in many studies.[21] Interestingly, the prevalence of celiac disease in patients with indigestion is twice that of the general population,[22] an indication that screening such patients for celiac might be warranted.

Bear in mind that, while symptoms may be severe, they may also be absent in celiac disease. New research shows that traditional gastrointestinal symptoms may be delayed for up to 8 years in some adults, with the first clinical signs being iron deficiency anemia, bone disease and sterility in women.[23]

A person with mild wheat intolerance (but not full-blown celiac disease) does not have the inflammation in the cells lining the intestine, but nevertheless may experience such symptoms as gas and bloating, distention and even diarrhea.[24]

How is it Diagnosed?

Diagnosis of celiac disease by symptoms alone is not possible with any degree of accuracy because of its similarity to aspects of other disorders: irritable bowel syndrome, gastric ulcers, anemia, intestinal infection, food allergy, gastroesophageal reflux disease, ulcerative colitis, Crohn's disease, lactose intolerance, HIV-related diseases and certain cancers.[25, 26, 27] It is common therefore to run certain tests to rule out or confirm the celiac disease diagnosis. A blood test to check for IgA and IgG antibodies to gliadin (a subfraction of gluten) and a tissue transglutaminase antibody is often done. The transglutaminase antibody is most specific (95%) and is related to destruction of the intestinal lining. If these tests yield a positive result, they would ideally be followed by a biopsy of the small intestine, which would reveal damage to the villi, if present, and give a definitive diagnosis. The biopsy is typically done in conjunction with endoscopy (see appendix). Some doctors may choose to forego the biopsy, basing their diagnosis instead upon blood test results and symptoms.

Lactose intolerance is common in those with celiac disease due to the fact that the damaged intestinal cells temporarily lose their lactase enzyme activity, making it impossible to digest the lactose in dairy products. Some doctors therefore may

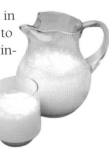

choose to test for lactose intolerance using a lactose breath test (see appendix), in addition to using the tests described above for celiac disease. Food allergy/sensitivity screening, using the ELISA blood test (described in appendix), may also be helpful in diagnosing gluten sensitivity. This test

Hidden Sources of Gluten

- Modified food starch
- Thickening agents
- Caramel coloring
- MSG
- Malted milk
- Flavored and instant coffees
- Soy sauce (some brands)
- Emulsifiers
- Stabilizers
- Hydrolyzed vegetable proteins
- Packaged rice mixes
- Creamed vegetables
- Some non-dairy creamers
- Prepared meats (like sandwich meats, hot dogs)
- Salad dressings
- Vodka, ale, whiskey, beer, gin, wine, malt
- Ovaltine
- Ice cream
- Soup
- Bouillon cubes
- Chocolate
- Catsup
- Pie fillings
- Baking powders
- Chewing gum
- Dry seasoning mixes
- Gravy mixes
- Processed cheeses
- Most dips
- Vanilla and flavorings made with alcohol
- Most condiments

Chart 1

Chapter 4

will reveal the presence of antibodies to gluten and other food components. A patient who is making antibodies to gluten but has no intestinal damage would be diagnosed with gluten intolerance rather than celiac disease. With either diagnosis, there is a probability of increased intestinal permeability (leaky gut). Therefore, physicians who are aware of this phenomenon may elect to order intestinal permeability screening (see appendix). It is also useful to assess digestive efficiency with the Comprehensive Digestive Stool Analysis and test for parasites (see testing information in appendix). Finally, since many patients with celiac disease have iron deficiency anemia, low levels of the fat-soluble vitamins (A, D, E and K), poor fat absorption and multiple mineral deficiencies, an assessment of nutrient status may be undertaken.

What is the Standard Medical Treatment?

Once diagnosed, prompt and thorough treatment of celiac disease is essential, for without treatment, the disease can result in malnourishment, which will adversely affect the entire body. There is no known cure for celiac disease, but it can be controlled by a lifelong adherence to a totally gluten-free diet. The removal of most grains and other gluten-containing foods from the diet eliminates irritation, giving the intestine a chance to heal. Strict adherence to a totally gluten-free diet results in disappearance of symptoms, prompt healing of the intestinal lining and the gaining back of lost weight. The problem is that it's not always easy to identify – much less avoid – all gluten-containing food products, particularly in a society like ours in the U.S. where there is such an abundance of processed and genetically modified foods that are wheat-based or wheat-containing. It has been shown that the closer a grain is related to wheat, the greater its ability to activate celiac disease.[28] There has been some controversy as to whether or not those with celiac disease can safely eat oats. Although several studies suggest that people with the disease can safely eat them, since oats are often processed along with other grains, it is difficult to determine whether oats are totally free of other grains.[29]

While those with mild gluten sensitivity may be able to tolerate such grains as millet, amaranth and buckwheat, those with severe gluten sensitivity will need to avoid wheat, oats, rye and barley and all related grains, which would include triticale, spelt, amaranth, buckwheat, spelt, kamut and millet. Aside from the obvious sources of these grains (breads, muffins, cereals, pastas, flours, crackers, etc.), there are many hidden sources of gluten, as indicated in chart 1.

The list in chart 1 is by no means comprehensive, but it gives a good idea of how much hidden gluten there is in commonly consumed foods. Add to this the fact that celiac disease patients may also need to avoid dairy products (and in some cases chicken and eggs), as well as any foods to which they may be allergic, and you can see that food selection and preparation can be quite problematic.

The good news for the patient with celiac disease is that there are many supportive organizations (see Resource Directory), periodicals and products to help make life easier. The magazine *Living Without* (www.livingwithout.com) carries current information about many lines of gluten-free products of all types, including baked goods and pastas made with safe grains — rice, soy, potato or corn. A "gluten home test" device is also advertised, which will help to quickly determine if there is any glucose in the food being tested. This instrument is made by ELISA Technologies (www.elisa-tek.com, 352-337-3929).

Some people with a severe or long-standing case of celiac disease may not respond to dietary management. In other words, their symptoms may not subside when they eliminate gluten. In such cases, doctors often prescribe corticosteroids to bring down the inflammation in the intestine. If damage to the small intestine is extensive, affected sections of tissue may have to be surgically removed.

Optional Nutritional Approaches

Both mainstream and holistic physicians would agree to the necessity of removing gluten-containing foods from the diet of the person with celiac disease. It could also be helpful to temporarily remove lactose-containing foods. The good news about strict adherence to a gluten-free diet is that most people tend to respond very quickly: 30% show improvements within 3 days, 50% respond within 1 month, 10% within another month and another 10% within 24 to 36 months.[30] The Digestive Care Diet in the appendix or the Candida Diet (in Chapter 4) can be followed (minus any gluten-containing foods). Again, refer to the Resource Directory for sourcing of foods that are gluten-free.

*** Please note: gluten (wheat) sensitivity is much more common than most people are aware. Most of us can benefit from a wheat-free, gluten-free diet regardless of whether or not we have celiac disease.

If celiac disease is suspected, your health care practitioner will want to rule out the following:

• Candida (see Chapter 4)
• Parasites (see Chapter 4)

SUPPLEMENTS

Care must be taken with supplements, as well as with foods, to avoid those containing hidden gluten. Look for supplements that say: "gluten free." Your supplement regime might include:

• Digestive enzymes - This supplement should include protease (at least 20,000 H.U.T.), amylase and lipase, as well as papaya and bromelain. Other ingredients in this formula might include soothing herbs like marshmallow and slippery elm. Additionally, a good digestive enzyme formula would contain glutamine (an amino acid) and N-acetyl-glucosamine, which helps soothe an irritated mucosal lining.

• EFAs (essential fatty acids) to lubricate the digestive tract. A combination of fish and flax (Omega-3) with borage oil (Omega-6) is good to reduce inflammation in the gastrointestinal tract. Absorption of the oils may be enhanced with the addition of lipase (a fat-digesting enzyme). Take three to six 1000 mg. capsules twice daily with food.

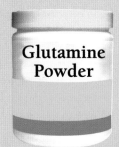

• A probiotic (good bacteria) supplement with multiple strains as a daily supplement; it should contain a minimum of two to six billion cultures. A prebiotic could be helpful (see appendix).

• A fiber supplement that provides a balance of both soluble and insoluble fibers. A flax/borage seed combination is a good choice, particularly one that contains other beneficial ingredients such as a probiotic blend with fructooligosaccharhides (FOS) and herbs like slippery elm bark, marshmallow and fennel seed. Another key ingredient would be L-glutamine, which the intestine uses as fuel to regenerate. This fiber supplement may be added to juices and taken any time of day. When beginning to add dietary fiber to the diet, remember to go slowly, as this can cause some gas if added too quickly.

• 10,000 mg. to 20,000 mg. of L-glutamine powder with N-acetyl-glucosamine (NAG) and gamma oryzanol once to twice daily on an empty stomach. This will help to rebuild the mucosal lining, which is damaged in celiac disease (see appendix).

• A multivitamin/mineral supplement (a liquid form could be helpful; find in health food store).

- Antioxidant supplements (vitamin C - 500 mg. to 3000 mg., vitamin A - 10,000 I.U. daily and zinc – 30 mg. to 60 mg. daily) with meals. Other antioxidants may also be taken with these (see appendix).

**Additionally, the following are essential:

- Vitamin K or alfalfa tablets
- B-12: 1,000 mcg. - 2000 mcg. daily (sublingual or injection from a doctor) and folic acid (400 mcg. - 800 mcg. daily).
- Extra B6 or B complex combination orally.
- Aloe, either as a drink or in capsule form. The mucilaginous polysaccharide molecules in aloe have a profound anti-inflammatory and healing effect on the intestinal lining.

Follow as much of this protocol as possible until you feel better or, if you are under the care of a doctor or practitioner, until you are told to discontinue. For maintenance (ongoing), the following are essential (all to be taken as indicated above):

- Digestive enzymes
- EFA's
- Fiber
- Probiotics
- Multivitamin/mineral
- Antioxidants

LIFESTYLE

- Learn to read labels carefully. This is the key to a lifetime of good health.
- When dining out, inquire about special sauces or secret ingredients. Let the waiter and cook know your needs and food requirements.
- Join support groups to help you with gluten intolerance. This is a lifelong issue. See our Resource Directory for relevant magazines and websites.
- Remember: Ale, beer, gin, whiskey and vodka are all distilled from grain. If you choose to drink alcohol, the following are safe: rum, tequila and sake.
- Exercise, in the form of walking or use of a

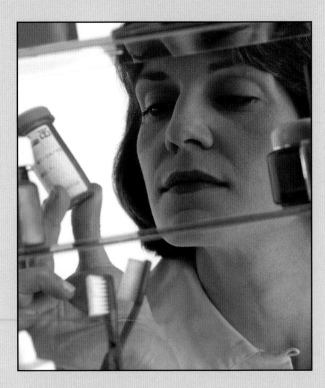

mini-trampoline (see appendix), should be incorporated into your daily routine.

COMPLEMENTARY MIND/BODY THERAPIES

- Colon hydrotherapy can be helpful in removing toxins from the colon in a very gentle way.
- Massage to help relax and assist in the healing process
- Yoga for exercise and healing
- Acupuncture
- Biofeedback
- Meditation/Prayer
- Music therapy
- Chiropractic

See appendix for information on the above herapies.

Dr Smith's Comments

I have personally seen patients with a wide variety of conditions in which gluten sensitivity has been implicated. One case was a 19-year old college student with a gradual history of pressure sensations in the back of his head and visual difficulties, especially pre-

cipitated by exercise. His MRI scan and neurologic exams were normal. ELISA food sensitivity testing showed 2-3+ sensitivity to wheat and dairy, and he was a blood type O. Strict removal of gluten and dairy foods, while adding antioxidants and fish oils, has decreased his symptoms considerably over several months.

Another case involved a 52-year old truck driver, who over a period of several years, noted increasing abdominal cramping and diarrhea, especially after eating pizza. He could relieve the symptoms somewhat if he took a probiotic product before eating pizza. He presented to the hospital with massive bloody diarrhea and toxic megacolon, and improved somewhat on strict hospital treatment; however, on colonoscopy, he had severe ulcerative colitis. He eventually had to have a subtotal abdominal colectomy.

What is the common link in these cases, as well as the many others with conditions ranging from childhood type I diabetes to multiple sclerosis and colon cancer? I believe it begins not with a sensitivity to wheat, but with a "leaky gut" or increased intestinal permeability. There are many causes of this that have nothing to do with wheat. Some common causes are:

- Excessive sugar and simple carbohydrates in the diet, which can promote an overgrowth of yeast, especially Candida, and pathogenic bacteria.
- Stress, dehydration, poor mucus production, nutrition, antioxidant status, and genetics
- Alcohol consumption and food sensitivities

It is known that a protein produced in the intestine called zonulin can, under certain conditions, increase the paracellular permeability. When this happens, the gliadin gets by the lining into the submucosal area, and it is here that a variety of severe immune events can take place. It could be that when children have a gastrointestinal flu syndrome with diarrhea, the resultant transient increased permeability may set the stage for serious sensitivities to wheat and dairy if they are introduced back into the diet before the intestinal tract has healed. This may be as long as 3-5 days, during

which time soups and cooked vegetables should be the diet of choice. Similarly, over-consumption of alcohol while eating commonly sensitive foods, such as wheat and dairy, could be the start of a sensitivity to a previously tolerated food. There is data in the pediatric literature showing that pretreating of wheat and dairy- sensitive children with sodium chromoglycate (a histamine blocker) will actually prevent the expected increase in intestinal permeability. In addition, there is data suggesting that the herb quercitin can block histamine release and prevent "leaky gut," as well. Any symptoms suggestive of gastrointestinal dysfunction, particularly in combination with inflammation in the body, such as arthritis or fibromyalgia, should warrant food sensitivity testing and elimination of sensitive foods as a starting point.

Chapter 4

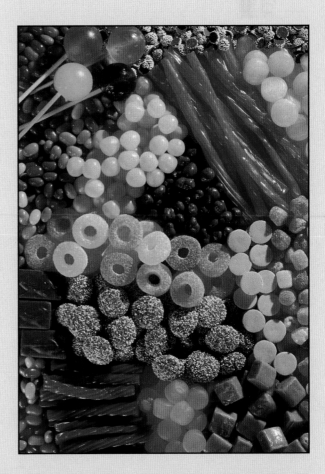

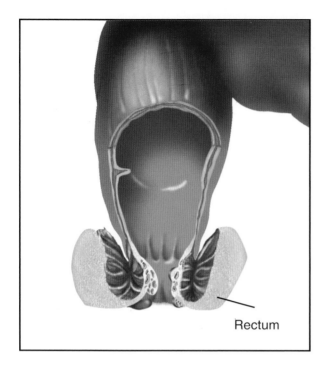

Rectum

HEMORRHOIDS
What is it?
Hemorrhoids (also known as piles) are swollen blood vessels in the anal area that stretch under pressure. They are much like varicose veins in the legs and may develop either inside the lower rectum (internal hemorrhoids) or under the skin around the anus (external hemorrhoids).

What Causes it?
There are two basic causes of hemorrhoids: (1) A genetic weakness in the wall of the veins and/or (2) Excessive pressure on those veins.[1] That pressure is often due to chronic constipation or straining during bowel movements but may also be caused and aggravated by chronic diarrhea. The most frequently recognized cause of constipation is a low-fiber diet; however, other factors such as lactose intolerance, inadequate water intake, low thyroid function and magnesium deficiency may also cause or contribute to the condition. (See "Constipation" in this chapter for more information on the subject.)

Excess pressure on the veins can also result from abdominal muscle strain stemming from heavy or improper lifting or from pushing during childbirth while in labor (thus placing a great deal of pressure on the anus). Pregnancy itself, due to the accompanying hormonal changes that cause blood vessels to expand, may cause hemorrhoids. The increased intra-abdominal pressure present in pregnancy as the fetus grows can also lead to development of hemorrhoids. This same type of increased intra-abdominal pressure can result from defecation, violent coughing, sneezing, vomiting, physical exertion or portal hypertension due to cirrhosis of the liver.[2] Prolonged sitting or standing also exerts excessive pressure on veins, which can cause them to weaken and herniate.

Other factors that can cause or contribute to development of hemorrhoids include obesity, lack of exercise, liver damage, food allergies or sensitivities and nutritional deficiencies.

Who Gets it?
About 89% of Americans will develop hemorrhoids at one time or another in their lives,[3] with the risk increasing with age so that half the population will have symptoms of the disorder by age 50.[4] It is interesting to note that the incidence of hemorrhoids increases up to age 70, at which time it decreases.[5] While they primarily affect older people, hemorrhoids can develop at any age. Those younger individuals who are most affected are pregnant woman and women with children. Some people may begin to develop hemorrhoids in their 20s, but usually there are no overt symptoms for another decade.[6] As noted, heredity can play a role in development of hemorrhoids.

While hemorrhoids are a very common complaint in the U.S. and in other industrialized nations, the condition is non-existent in indigenous cultures that have no access to processed foods. The processing of our foods results in removal of fiber and important nutrients, causing constipation and digestive problems.

While hemorrhoids are not life-threatening, they can be quite uncomfortable. Since diet and lifestyle play a prominent role in their development, hemorrhoids can be prevented by appropriately modifying these.

What Are the Signs and Symptoms?

Not everyone who has hemorrhoids will have symptoms. When present, hemorrhoids may cause or display any or all of the following signs and symptoms:

- Rectal bleeding
- Rectal pain
- Burning
- Swelling of tissue/inflammation
- Protrusion of tissue (prolapse)
- Painful bowel movements
- Engorgement with blood
- Sensation of incomplete evacuation
- Mucous discharge
- Itching

When bleeding occurs, it is generally bright red (a sign of fresh blood) and usually indicative of internal hemorrhoids, which occur in the anal canal, out of view. This may be the only symptom displayed with internal hemorrhoids. Some bleeding should not be cause for alarm unless the bleeding is dark and/or lasts for more than a few days, in which case medical help should be sought. Bleeding can also be a sign of other conditions such as polyps, ulcerative colitis or even rectal or colon cancer and so should be thoroughly investigated.

Internal hemorrhoids can cause a great deal of pain when they herniate (prolapse) or collapse and protrude below the anal sphincter when straining to pass stools. A mucous discharge and itching may accompany the prolapsed hemorrhoid. This is generally the only time that itching is experienced as a result of hemorrhoids. Anal itching can be a sign of other problems, however, such as parasites, Candida albicans, food allergy or tissue irritation from the vigorous use of harsh toilet paper.

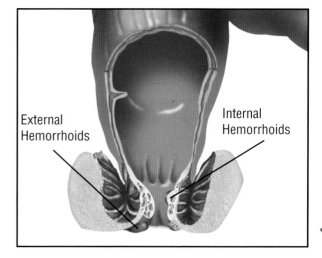

External hemorrhoids are visible to the eye, since they occur in veins outside the anus. These ballooned, skin-covered veins often appear as hard bluish lumps. There is generally no pain with an external hemorrhoid unless it ruptures and forms a blood clot (thrombus). This clotting can also occur with prolapsed internal hemorrhoids. In time, the clot is replaced by fibrous connective tissue, and the hemorrhoid may shrink and not be detectable..

Where there is no prolapse, there may be bleeding from a hemorrhoid, but there is no pain; with prolapse, there is pain and possibly bleeding. Occasionally, a hemorrhoid will prolapse to such a degree and for so long that its blood supply is blocked by constriction of the anal sphincter. Such a strangulated hemorrhoid usually thromboses (fills with blood) and is very painful.

How is it Diagnosed?

Diagnosis is based upon the doctor's examination of the anus and rectum for signs of swollen blood vessels. He or she will also do a digital rectal exam, using the fingers of a gloved hand. Closer inspection of the rectum is possible with the aid of an anoscope, a flexible, lighted tube. The tube is inserted in the rectum, and internal hemorrhoids may be viewed. A proctoscope is used for a more extensive examination of the entire rectum, if needed. A sigmoidoscopy or colonoscopy

Chapter 4

(described in the appendix) may be performed to rule out gastrointestinal bleeding or find its source. If necessary, tissue may be cauterized through the scope to stop the bleeding.

What is the Standard Medical Treatment?

Standard treatment of hemorrhoids consists of relieving and preventing through such measures as:

- Tub or sitz baths (in 3" - 4" of warm water) for 10 minutes several times daily (Baking soda or Epsom salts - 1/4 cup - may be added to the water.)
- Local applications of creams, suppositories, ointments, anorectal pads sold over-the-counter for temporary relief of pain (Note: These do not shrink hemorrhoids.)
- High dietary fiber intake (fruits, vegetables, whole grains and bulk fiber supplements) to promote peristalsis and soften stools
- Adequate water consumption – 6 to 8 glasses per day
- Local application of ice packs to reduce swelling of hemorrhoids
- Use of stool softeners
- Frequent cleansing of anal area with warm water (no soap)
- No sitting on hard surfaces; use a soft cushion.
- Use of proper lifting technique (Bend at knees, not at waist. Exhale while lifting; don't hold breath.)
- No heavy lifting.
- No use of rough toilet paper; use damp toilet paper.
- Regular exercise
- No sitting on toilet for long periods of time (over 10 minutes), as blood will pool in the hemorrhoidal veins.

Although some cases of hemorrhoids may be successfully treated using the above conservative methods, at times doctors will elect to use more aggressive treatments aimed at shrinking and destroying hemorrhoidal tissues. These treatments may include:[7]

Rubber band ligation – Here a rubber band is placed around the base of an internal hemorrhoid to cut off its circulation. The result is that the hemorrhoid withers and drops off within a few days. Although ligation is the most common treatment used today, it can be painful and may require repeat treatments.

Infrared photocoagulation – involves the use of infrared heat to treat minor internal hemorrhoids. It is less painful than ligation but is not always as effective.

Bipolar electrocoagulation – uses intermittent electrical current to shrink hemorrhoids and is comparable to infrared photocoagulation in terms of pros and cons.

Sclerotherapy – involves injection of a solution containing either quinine and urea or phenol directly into the hemorrhoid for the purpose of shrinking it and stopping any bleeding that may be present.

Laser – heat (laser coagulation) is used to burn off hemorrhoidal tissue. This is the easiest and least painful way of medically dealing with internal hemorrhoids. However, there is controversy about its use, with some researchers believing that more study to improve effectiveness of the technique is needed before it is routinely recommended.

Hemorrhoidectomy – This surgical removal of hemorrhoidal tissue is occasionally used in severe cases. Although the surgery is considered "completely effective" in 95% of cases, additional surgery is needed should the hemorrhoids recur.

Optional Nutritional Approaches

If there is rectal itching and burning, it will also be necessary to rule out the following:

- Parasites (see Chapter 4), especially pinworms
- Candida (see Chapter 4)

DIET

Follow the Digestive Care Diet in the appendix of this book. Make sure there are plenty of green leafy vegetables in the diet. Black strap molasses is also highly recommended. Juicing of fresh vegetables, especially green ones (see recipes in the appendix), can be helpful in maintaining digestive health.

SUPPLEMENTS

**A 30-day herbal detox (see appendix) biannually to support the liver and colon is suggested to prevent recurrence of hemorrhoids.

*** A good specific liver cleanse (see appendix), done at least once or twice a year, can help keep hemorrhoids from reoccurring.

- Take EFAs (essential fatty acids) to lubricate the digestive tract. A combination of fish and flax (Omega-3) with borage oil (Omega-6) is good to reduce inflammation in the gastrointestinal tract. Absorption of the oils may be enhanced with the addition of lipase (a fat-digesting enzyme). Take three 1000 mg. capsules twice daily with food.
- Take a fiber supplement that provides a balance of both soluble and insoluble fibers. A flax/borage seed combination is a good choice, particularly one that contains other beneficial ingredients such as a probiotic blend with fructooligosaccharides (FOS) and herbs like slippery elm bark, marshmallow and fennel seed. Another key ingredient would be L-glutamine, which the intestine uses as fuel to regenerate. This fiber supplement may be added to juices and taken any time of day. When beginning to add dietary fiber to the diet, remember to go slowly, as this can cause some gas if added too quickly.

- Take antioxidant supplements (vitamin C with bioflavonoids - 500 mg. to 3000 mg., vitamin A - 10,000 I.U. daily, vitamin E – 400 I.U. to 800 I.U. and zinc – 30 mg. to 60 mg. daily) after meals. Other antioxidants may also be taken with these. (See appendix for specification on antioxidants.)
- Take a B complex vitamin, including B6.
- Take a calcium/magnesium supplement. Try a liquid (see appendix and Resource Directory).

*** Please note: It is very important not to become constipated. Keep a colon cleanse formula on hand to use as needed. Try one containing herbs like cape aloe and rhubarb (that will gently stimulate peristalsis), as well as magnesium oxide to bring water to the bowel. Start with one capsule before bed, and increase by one capsule each night until bowel elimination occurs. Drink plenty of water during the day.

The following topical applications can be helpful for inflamed hemorrhoids:

- Vitamin E suppositories (see Resource Directory)
- Aloe vera/Neem gel can be applied directly to hemorrhoids.
- Witch hazel can be applied directly. It will help shrink hemorrhoids due to its astringent nature.
- Make a poultice of L-glutamine powder, gamma oryzanol, N-acetyl-glucosamine and water (see appendix). Apply directly to hemorrhoids.

Folk remedies include:

- Core out the center of an Idaho potato, and put in rectum before bed. Take out in the morning.
- Use a peeled garlic clove as a suppository.

Take the following orally:

- An effective herbal formula known as Pilex has its origin in ancient Hindu medicine. It is a patented blend of three herbs from India

Chapter 4

(neem, nagkesar and barberry). It can be taken to stop itching, burning and bleeding of hemorrhoids (see Resource Directory).

Warm sitz baths can be beneficial. Take one daily. Find a good mineral bath in your health food store.

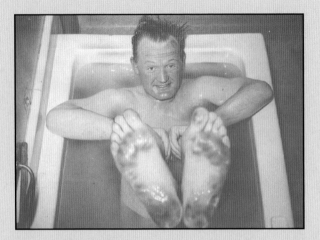

LIFESTYLE
- Chew foods to mush.
- Eat slowly.
- Drink plenty of water daily.
- Avoid wearing tight-fitting clothes that constrict the abdomen.
- Assume a squatting posture to ensure good bowel elimination. This will help prevent hemorrhoids or keep them from reoccurring. Pressure in the lower bowel area is a contributing factor to hemorrhoid formation. Use the LifeStep™ (see Resource Directory).
- Use a slant board to position the legs and pelvis higher than the heart (see Resource Directory).
- After hemorrhoids have healed, start an exercise program.

COMPLEMENTARY MIND/BODY THERAPIES
- Colon hydrotherapy is indicated for hemorrhoids because it decreases abdominal pressure and cleans out the colon in cases of constipation. It would also be good to do colon hydrotherapy during your biannual 30-day herbal detox program or your liver detox program. Colon hydrotherapy should not be used when hemorrhoids are bleeding.
- Massage
- Yoga
- Acupuncture
- Chiropractic
- Meditation/Prayer
- Music therapy
- Biofeedback

See appendix for information on the above therapies.

Dr. Smith's Comments
I would have to say that most patients whom I have treated for hemorrhoids are women who have had children and patients with a history of constipation, with a low-fiber diet and inadequate water intake. Stress is another important factor. I have seen healthy young college students present with acute prolapsed or thrombosed (clotted) hemorrhoids, and anal fissures (crack in the anal lining, due to tight anal sphincters very similar to a chapped lip), especially near the time of their final exams. Often, people who are chronically anxious with tight jaw muscles and teeth grinding will also have tight anal sphincters, which impede venous drainage and result in hemorrhoids. These can at times be treated with gentle self-anal dilation with aloe gel, and muscle relaxants and anti-anxiety medications. With time, lifestyle changes and patience, many of these people can avoid surgery.

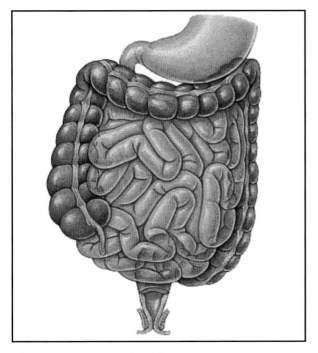

This is a photo of the small and large intestines.

INFLAMMATORY BOWEL DISEASE

What is it?

Inflammatory bowel disease (IBD) is the overall name given to those diseases that cause inflammation in the gastrointestinal tract, especially in the large and small intestines. These diseases are classified as either ulcerative colitis or Crohn's disease, terms which may encompass or may be used interchangeably for such labels as enteritis, ileitis, proctitis and colitis. Ulcerative colitis and Crohn's disease are potentially serious inflammatory bowel diseases. They are treated separately in the pages that follow. Although they share many symptoms, there are significant differences in the two diseases, as chart 1 indicates.

IBD can cause malnutrition for many reasons:[1]

- Inadequate food intake due to loss of appetite or to the symptoms of the disease process
- Malabsorption – (lack of absorption of food and nutrients) with small intestine involvement or surgical resection of the small bowel
- Failure to use nutritional supplements when on restricted diets
- Reduced absorptive surface resulting from previous surgical resections of the small bowel
- Bile deficiency resulting from previous resections of the small bowel
- Bacterial overgrowth of the small intestine
- Drug-induced nutritional deficiency
- Protein loss due to shedding of intestinal cells
- Mineral loss/electrolyte imbalance from diarrhea
- Inflammation, fever, infection
- Increased turnover of intestinal cells
- Increased utilization of nutrients, along with increased requirements for them
- Increased secretions and nutrient loss (especially blood proteins)

The nutritional deficiencies caused by IBD lead in turn to altered functioning of gastrointestinal tract, resulting in further increases in malabsorption, so that the patient is caught in a vicious cycle. See more detail about the cause, effect and treatment of Crohn's disease and ulcerative colitis in the next two sections.

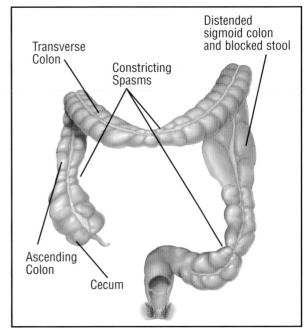

Transverse Colon

Constricting Spasms

Distended sigmoid colon and blocked stool

Ascending Colon

Cecum

Chapter 4

The Differences Between Ulcerative Colitis and Crohn's Disease

General	Ulcerative colitis	Crohn's disease
Age at onset	any, usually 15 to 30	any, usually 15-30
Organs involved	rectum, sigmoid colon	entire GI tract (usually ileum and/or colon)
Tissue layers involved	surface membrane	all layers of bowel wall
Distribution of disease	continuous	in segments
More common in	non-smokers	smokers
Symptoms/complications		
Fistulas (ulcer tunnels)	no	yes
Dehydration risk	yes	yes
Abdominal cramps	yes	yes
Steatorrhea (fat malasbsorption)	no	often
Weight loss	yes	yes
Diarrhea	yes, frequent	yes, frequent
Inflammation outside GI tract	yes	yes
Vomiting	yes	yes
Fever	not usually (only with toxic megacolon)	yes
Short bowel syndrome	no	yes
Nutritional Problems		
Protein	lost due to diarrhea or inflammation	lost due to diarrhea or inflammation
	Inadequate intake	Inadequate intake
Fat	no	malabsorption
Vitamin B12	No	yes, if terminal ileum is involved
Vitamins A, D, E, K	Yes, medications interfere	Yes, medications interfere
Copper, zinc, selenium	yes, losses from diarrhea	yes, losses from diarrhea and malabsorption
Iron	yes, due to bleeding	yes, if duodenum is affected, bleeding

Chart 1

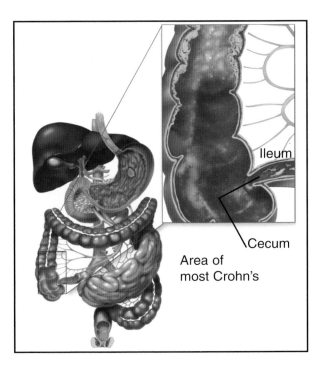

Ileum

Cecum

Area of
most Crohn's

CROHN'S DISEASE
What is it?

Crohn's disease is an inflammatory bowel disease (IBD) that can affect tissue anywhere along the gastrointestinal tract from mouth to rectum, but it most commonly involves the intestines, particularly the last section of the small intestine, the ileum. Crohn's disease causes the bowel wall to thicken and may cause a narrowing of the bowel channel. Unlike ulcerative colitis and some other intestinal conditions, all layers of the bowel wall are affected, not just the inner lining. Adjacent organs can be affected as well, since ulcerated lesions may spread into them forming unnatural tunnels called fistulas. The inflammation characteristic of Crohn's tends to develop in a skip pattern (i.e., it is not continuous, but may skip areas of tissue).

Dr. Burrill Crohn, for whom the disease is named, is generally credited with first describing Crohn's disease in 1932. He called it regional ileitis because, at that time, it was considered to be a localized disease. When it was later discovered that any portion of the GI tract could be affected by Crohn's disease, new names for it cropped up; these names often described the disease by location: enteritis (indicating intestinal involvement), ileitis (ileum involvement), proctitis (rectum involvement), colitis (colon involvement), ileocolitis (involvement of both the ileum and the colon) and granulomatous ileitis or granulomatous colitis. Granulomas are inflammatory lesions made up of masses of capillaries and collagen. They appear as small nodules in the intestinal wall, giving it a cobblestone appearance. They form as the affected tissues go through cycles of inflammation, damage and healing. These cycles are common, as the disease is characterized by periods of remission and flare-ups. Of those who suffer from Crohn's disease, 35% have only the ileum affected; 20% have only the colon affected; 45% have both ileum and colon affected,[1] making it primarily a "right-sided" disease.

What Causes it?

The cause of Crohn's disease, like so many gastrointestinal disorders, is officially unknown. However, there are many clues and theories. Perhaps our biggest clue is the fact that the disease is virtually non-existent in cultures where people consume their native diet in a natural, unprocessed form, but it is increasing rapidly in Western countries where processed foods are the norm.[2] With regard to diet and lifestyle factors, the following have been found to contribute to Crohn's disease:

• Low fiber diets[3]
• Fast foods[4]
• Cigarette smoking[5]
• Birth control pills[6]
• High consumption of refined carbohydrates and sugar[7]
• High intake of animal protein[8]
• Low intake of Omega-3 fatty acids (found in flaxseed oil and fish)[9]
• Antibiotic use (The annual increase in prescriptions for antibiotics parallels the annual increase in the incidence of Crohn's disease.)[10]

Chapter 4

- Food allergies and sensitivities (especially to wheat and dairy)[11]
- Low vitamin D levels (inadequate sun exposure)

Many of the practices listed above contribute to leaky gut syndrome, which is prevalent in IBD sufferers.[12] With leaky gut syndrome, the bowel wall becomes hyper-porous, allowing undigested food particles and microorganisms to pass into the bloodstream. Food allergies can develop when the body launches an immune reaction in response to the presence of undigested food particles in the blood because these particles are seen as foreign bodies. As such, food allergy, highly implicated in Crohn's disease, is considered to be an autoimmune disease. So is Crohn's disease itself. Not surprisingly, friendly flora (good bacteria) are found to be significantly out of balance in IBD patients.[13] This imbalance can be caused by antibiotic use, a diet high in refined sugar and/or an infectious agent.

It is known that infections commonly cause flare-ups of Crohn's disease. Many believe that an infectious agent may be involved in the development of the disease, that the inflammation of Crohn's disease is the body's reaction to the presence of a foreign agent, a virus, bacteria or fungus. That inflammation is then accelerated when the immune system attacks its own tissues where the microorganism resides.[14]

There is thought to be a genetic component to Crohn's disease, though no genetic markers have been identified. It is possible that this genetic predisposition is one that may lay dormant until activated by the presence of a pathogen.[15] Whether onset of Crohn's disease is the result of an overactive immune system response to bacteria and other microbes that are normally present in the intestine or to a microbial infection is a matter of speculation. It is known that bacteria can stimulate the production of proteins called cytokines that cause inflammation.[16] And there is some compelling evidence that a particular bacterium, mycobacterium paratuberculosis, may be the culprit.

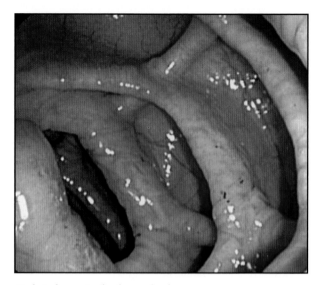

Crohn's disease in the ileocecal valve

Mycobacterium paratuberculosis, also known as Mycobacterium avium subspecies paratuberculosis (MAP), affects cattle, giving them Johne's disease, which produces symptoms that are virtually identical to Crohn's disease in humans. Interestingly, MAP triggers a massive immune reaction against the body's affected tissue (the gut), but cannot be detected using standard testing procedures. It is the only one of all the pathogens once believed to be associated with Crohn's disease that, when directly cultured from cattle, is capable of causing pathologically indistinguishable diseases in other animals. This information would raise the possibility that humans may become infected with MAP by drinking cow's milk or eating beef. This suspicion seems to be confirmed by the fact that Crohn's disease is only seen in milk-drinking areas of the world. Since the bacterium is extremely heat-resistant, it is not destroyed by pasteurization. It seems to be no coincidence that the U.S. has the worst MAP problem in the world and also has the highest incidence of Crohn's disease. Unfortunately, since MAP is not considered a human pathogen, there are no efforts to keep dairy products from infected cattle out of the food supply. (For more information on the link between MAP and Crohn's disease and full documentation of the data presented in this paragraph, visit the web site from which it comes, www.veganoutreach.org/health/gotmilk-intro.html, and see the article "Paratuberculosis and Crohn's Disease: Got Milk?")

Carrageenan is a compound extracted from red seaweeds, and it is often used to induce ulcerative colitis (another form of IBD) in experimental animals.[17] This compound is also used widely in the food industry as a stabilizing and suspending agent, most particularly in dairy products to stabilize the protein in milk. The interesting thing is that when healthy people and germ-free animals are fed large amounts of carrageenan, they do not develop IBD. It is thought that the presence of a particular bacterium is needed in order for carrageenan to cause the inflammatory lesions typical of ulcerative colitis.[18] The bacterium that has been linked to facilitating the carrageenan-induced damage in animals is a strain of Bacteroides vulgatus,[19] an organism that is six times more prevalent in people with ulcerative colitis than in healthy people. Could it be that a different bacterium, MAP, causes another form of IBD (Crohn's disease) in the presence of carrageenan found in dairy products? Although evidence from animal models has demonstrated that degraded carrageenan causes ulcerations and malignancies in the gastrointestinal tract, there is no Food and Drug Administration restriction on the use of the substance in the food supply in the U.S.[20]

People with both forms of inflammatory bowel disease, Crohn's disease and ulcerative colitis, show an increase in the synthesis of inflammatory compounds called leukotrienes. Like histamines, leukotrienes respond to allergens in the body. Therefore, they can be reduced by eliminating or reducing consumption of foods to which the body is sensitive, such as meat and dairy products. Increasing consumption of Omega-3 fatty acids (found in ocean fish and flaxseed oil) is also effective in managing leukotrienes.[21] This fact, coupled with knowledge of the high allergic potential of dairy products and the possible presence of pathogens in them that could trigger inflammatory reactions in the gut, would seem to give the IBD sufferer ample reason to eliminate dairy products and reduce or eliminate red meat consumption.

IBD is not just about what is put in the body, but also what is taken out of it. Several studies have shown reduced antioxidant concentrations (vitamins A, C and E and the minerals selenium and zinc) in patient groups with both active and inactive Crohn's disease compared to control groups.[22] This may be both a result of, as well as a contributing factor in the disease, however, as inflammation increases the production of free radicals, which will consume the antioxidants. Lower tissue antioxidant levels negatively affect cell functions and hasten tissue damage if inflammation continues unabated.

Who Gets it?

Crohn's disease is considered a "disease of affluence" in that it is concentrated in developed countries, particularly in urban rather than rural areas.[23] Although it affects all age groups, onset of the disease generally occurs between the ages 15 and 30 or, less often, after age 50.[24]

Crohn's disease is thought to affect somewhere between 400,000 and 1,000,000 Americans,[25] and it has spread like an epidemic since 1950.[26] Males and females are equally affected.[27] Crohn's is four times more common in Caucasians and Jewish people than in people of other ethnic backgrounds.[28]

This disease appears to run in families. Of all people with Crohn's, 20% have a close blood relative with the disease.[29] It is unknown whether the connection is environmental or genetic. People who have a relative with Crohn's have at least ten times the risk of developing it compared with the general population.[30] Interestingly, people who have a family member who has either Crohn's disease or ulcerative colitis are at higher risk for developing Crohn's disease than those who do not.[31]

People who smoke cigarettes, have other autoimmune diseases, eat processed foods and/or have a high intake of animal proteins and sugar-containing products are also at increased risk for developing Crohn's disease.

What Are the Signs and Symptoms?

The symptoms of Crohn's disease are similar to those of other intestinal disorders, especially ulcerative colitis. They generally occur intermittently – every few months to every few years in some people; however, in rare case, symptoms may appear once or twice and never return.[32] They can range from mild to severe. While Crohn's disease is generally characterized by inflammatory lesions (granulomas) throughout the entire thickness of the bowel wall, in 40% of cases, these lesions are either poorly developed or totally absent.[34]

Gastrointestinal signs and symptoms of Crohn's disease may include:

• Abdominal pain (usually right-sided)
• Diarrhea (may alternate with constipation)
• Loss of appetite
• Weight loss
• Nausea/vomiting
• Blood in stool
• Mucus in stool
• Fever
• Flatulence
• Malaise
• Bouts of severe fatigue
• Delayed development/stunted growth in children
• Steatorrhea (excess fat in feces) from fat malabsorption

Fat malabsorption occurs because the last section of the small intestine, the ileum, is where reabsorption of bile salts occurs. Since the ileum is the intestinal site most often affected by Crohn's disease, the condition has a negative impact on the organ's function. With an ileum that is functioning normally, bile is absorbed and recycled so that it can emulsify fats for digestion. If the level of bile salts is low, fat cannot be digested and is instead excreted in the stools. Along with the fat, go the fat-soluble nutrients.[35]

Some of the more severe symptoms listed above are a result of gastrointestinal complications such as development of:

• Fistulas (ulcer tunnels) connecting loops of the intestine or bridging the intestine and an adjacent organ (often the urinary bladder or vagina) or the skin
• Abscesses (pus-filled pockets of infection)
• Anal fissures (cracks in the tissue)
• Intestinal obstruction (develops slowly after many years of diarrhea; results from narrowing and scarring of the intestine, which occurs during healing)
• Strictures (narrowing of the lumen – opening of the intestinal passageway – due to inflammation and scar tissue)
• Rupture (can lead to a fatal infection called peritonitis)
• Nutritional deficiencies (as a result of malabsorption when there is small intestine involvement)
• Colon cancer (increased risk, except where rectum and distal end of the colon are the only affected areas[35])

Abscesses develop in 20% of those with Crohn's disease, while about 30% develop a fistula.[36]

Systemic complications often occur as a result of Crohn's disease. In fact, there are over 100 systemic disorders that may result from inflammatory bowel disease.[37] The most common of these is arthritis, occurring in 25% of Crohn's disease patients, usually those with colon involvement.[38] Fifteen percent will develop skin lesions, while 3-7% will have serious liver disease.[39]

Other systemic complications may include:

• Inflammation of blood vessels
• Impaired blood flow to fingers and toes

- Kidney stones
- Gallstones
- Inflammation of eyes or mouth
- Inflammation of spine
- Inflammation elsewhere in the body

The nutritional deficiencies caused by Crohn's may also result in such problems as osteoporosis, neurological dysfunction and Alzheimer's disease.[40]

Side Effects of Corticosteroids

- Depression of protein synthesis
- Inhibition of calcium absorption (by increasing excretion of vitamin C in the urine)
- Bone thinning
- Skin problems
- Muscle deterioration
- Infections
- Pancreatic damage
- Neurological problems
- Stimulation of protein breakdown
- Decreased absorption of phosphorus
- Urinary excretion of vitamin C, vitamin K, calcium and zinc
- Increased levels of blood glucose, serum triglycerides and serum cholesterol
- Increased requirements for vitamin B6, vitamin C, folate and vitamin D
- Impairment of wound healing
- Electrolyte imbalances
- Cataracts
- Weight gain
- Bone mineral depletion
- Ulcers
- Congestive heart failure
- Diabetes
- Hypertension
- Facial hair growth
- Obesity of the upper torso

Chart 1

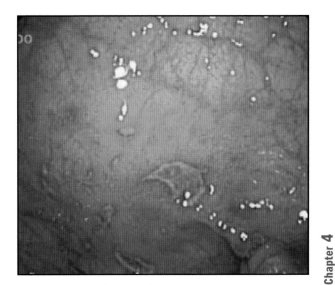

Crohn's disease in the sigmoid colon

Chapter 4

How is it Diagnosed?

As stated, symptoms of Crohn's disease are similar to those of other gastrointestinal disorders, especially ulcerative colitis. When inflammation is present elsewhere in the body – often in the joints, skin or eyes – the doctor will most likely suspect Crohn's disease. Accurate diagnosis may be difficult, especially early in the disease process. It may be necessary to watch and wait – until the course of the disease makes it possible to differentiate between Crohn's disease and ulcerative colitis. Endoscopic evaluation of the colon with tissue biopsy may be necessary (see "sigmoidoscopy" and "colonoscopy" in the appendix). A telltale sign of Crohn's disease is the presence of patches of inflamed tissue with a cobblestone appearance. The endoscope is equipped to take a tissue specimen that will later be examined microscopically.

A lower GI series (barium enema) of x-rays (described in the appendix) may be ordered to help distinguish between ulcerative colitis and Crohn's disease. An upper GI series of x-rays (see appendix) with small bowel study may be ordered to see if the ileum is involved.

These tests will, of course, be preceded by a

thorough physical examination (including rectal exam to rule out cancer of the rectum) and health history. Proctoscopy, an in-office procedure, may also be performed, allowing the doctor to examine the mucosal lining of the rectum, if necessary.

Blood tests are typically done to find clues in the body's chemistry. These tests allow physicians to detect anemia based on iron levels, to assess protein status and to spot inflammation based on an elevated erythrocyte sedimentation rate and white blood cell count. Stool analysis can be useful to detect the presence of hidden (occult) blood, as well as bacteria and parasites. To detect parasites with any degree of accuracy, specialized tests (see appendix) are needed. Many holistic physicians will use the Complete Digestive Stool Analysis with parasitology, which will also give helpful information on the patient's digestive and absorptive capabilities, as well as intestinal flora (bacteria) balance (or imbalance).

Further tests that may be ordered (typically by nutritionally-oriented doctors) are:

- ELISA food and environmental sensitivity test (see appendix)
- Lactose breath test (see appendix)
- Intestinal permeability screening (see appendix)
- Nutritional analysis (of blood and/or hair)
- Antioxidant analysis

What is the Standard Medical Treatment?

Exact treatment protocol would depend upon the severity of the Crohn's disease, the phase of the disease and its location in the body. Medical treatment goals ideally would be to:

- Control inflammation
- Relieve symptoms
- Control infection, if present
- Prevent stimulation/irritation of the GI tract
- Correct nutritional deficiencies

The first three of these goals would generally be

addressed through drug therapy, which may include use of:

- Mild anti-inflammatory drugs (often salicylates like sulfasalazine) to prevent flare-ups
- Corticosteroids (like prednisone or hydrocortisone) to treat flare-ups
- Antibiotics (Flagyl and Cipro are often used in serious cases, especially if abscess or fistula is present.)
- Immunosuppressive drugs – (like methotrexate, cyclosporine and Remicade, which is genetically-engineered from human and mouse cells[41]) used on the theory that IBD is an autoimmune disease
- Anti-spasmodic drugs (opium derivatives to slow down diarrhea)
- Pain killers

The most commonly used drugs, sulfasalazine and corticosteroids, have a host of side effects: The former inhibits the transport of folic acid (a B vitamin) and iron, causing anemia;[42] increases urinary excretion of vitamin C; and may cause nausea, vomiting, weight loss, heartburn and/or diarrhea, among other side effects.[43] See chart 1 for a partial list of side effects from corticosteroids. Crohn's disease patients typically take a lot of prescription drugs. It's not unusual for them to take ten or more daily.[44]

All drugs cause some degree of nutritional deficiency or imbalance. For the Crohn's disease patient, who may already be suffering from malnutrition as a consequence of the disease process itself, the added nutritional depletion of constant drug therapy can create serious nutritional deficiencies. For these reasons, nutritional supplementation, along with a balanced and appropriate diet, is absolutely vital.

Unfortunately, the nutritional awareness and knowledge of the traditional medical doctor may be limited. His dietary counseling is likely to be limited to advising the patient to eat whatever can be tolerated. He will be aware of the most important aspect of nutritional therapy, which is to provide adequate caloric intake, and he will probably be aware of the need to increase protein intake (because of blood loss and damaged intestinal mucosal tissue). He may even be aware of the probability of secondary lactose intolerance with Crohn's disease. Unfortunately, his awareness of nutritional matters may not extend any further, though he will likely counsel his patient to avoid alcohol, tobacco and caffeine or to use them moderately. Some doctors may recommend an increase in dietary fiber and a fiber supplement to control diarrhea; most will rely on anti-diarrhea medications.

In severe cases, patients may require surgery (a bowel resection) where inflamed segments of the intestine are removed and the remaining ones connected. Surgery, like drug therapy, cannot cure Crohn's disease. It is typically done when blockages, perforation, abdominal abscesses or fistulas are present. Once a resection is done, the possibility of an adjacent area of the intestine being affected by the disease, requiring another resection, exists. When repeated resections are done on the small intestine, "short bowel syndrome," a condition in which absorption of nutrients declines even further, develops. This is a critical situation; in fact, it is unlikely that the patient will survive when as much as 75% of the small intestine is removed.[45]

As regards the goal of preventing stimulation and irritation of the GI tract, this is generally done through total bowel rest at the onset of a flare-up. If it is severe, and the patient is hospitalized, all food and beverages will be withheld for a short time, with fluids, electrolytes and glucose being administered intravenously to prevent dehydration. At the appropriate time, food will be either introduced orally, through a tube (enteral nutrition) or intravenously (parenteral nutrition), depending upon the condition of the patient. Parenteral or IV feedings deliver nutrients directly into the bloodstream. They are generally used when a fistula or obstruction is present, and the

patient is malnourished. Enteral feedings are used if the patient is not well enough to drink. They provide nutrients in a predigested (elemental) or partially hydrolyzed form. As healing progresses, the patient will move to a liquid diet, then to a soft diet and then on to regular eating.

Those patients experiencing mild flare-ups who do not require hospitalization will still need to rest the bowel initially, then ease into regular eating as described above. Some have obtained benefit from drinking enteral formulas. The use of elemental diets has been found to be effective in delaying the time between onset of Crohn's disease and the first bowel resection. In addition, such a diet reduced the need for a second resection.[46] The benefits seen from such a diet may be attributable to the fact that it has a very low allergenic potential. Still, this approach isn't perfect. While enteral formulas provide readily utilized nutrients, they are costly and unpalatable.

Patients with steatorrhea (fat loss in stools) may benefit from a decreased intake of dietary fat, as well as supplementation with medium-chain triglycerides, a form of fat that does not require emulsification and requires minimal digestion to be absorbed.[47]

As Crohn's disease patients recover from flare-ups, they will need to adhere to a low-fiber diet for a time to reduce gastrointestinal stimulation. Once able to return to normal eating, however, a high intake of dietary fiber is recommended to optimize bowel function.

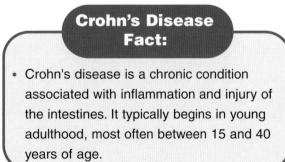

Crohn's Disease Fact:

- Crohn's disease is a chronic condition associated with inflammation and injury of the intestines. It typically begins in young adulthood, most often between 15 and 40 years of age.

Chapter 4

Optional Nutritional Approaches

The treatment of Crohn's depends on the phase of the disease and where you are in that process. If you are experiencing a flare-up (or active Crohn's), treatment usually focuses on anti-inflammatory medication and handling symptoms of pain, diarrhea and GI tract irritation. In addition, if infection is present, antibiotics will be of extreme importance. Prescription drugs are standard treatment for this disease due to their fast-acting nature. The problem is that the many side effects can be severe. Nutritional therapies have been shown to be effective without the side effects. The suggestions below are not to be implemented without the consent of your medical doctor.

The following tests (ordered by a health care practitioner) could be helpful in identifying underlying conditions:

- CDSA (Complete Digestive Stool Analysis) - for Candida (see appendix)
- Parasite test (see Chapter 4 on parasites) - See appendix for test
- Gut permeability test (see appendix)
- Heidelberg test for low or excess stomach acid (see appendix)
- Food sensitivity test - ELISA (see appendix)

DIET

Most people do well on a yeast-free diet (see Candida Section, Chapter 4), minus wheat and dairy, for a period of one month, after which time the Digestive Care Diet in the appendix of this book (minus wheat and dairy) may be followed. See wheat and dairy substitutes in the diet.

Should surgery prove necessary, after surgery, you may want to follow a liquid or soft food diet for awhile. Include broth, bouillon, herbal teas and green drinks. A good liquid meal replacement would be Living Fuel (see Resource Directory). Sports drinks can help with electrolyte replacement. Include such soft foods as bananas, rice, potatoes, soups, squashes and steamed vegetables, and be sure to drink plenty of water.

Persons with IBD will want to use caution with the following: raw vegetables, raw vegetable skins, raw fruit, seeds and nuts. These can be hard to digest. Wait until the digestive tract is healed to eat them. Steamed vegetables would be easier to digest.

Fat can be a powerful stimulant of the GI tract, and thus should be avoided in Crohn's patients. It is the "bad" fats, not the "good" ones (like essential fatty acids, as recommended) that are to be avoided. These bad fats would include fried foods, egg yolks, mayonnaise, margarine and dairy products.

Caffeine is stimulating to the digestive tract. Many people rely on a morning cup of coffee for bowel elimination. People with Crohn's will need to avoid such stimulation.

Alcohol is an irritant to the GI tract. Some people will be reactive to it, and others will experience no ill effect, depending on the amount ingested and whether or not it is taken with food.

Avoid carbonated drinks like soda and beer. Gas-producing foods like broccoli, beans, garlic, onions, leeks, cabbage, and cauliflower produce sulfur and can create gas, which can be painful. Drink herbal teas like chamomile, peppermint, ginger, fennel or slippery elm.

Red meat should be avoided, as it can be hard to digest and contains arachidonic acid (inflammation promoter) and elevates hydrogen sulfide levels, which negatively affects the digestive tract.

Avoid artificial sweeteners like sorbitol, sucralose and Nutrasweet because of possible sensitivity. Natural sweeteners such as lohan and stevia may be used. It is wise to avoid sugar in most gastrointestinal conditions.

SUPPLEMENTS

The following should be discussed with your doctor or holistic practitioner:

- A plant enzyme blend: This supplement should include protease (at least 20,000 H.U.T.), amylase and lipase, as well as papaya and bromelain. Other ingredients in this formula might include soothing herbs like marshmallow and slippery elm. Additionally, a good digestive enzyme formula would contain glutamine (an amino acid) and N-acetyl-glucosamine, which helps soothe an irritated mucosal lining.
- Take HCl/pepsin supplements before meals if stomach acid levels are low. Start with one capsule, and increase by one capsule daily with meals until symptoms are gone. (If you feel a burning sensation, back off to previous dose.) The supplement may contain other soothing ingredients like quercitin, bromelain, gamma oryzanol, L-glutamine and N-acetyl-glucosamine.

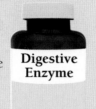

Choose one or the other of the above to take with meals.

- Take essential fatty acids (EFA's) to lubricate the digestive tract. A combination of fish and flax (Omega-3) oils with borage oil (Omega-6) is good to reduce inflammation in the gastrointestinal tract. Absorption of the oils may be enhanced with the addition of lipase (a fat-digesting enzyme). Take three to six 1000 mg. capsules twice daily with food. Daily doses of 3,000 mg. of EPA and 2,000 mg. of DHA (from fish oil) have been shown to be helpful in reducing inflammation.

- Take a probiotic (good bacteria) supplement with multiple strains as a daily supplement. It should contain a minimum of two to six billion cultures. A prebiotic could be helpful (see appendix).
- Take a fiber supplement that provides a balance of both soluble and insoluble fibers. A flax/borage seed combination is a good choice, particularly one that contains other beneficial ingredients such as a probiotic blend with fructooligosaccharides (FOS) and herbs like slippery elm bark, marshmallow and fennel seed. Another key ingredient would be L-glutamine, which the intestine uses as fuel to regenerate. This fiber supplement may be added to juices and taken any time of day. When beginning to add dietary fiber to the diet, remember to go slowly, as this can cause some gas if added too quickly. Insoluble rice fiber for adding bulk to stool may be helpful (see appendix).

- Take 5,000 mg. to 20,000 mg. of L-glutamine powder with N-acetyl-glucosamine (NAG) and gamma oryzanol once to twice daily on an empty stomach (see appendix).
- Multivitamin/mineral supplement (see appendix). Please note: a liquid supplement from your health food store could be extremely beneficial. It should contain vitamin E - 800 I.U., folic acid – 1 mg. to 10 mg., zinc 30 mg. to 60 mg.
- B complex vitamin daily, plus B12 injection or sublingual tablet
- A liquid calcium/magnesium supplement (see appendix)
- A liquid iron supplement (Floradix – see appendix) - Take only if iron levels are low.
- Antioxidant supplement: Take vitamin C at 500 mg. doses 2 to 4 times daily (if stools gets loose, back off and go slower) and vitamin A (from beta-carotene) - 5,000 mg. to 25,000 mg. per day.

Start your supplementation program slowly. After your body has healed, stay on a maintenance

Chapter 4

program of the following:

- Digestive enzymes
- Essential fatty acids
- Probiotics
- Fiber
- Multivitamin/mineral
- Antioxidants.

In cases of inflammation, enemas could be helpful. Fill an enema bag with the following:

- 2 to 3 capsules of acidophilus and bifidus bacteria
- 1/4 cup of warm olive oil
- The contents of 2 vitamin E capsules
- 1/2 tsp. L-glutamine powder (empty capsules, using the oral supplement recommended in the appendix) – See appendix (glutamine powder).
- 10 drops of any of the following: marshmallow root, echinacea, geranium, goldenseal, comfrey or slippery elm (in liquid tinctures at the health food store)

Fill a small enema bulb with this mixture (or empty a Fleet enema syringe, and fill it with the mixture); put small amount in the rectum, and hold as long as possible. REMEMBER: if you put too much fluid in at one time, you will not be able to hold it as long.

LIFESTYLE

- Stress is a major component of this disease, so it is of the utmost importance to find ways to reduce it. It may be advisable to start journaling as a way to determine if certain situations trigger stress. Check also into some type of counseling with a professional therapist or with a spiritual advisor.
- It is also important when away from home to know the locations of all bathrooms wherever you are going. When on the road, the best places to stop (not to eat but to use the restroom) are fast food establishments.
- During social events like going to a theatre, always sit near the aisle so you can get out

quickly.
- When dining out, try to call ahead, find out the choices available on the menu, and let the cook know of your diet restriction. If this is not possible, choice an entrée that is steamed, baked or broiled rather than fried. Avoid sauces, as there can be hidden ingredients in them that could trigger symptoms.
- Exercise is very important. The following could be very beneficial in helping restore your health: walking, low impact aerobics or weight training.

COMPLEMENTARY MIND/BODY THERAPIES

- Yoga could be beneficial for Crohn's, both for exercise and stress reduction.
- Massage therapy can help with relaxing the body and mind, as this is needed, especially during times of flare-ups.
- Acupuncture would be good with people with Crohn's, as it targets the energy meridians (channels) associated with the digestive system, and it is also a stress reducer.
- Colon hydrotherapy is not suggested in Crohns disease. If Crohn's is in remission, please consult your holistic doctor before proceeding with this therapy.
- Meditation/Prayer
- Biofeedback
- Chiropractic
- Music therapy

See appendix for above therapies.

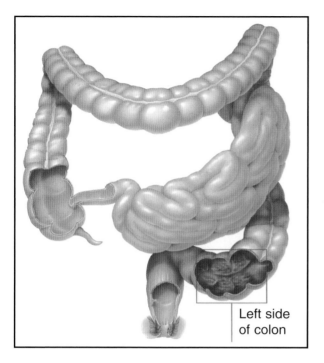

Left side
of colon

ULCERATIVE COLITIS

What is it?

Ulcerative colitis is an inflammatory bowel disease (IBD) that generally affects the rectum (proctitis) and the lower left portion of the colon, the sigmoid area, though it may spread throughout the entire colon (pancolitis). With this chronic condition, there are ulcers, along with inflammation. Also, there is usually blood in the stool, as well as diarrhea and cramping. Unlike Crohn's disease, which involves the entire thickness of the bowel wall, the inflammation of ulcerative colitis is generally confined to the first layer of the colon lining, the mucosal membrane. It spreads in a continuous fashion rather than in patches like Crohn's disease. Ulcerative colitis does not involve the small intestine – except in those few cases when it backs up into the ileum (lower portion of the small bowel).[1]

What Causes it?

While the cause of ulcerative colitis is unknown, many theories have been put forth, and a number of contributing factors have been identified.

Among the proposed contributing factors are poor eating habits, stress, food allergies and infectious agents.[2] Involvement of microbes like bacteria, although not proven, is often associated with the use of antibiotics, which alter the normal bacterial balance in the intestines and permit microorganisms that are normally held in check to proliferate.[3]

A dominant theory as to cause of ulcerative colitis is an over-reaction of the immune system to the presence of microbes, toxins or other stress factors (like irritating or allergenic foods). What is unknown, however, is whether the immune system disturbances found in the disease are the cause or the result of ulcerative colitis.[4] For a more in-depth discussion of possible microbial involvement in IBD, see the section on Crohn's disease.

Who Gets it?

Like Crohn's disease, ulcerative colitis symptoms generally first appear between ages 15 and 30, with a second peak between ages 50 and 70.[5] Also like Crohn's, there is a higher incidence – 4 to 5 times higher – of the disease among people of Jewish ancestry than among other people.[6] Other similarities to Crohn's are the facts that ulcerative colitis affects men and women equally, and the disease appears to run in families, though no genetic markers have been identified.

Most studies show that ulcerative colitis is more common than Crohn's disease.[7] In the United States, 5 to 7 Americans out of 100,000 develop ulcerative colitis.[8]

What are the Signs and Symptoms?

The symptoms of ulcerative colitis often resemble those of Crohn's disease or irritable bowel syndrome. Microscopically however, the superficial inflammation of ulcerative colitis gives a different appearance than the deep lesions of Crohn's disease. Still, ulcerative colitis, like Crohn's disease, usually lasts a lifetime, but may go into remission for long periods of time. Those with ulcerative colitis may experience any of the following symptoms:

Chapter 4

- Diarrhea, which is often bloody (and may lead to iron-deficiency anemia)
- Pain in the low abdomen (especially in the lower left quadrant)
- Weight loss
- Fever
- Fatigue
- Nausea

Because of rectal involvement, fissures, hemorrhoids and abscesses may develop. With ulcerative colitis, however, fistulae (ulcer tunnels connecting organs or parts of an organ) generally do not form because the inflammation does not typically extend throughout the entire thickness of the bowel wall.[9]

Like Crohn's disease, the diarrhea of ulcerative colitis can lead to dehydration and electrolyte disturbances. Unlike Crohn's, the malnutrition that may result from ulcerative colitis is not directly due to malabsorption (because the small intestine is not generally involved) but rather due to loss of appetite and fear of eating stemming from the discomfort of the symptoms.[10]

Another similarity between ulcerative colitis and Crohn's disease is that both may produce systemic problems such as:

- Inflammation of the joints
- Inflammation of the eyes
- Inflammation of the spine
- Inflammation of the liver/gallbladder

These symptoms are usually mild and disappear when the colitis is treated.[11] Having ulcerative colitis also increases the risk of developing other serious conditions, such as osteoporosis and kidney stones.

A rare but serious complication of ulcerative colitis is toxic colitis, which can develop into a condition known as toxic megacolon. Toxic megacolon is a condition in which the entire colon is damaged and loses its ability to contract. In time,

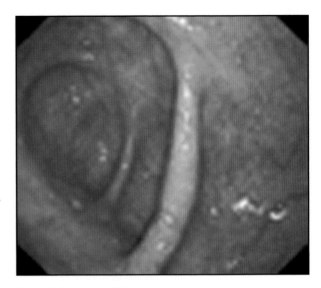

Scope of ulcerative colitis.

it will dilate, or expand, due to loss of muscle tone. Toxic megacolon can lead quickly to perforation, a life-threatening complication. Another possible complication of ulcerative colitis is the development of dysplasia, abnormal cell changes, which increases the risk of cancer.

How is it Diagnosed?

In addition to physical examination and thorough health history, a colonoscopy with biopsy (described in the appendix) can help doctors to diagnose ulcerative colitis and assess its severity. A sigmoidoscopy (see appendix) may alternatively be used if complaints are confined to the rectal area. These types of endoscopic exams allow the doctor to take a biopsy – tissue sample – that can later be microscopically evaluated for a definitive differential diagnosis. They also look for dysplasia.

A barium enema (lower GI series of x-rays) may also be used to reveal abnormalities in colonic tissue. See the appendix for a description of this test.

In addition to endoscopic evaluation – and possibly barium enema – blood tests are normally ordered for the purposes of detecting iron-deficiency anemia, signs of inflammation and protein status. Finally, a stool analysis can be helpful in detecting infection and/or parasites Specialized testing, involving more than one stool sample, is needed to accurately detect parasites (see appendix).

What is the Standard Medical Treatment?

Treatment depends upon the severity and extent of the ulcerative colitis. It would ideally be tailored to meet the individual needs of the patients.

Most doctors will recommend the avoidance of irritating substances, which may include highly seasoned foods, alcohol, caffeine and sugar. Interestingly, ciga-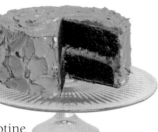rette smoking may not appear on the "to be avoided" list, for some studies have found (and some have not) that nicotine patches may help induce remission, or at least reduce symptoms, in approximately 40% of patients who used the patch for more than four weeks.[12]

The nutrition-oriented MD would most likely expand the list of offending foods to include those to which the patient is sensitive or allergic as established through ELISA blood testing (see appendix) or through a trial on an elimination diet. Even without testing, some doctors may advise the avoidance of milk and wheat, since these foods have the highest allergy potential.

Traditional dietary treatment of serious cases of IBD (both Crohn's disease and ulcerative colitis) often involves use of an elemental (predigested) diet or one that is administered intravenously. These approaches, as well as the exclusion diet (to treat allergies) have been quite successful in managing inflammatory bowel diseases. Medical management, however, relies very heavily on drug therapy to achieve this end, and these treatments can be extremely problematic.

The most widely used drugs in treatment of both Crohn's disease and ulcerative colitis are corticosteroids and sulfasalazine. The side effects of both of these medications are discussed in the section on Crohn's disease. Additionally, ulcerative colitis patients may be placed on medications to relax them, relieve their pain, suppress their immune systems (due to the suspected auto-immune nature of the disease) and to counter infection and diarrhea. All these drugs contribute to nutrient depletion, already an issue with IBD patients. Protein depletion is of particular concern due to tissue damage in the bowel, which is sometimes extensive. Ongoing diarrhea raises concerns about iron and trace mineral status. Those on sulfa drugs (like sulfasalazine and related 5-ASA agents) are depleting vitamin K as well. Supplementation with a good multiple vitamin/mineral is therefore needed, though this need may go unrecognized by some traditional physicians whose knowledge of nutrition is limited.

Mild cases of ulcerative colitis, such as proctitis (inflammation of the rectum), may be treated with a mesalamine (Rowasa) suppository at bedtime or enemas using the same medication if the inflammation extends beyond the rectum. Alternatively, steroid enemas may be used. However, here there is some danger of absorption of the medication into the body, with the accompanying side effects (see chart 1 in Crohn's disease section). The holistic physician would be more likely to prescribe a butyrate enema. Butyrate is a short-chain fatty acid, a product of bacterial fermentation of dietary fiber that serves as food for the cells of the colon, helping to heal the colitis. Omega-3 essential fatty acids, found in fish oil and flax, are also helpful in reducing inflammation.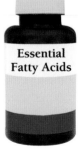

Essential Fatty Acids

More involved cases may be treated with oral administration of a 5-ASA drug (like sulfasalazine) or a steroid. At times, both are used concurrently.

Chapter 4

Immunosuppressive drugs may be added to the mix as the patient is being weaned off the steroids (a necessary process, as these drugs cannot be abruptly discontinued).

Hospitalization is required for those with severe cases of ulcerative colitis. Here nutrients, antibiotics and steroids are administered intravenously. If these treatments are not effective, then immunosuppressive drugs like cyclosporine may be added, first intravenously, then orally. In patients with severe colitis, anti-diarrheal drugs like Lomotil and Imodium AD and narcotics are generally avoided since they can precipitate the development of toxic megacolon.[13] To treat toxic megacolon, the bowel is compressed by inserting a tube through the nose into the stomach so that air and stomach contents may be aspirated on a continuous basis; a rectal tube may also be placed to decompress the colon.[14]

A low-fiber diet is necessary during the initial stages of recovery in the disease process, to be replaced with a higher-fiber diet later, if tolerated.

Treatment goals for the hospitalized patient are to:

• Correct malnutrition (often through administration of an elemental diet, which is pre-digested)
• Stop diarrhea
• Stop blood loss
• Stop loss of fluids and minerals

If these conservative measures fail, surgery may be recommended. Although the majority of patients with ulcerative colitis will never require surgical intervention, about 20 to 25% will eventually require removal of their colon due to one or more of the following:[15]

• Massive bleeding
• Chronic debilitating illness
• Perforation of the colon
• Cancer risk (which may be as much as 32 times normal, especially if the whole colon is involved and the disease has been long-standing. But if only the rectum and sigmoid

are involved, there's no elevated risk.)[16]
• Failure of drug treatment (as described above)
• Side effects of steroids (or other medications)

There are basically three surgical options for removal of the colon. The first (and most common) is the proctocolectomy with ileostomy. Here the entire colon and rectum are removed, and a small opening is made in the abdominal wall, through which the tip of the ileum is brought to the surface of the skin. A pouch is worn over the opening to collect waste. The patient will ultimately empty this pouch on his or her own.

A second surgical option is proctocolectomy with continent ileostomy. Here a pouch is surgically created out of the ileum inside the wall of the lower abdomen. The patient empties the pouch by inserting a tube through a small leak-proof opening in the side of his body.

The last option is an ileoanal anastomosis. Here the diseased portion of the colon is removed, but the outer muscles of the rectum are not. The surgeon attaches the ileum to the inside of the rectum, forming a "J-pouch" that holds the waste. With this procedure, which requires a temporary ileostomy, the patient is able to pass stool through the anus, though bowel movements are more frequent and watery than normal.

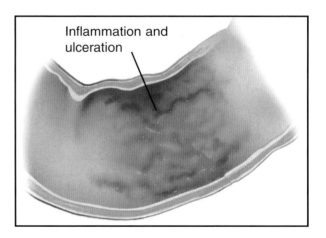

Inflammation and ulceration

Optional Nutritional Approaches

The treatment of colitis depends on the severity of the condition. There is "mild to moderate" colitis in which the person experiences loose stool and mucus in the stool with inflammation. Colitis is the inflammation of the colon, usually affecting the left side. As the condition worsens and the bowel becomes more inflamed, it becomes known as ulcerative colitis. Prescription drugs are standard treatment for this condition due to their fast-acting nature. The problem is that there can be many severe side effects. Nutritional therapies have been shown to be effective without side effects. The suggestions below are to be implemented with consent of your medical doctor.

In mild to moderate colitis, the symptoms may include cramps, diarrhea with mucus and an urgent need to eliminate several times a day. Gas, bloating and abdominal pain are often present as well.

The following suggestions are similar to suggestions for Crohn's since the two conditions are so similar in nature. Whether you have mild, moderate or ulcerative colitis, the information below could be extremely helpful.

The following tests (ordered by a health care practitioner) could be helpful in determining underlying conditions:

* CDSA (Complete Digestive Stool Analysis) to rule out Candida (see appendix)
* Parasite test (see Chapter 4 on parasites) - See appendix for test.
* Gut permeability test (see appendix)
* Heidelberg test for low or excess stomach acid (see appendix)
* Food sensitivity test - ELISA (see appendix)

DIET

Follow the Digestive Care Diet in the appendix of this book, or go on the Candida Diet in Chapter 4 of this book (the Candida section) for one month, and then go on the Digestive Care Diet in the appendix. ***Please note: After going on the Digestive Care Diet, limit fruit to one piece per day for the first month. Stay off wheat and dairy (see appendix for substitutes) for at least 60 days.

If surgery proves necessary, after surgery, you may want to follow a liquid or soft foods diet for awhile. Include broth, bouillon, herbal teas and green drinks. A complete liquid meal replacement, Living Fuel (see Resource Directory), can be beneficial. Sports drinks can help with electrolyte replacement. Include such soft foods as bananas, rice, potatoes, soups, squashes and steamed vegetables, and be sure to drink plenty of water.

Persons with IBD will want to use caution with the following: raw vegetables, raw vegetable skins, raw fruit, seeds and nuts. These can be difficult to digest. Wait until the digestive tract is healed to eat them. Steamed vegetables would be easier to digest.

Fat can be a powerful stimulant of the GI tract, and thus should be avoided in ulcerative colitis patients. It is the "bad" fats, not the "good" ones (like essential fatty acids, as recommended) that are to be avoided. These bad fats would include fried foods, margarine, mayonnaise, cooking oil and dairy products.

Caffeine is stimulating to the digestive tract and should therefore be avoided.

Alcohol is an irritant to the GI tract. Some people will be reactive to it, and others will experience no ill effect, depending on the amount ingested and whether or not it is taken with food.

Avoid carbonated drinks like soda and beer. Foods like broccoli, beans, garlic, onions, leeks, cabbage, and cauliflower produce sulfur and can create gas, which can be painful. Drink herbal teas like chamomile, peppermint, ginger, fennel or slippery elm.

Red meat should be avoided, as it can lead to

Chapter 4

inflammatory reactions and elevate hydrogen sulfide levels, which negatively affects the digestive tract.

Avoid artificial sweeteners like sorbitol, sucralose and Nutrasweet. Small amounts of sugar would be better than substitutes.

SUPPLEMENTS

The following should be discussed with your doctor or holistic practitioner:

• A plant enzyme blend: This supplement should include protease (at least 20,000 H.U.T.), amylase and lipase, as well as papaya and bromelain. Other ingredients in this formula might include soothing herbs like marshmallow and slippery elm. Additionally, a good digestive enzyme formula would contain glutamine (an amino acid) and N-acetyl-glucosamine, which helps soothe an irritated mucosal lining.

• Take HCl/pepsin supplements before meals if stomach acid levels are low. Start with one capsule, and increase by one capsule daily with meals until symptoms are gone. (If you feel a burning sensation, back off to previous dose.) The supplement may contain other soothing ingredients like quercitin, bromelain, gamma oryzanol, L-glutamine and N-acetyl-glucosamine.

Choose one or the other of the above to take with meals.

• Take essential fatty acids (EFAs) to lubricate the digestive tract. A combination of fish and flax (Omega-3) with borage oil (Omega-6) is good to reduce inflammation in the gastrointestinal tract. Absorption of the oils may be enhanced with the addition of lipase (a fat-digesting enzyme). Take three to six 1000 mg. capsules twice daily with food. A daily dose of 3,000 mg. of EPA and 2,000 mg. of DHA (from fish oil) has been shown to decrease the symptoms of ulcerative colitis.

• Take a probiotic (good bacteria) supplement with multiple strains as a daily supplement. It should contain a minimum of two to six billion cultures. A prebiotic could be helpful (see appendix).

• Take a fiber supplement that provides a balance of both soluble and insoluble fibers. A flax/borage seed combination is a good choice, particularly one that contains other beneficial ingredients such as a probiotic blend with fructooligosaccharides (FOS) and herbs like slippery elm bark, marshmallow and fennel seed. Another key ingredient would be L-glutamine, which the intestine uses as fuel to regenerate. This fiber supplement may be added to juices and taken any time of day. When beginning to add dietary fiber to the diet, remember to go slowly, as this can cause some gas if added too quickly. Additionally, an insoluble fiber product from rice bran (see appendix) may be helpful.

• Take 5,000 mg. to 20,000 mg. of L-glutamine powder with N-acetyl-glucosamine (NAG) and gamma oryzanol once to twice daily on an empty stomach (see appendix).

• Multivitamin/mineral supplement (see appendix). Please note: a liquid supplement from your health food store could be extremely beneficial. It should contain vitamin E - 800 I.U., folic acid – 1 mg. to 10 mg., zinc 30 mg. to 60 mg.

• B complex vitamin daily, plus B12 injection or sublingual tablet

• A liquid calcium/magnesium supplement (see appendix)

• A liquid iron supplement (Floradix – see appendix)

• Antioxidant supplement: Take vitamin C at 500 mg. doses 2 to 4 times daily (if stool gets loose, back off and go slower) and vitamin A (from beta-carotene) - 5,000 mg. to 25,000 mg. per day.

Start your supplementation program slowly. After your body has healed, stay on a maintenance program of the following:

- Digestive enzymes
- Essential fatty acids
- Probiotics
- Fiber
- Multivitamin/mineral
- Antioxidants.

In cases of inflammation, enemas could be helpful. Fill an enema bag with the following:

- 2 to 3 capsules of acidophilus and bifidus bacteria
- 1/4 cup of warm olive oil
- The contents of two vitamin E capsules
- 1/2 tsp. L-glutamine powder (empty capsule/s, using the oral supplement recommended in the appendix) – See appendix (glutamine powder).
- 10 drops of any of the following: marshmallow root, echinacea, geranium, goldenseal, comfrey or slippery elm (in liquid tinctures at the health food store)

Fill a small enema bulb with this mixture (or empty a Fleet enema syringe and fill with the mixture), put small amount in the rectum, and hold as long as possible. REMEMBER: if you put too much fluid in at one time, you will not be able to hold it as long.

Another enema that can be healing in ulcerative colitis is a butyrate enema. Butyrate is formed in the colon as a result of the fermentation of bacteria. It is the nutrient the cells that line the colon use for fuel. People with ulcerative colitis have been found to have low levels of butyrate in their stool. Stool analysis (see appendix) will show butyrate levels in test results. Butyrate enemas are available by prescription from compounding pharmacies (see appendix).

LIFESTYLE

- Stress is a major component of this disease, so it is of the utmost importance to find ways to reduce it. It may be advisable to start journaling as a way to determine if certain situations trigger attacks. Check also into some type of counseling with a professional therapist or with a spiritual advisor.
- It is also important when away from home to know the locations of all bathrooms wherever you are going. When on the road, the best places to stop (not to eat but to use the restroom) are fast food establishments.
- During social events like going to a theatre, always sit near the aisle so you can get out quickly.
- When dining out, try to call ahead, find out the choices available on the menu, and let the cook know of your diet restriction. If this is not possible, choice an entrée that is steamed, baked or broiled rather than fried. Avoid sauces, as there can be hidden ingredients in them that could trigger symptoms.
- Exercise is very important. The following could be very beneficial in helping restore your health: Walking, low impact aerobics or weight training.
- Do not wear tight-fitting clothing around the waist.
- Undergo regular colonoscopy. You are at an increased risk for colon cancer.

COMPLEMENTARY MIND/BODY THERAPIES
- Yoga could be beneficial for ulcerative colitis, not only as a form of exercise but also as stress reduction.
- Massage therapy can help with relaxing the body and mind, as this is needed, especially during times of flare-ups.
- Acupuncture would be good for people with ulcerative colitis.
- Colon hydrotherapy should be performed only under a physician's supervision in cases of ulcerative colitis.
- Meditation/Prayer
- Biofeedback
- Chiropractic
- Music therapy

See appendix for information on the above therapies.

Chapter 4

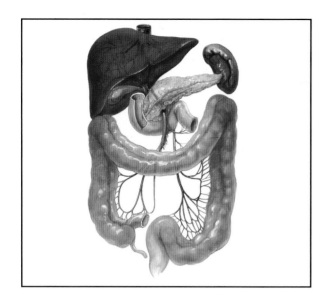

IRRITABLE BOWEL SYNDROME

What is it?

Irritable Bowel Syndrome (IBS), not to be confused with the more serious IBD (inflammatory bowel disease), is considered a "functional disorder" of the colon, which is to say that the large intestine in not functioning properly, although there is no evidence of any organic structural abnormality. Over the years, IBS has been known by a variety of different names: spastic colon, intestinal neurosis, irritable colon, mucous colon, nervous colon, laxative colon, cathartic colon, nervous diarrhea, spastic bowel, functional dyspepsia, nervous indigestion, spastic colitis, mucous colitis, functional colitis and colitis. Reference to the disorder as any type of colitis is technically incorrect, for with it there is no inflammation, no ulceration or other tissue changes. Use of the words "neurosis" and "nervous" imply that IBS is a psychological disorder – another inaccuracy. It is a very real physiological disorder, not a psychosomatic ailment, as once believed,[1] although not one that is entirely understood at present. In truth, more is known about what IBS isn't than what it is. Some think that IBS is a disorder of the enteric nervous system; that is to say that the nerve supply in the 'brain in the gut' alters normal pain perception,[2] so that the bowel becomes oversensitive to normal stimuli.

What Causes it?

The cause of IBS is uncertain, although the following factors may well play a causative role:

- Irregularities in intestinal hormones and nerves responsible for bowel motility (muscle contraction)
- Bacterial, fungal or parasitic involvement
- Stress
- Dietary inadequacies
- Food intolerances (allergies and sensitivities)
- Inadequate enzyme production
- Dysbiosis (imbalance in intestinal flora – too many bad bacteria, not enough good ones)
- Reaction to medications (such as destruction of intestinal flora by antibiotics)
- Undiagnosed lactose intolerance

IBS is at least partially a disorder of colon motility. In it, the normally rhythmic muscular contractions of the digestive tract become irregular and uncoordinated. This interferes with the normal movement of food and waste material and leads to the accumulation of mucus and toxins in the intestine. This accumulated material sets up a partial obstruction of the digestive tract, trapping gas and stools, which in turn causes bloating, distention and constipation.[3]

The colon of the IBS sufferer seems to be more sensitive and reactive to stimulation than that of most people. Intestinal spasms may result from ingestion of certain foods or medicines and from abdominal distention caused by gas. While these factors would not cause undue gastrointestinal stress for the average person, for the IBS sufferer, they can be triggers of painful abdominal spasms.

It is normal for eating to cause contractions in the colon. Normally, these contractions would result in the urge to defecate within an hour after eating. For the person with IBS however, the urge may come sooner, accompanied often with cramps and

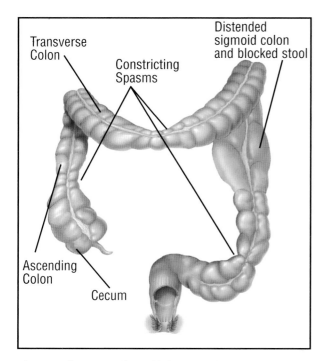

This is an illustration of irritable bowel syndrome.

diarrhea. This is especially true if the meal is large and/or contains a high percentage of fat. Fatty foods such as meat, dairy products, oils and avocados provide a strong stimulus for colonic contractions after a meal for the person with IBS. Stress has the same effect.

There is evidence that food sensitivities and allergies may play a major causative role in IBS, for they are found in 1/2 to 2/3 of those afflicted with the disorder.[4] The most common allergens are dairy products and grains (especially wheat and corn). Other foods that often trigger episodes of IBS are coffee, tea, citrus and chocolate.[5] Caffeine in any form may serve as a gut irritant, as may nicotine. Over-consumption of alcohol may also trigger intestinal spasms in the person with IBS. Meals high in sugar can also contribute to IBS by decreasing intestinal motility.[6] A high percentage of people with IBS are intolerant not only to sucrose (table sugar), but also to other forms of sugar like mannitol, sorbitol and fructose.[7] Foods from the cabbage family (broccoli, Brussels sprouts, cauli-

flower) may be irritating to the IBS sufferer because of their tendency to cause gas.

Other factors that appear to play a role in IBS include hormonal changes (women tend to have flare-ups around the time of their menstrual cycle), low-fiber diets and infection. Many patients have reported onset of symptoms during or soon after recovery from gastrointestinal infection (such as an episode of food poisoning), abdominal surgery or treatment with antibiotics.

The true cause of IBS symptoms in some cases may be an undetected parasitic infection, especially giardiasis or amebiasis. Because of the similarity in symptoms, it is not uncommon for giardial infection to be mistaken for IBS.[8] There also may be an underlying problem with overgrowth of the yeast Candida albicans.

Who Gets it?

An estimated one out of five Americans suffers from irritable bowel syndrome (IBS).[9] The average age of onset is between 25 and 45, with prevalence of the disease declining with age. It is not uncommon for IBS symptoms to surface during teen years, though the disease may be present from infancy.[10] At least twice as many women as men are diagnosed with it.[11] More men may suffer from the disease than reported, however, for many with IBS (an estimated 90%) never consult a physician – at least in Western cultures. Interestingly, the incidence of IBS is

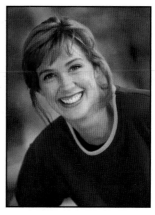

reversed in India (twice as many men affected as women) where men are more apt than women to seek medical care.[12] Although once thought to be a disease of the white middle class, recent studies have established that the prevalence of IBS seems to be independent of race, with Japanese, Chinese,

African Americans and Hispanics having the same incidence of the disease as Caucasians.[13]

IBS is the most common gastrointestinal disorder seen by physicians and makes up 40% of all visits to gastroenterologists (GI disorder specialists).[14] Three and a half million office visits are made to doctors every year for IBS in the United States, making it the 7th leading diagnosis overall.[15]

What are the Signs and Symptoms?
International conferences have actually been held to establish agreed-upon criteria by which function bowel disease can be recognized. These conferences have produced the "Manning criteria" (named after Adrian Manning who proposed one set of criteria) and the "Rome criteria" (named for the location of one of the conferences). The Manning criteria are: [16]

* Stools that are more frequent and looser at the start of episodes of abdominal pain
* Relief of pain after defecating
* A sense of incomplete rectal evacuation
* Passage of mucus with the stool
* A sense of abdominal bloating

The Rome criteria added to the above:

* Constant presence of abdominal pain and altered bowel habits
* Presence of remaining symptoms 25% of the time

Although the above criteria are the "official" ones, in reality, patients presenting with variations of these symptoms may be diagnosed with IBS;[17] these variations may include:

* Constipation with or without pain
* Pain associated with bowel movements
* Painless diarrhea only
* Alternating constipation and diarrhea

IBS sufferers may also experience other symptoms, including:

* Flatulence
* Nausea
* Vomiting
* Headaches
* Loss of appetite
* Anxiety
* Depression
* Poor nutrient absorption (if diarrhea is severe)

The abdominal pain associated with IBS is often triggered by eating and accompanied by abdominal spasms. The person with IBS may feel an urgent need to move the bowels but be unable to do so.

Rectal bleeding is not a typical sign of IBS. If it is present in an IBS sufferer (who is correctly diagnosed), it will be due to a minor disorder such as hemorrhoids or a fissure (a crack in the lining where the rectum joins the skin around the anus).

How is it Diagnosed?
IBS is basically a "diagnosis of exclusion," which is to say, the diagnosis is largely the result of ruling out other disorders that may have the same or similar symptoms. These include:

* Colon cancer
* Diverticular disease
* Infectious diarrhea
* Inflammatory bowel disease (Crohn's disease and ulcerative colitis)
* Candidiasis
* Lactose intolerance
* Laxative abuse
* Pancreatic insufficiency
* Celiac disease
* Fecal impaction
* Adrenal insufficiency
* Diabetes
* Hyperthyroidism
* Ulcers
* Parasites
* Gallbladder disease
* Endometriosis

A thorough medical history and physical examination, along with appropriate laboratory tests (blood tests and stool exam), will help to rule out disorders such as those listed above. At times it may be necessary for the physician to do an endoscopic procedure, which allows him or her to visually inspect the colon (or parts of it). (See "colonoscopy" and "sigmoidoscopy" in the appendix.) A tissue biopsy may be taken in conjunction with the endoscopic procedure and, as mentioned, a significant percentage of patients will have immunologic evidence of inflammation. "Occasionally, patients with chronic diarrhea and abdominal pain who have a normal-appearing colon have a condition called microscopic colitis rather than IBS. Biopsy of the normal-looking colon affected by microscopic colitis will show inflammation similar to patients with ulcerative colitis."[18]

What is the Standard Medical Treatment?

The conventional approach to controlling IBS is through:

• Dietary restrictions
• Stress management
• Medications

Some doctors may limit their dietary advice to avoidance of caffeine-containing foods and beverages (coffee, tea, chocolate, colas) and reduced alcohol consumption. Others, recognizing the role of individual food allergies (involving an immediate allergic response) and food sensitivities (involving a delayed response) may order special blood tests, such as the ELISA (see appendix), which measures antibodies, to identify offending foods.

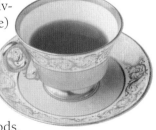

An alternative way of identifying food allergens and sensitivities would be through use of an elimination diet, where the patient is placed on a diet of a few select foods that have a low allergic potential and then slowly adds suspected allergens back into the diet, one food at a time, observing and recording the body's reaction to them. The simple act of keeping a diet journal can help identify irritating foods. The journal approach is most effective for identifying intolerances to specific foods when used in conjunction with the elimination diet. Once offending foods are identified, they must be avoided for a lengthy period of time (at least two months), then added back into the diet on a rotating basis.

Many doctors, while unaware of the role food allergies and sensitivities may play in IBS, may nonetheless recommend that their patients eliminate dairy products on a 2-week trial basis. This recommendation is based on the recognition that lactose intolerance may play a role in the patient's symptoms. Some may also advise a 2-week trial elimination of grains, based on the role that celiac disease or gluten sensitivity may play.

Most doctors, regardless of the level of their understanding of nutrition, will advise the IBS patient to increase intake of dietary fiber (whole grains, fruits and vegetables), because high-fiber diets keep the colon mildly distended, which helps prevent spasms from developing.[19] Some may additionally advise the use of a bulk-forming fiber supplement, such as psyllium (often in the form of Metamucil).

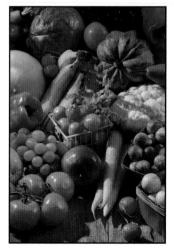

Such an increase in fiber may aggravate symptoms if it is done too suddenly; a slow, gradual increase in dietary fiber is advised to avoid irritation from it. Some IBS patients may not be able to handle the increase, however, even when the transition is made slowly. One potential problem with fiber supplements is that wheat bran is often used, and wheat is a grain with a high allergy potential.

A standard treatment for diarrhea has been to place the patient on the BRAT diet, which consists of bananas, rice, applesauce and tea. The patient may then transition into a regular diet as the diarrhea subsides. Nutritionally aware doctors may avoid use of such a diet, however, due to the high carbohydrate content.

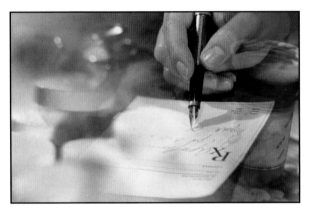

Doctors have prescribed several types of drugs to help alleviate IBS symptoms. These have included:

- Anti-cholinergic drugs (atropine preparations like belladonna) to block one portion of the autonomic nerves that regulate contractions of the intestine
- Tranquilizing drugs or general relaxers
- Antispasmodics (like Bentyl) that block nerve impulses to the intestinal muscles
- Anti-depressants/mood elevators (like Elavil)- seem to work by filtering out painful stimuli from the gut to the brain
- Antibiotics to treat infection, if present
- Antacids – to slow the movement of food through the GI tract (See GERD section for discussion of the adverse effects of antacids.)
- Stool softeners/laxatives – to combat constipation, if present

The above drugs all have adverse side effects (some

of which may make GI symptoms worse), and they are expensive and only moderately effective.[20] Often herbs can be used with equal benefit (and without unwanted side effects). These can be quite effective in combination with dietary management and regular exercise to help control the symptoms of IBS.

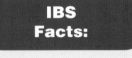

IBS Facts:

- According to the National Institute of Diabetes and Digestive and Kidney Diseases, irritable bowel syndrome (IBS) is one of the most frequently occurring gastrointestinal disorders and accounts for 41% of all visits to gastroenterology practices.

- It is estimated today that one in five Americans has IBS symptoms, making it second only to the common cold as the most frequent cause of absenteeism from work and school.

- Most people with IBS have such mild symptoms that they do not seek medical care for it, and those that do are seldom hospitalized.

Optional Nutritional Approaches

Depending upon their level of awareness, doctors may also advise their IBS patients to eat smaller meals, chew thoroughly, reduce fat intake, increase water consumption, eliminate gas-forming foods, refined foods and sugar. Some may recommend the use of digestive enzymes with meals, probiotics (to increase friendly bacteria), glutamine (to help heal the bowel wall) and peppermint oil (enteric-coated capsules have been used to help soothe and relax intestinal muscles[21]).

Most IBS sufferers report having mental/emotional problems, though it is unknown whether such problems are a cause or a result of the IBS.[22] Nonetheless, "psychotherapy in the form of relaxation therapy, biofeedback, hypnosis, counseling or stress management training, has been shown to reduce symptom frequency and severity and enhance the results of standard medical treatment of IBS."[23] Such therapies, moreover, have shown a greater benefit than drug therapies[24] as described below.

Rule out the following as these could be underlying problem.

- Food sensitivities - ELISA test (see appendix)
- Parasites - See Parasite section.
- Candida - CDSA (Complete Digestive Stool Analysis) See Candida, Chapter 4.
- H-pylori infection

DIET

Regardless of the type of IBS you have (constipation, diarrhea or spastic), diet is a major consideration in the treatment. Follow the Digestive Care Diet in the appendix of this book, or you may want to go on the Candida Diet in Chapter 4 (candidiasis) for one month, and then go to the Digestive Care Diet. The following foods should be temporarily eliminated from the diet, as they are considered trigger foods.

- High-fat foods (fried)
- Red meat

- Dairy
- Egg yolks
- Coffee, soda and alcohol
- Chocolate
- Sugars, like mannitol, sucrose, sorbitol and fructose
- High sulfur foods - garlic, onions, leeks, broccoli, cauliflower, cabbage, Brussels sprouts

If raw foods are a problem, lightly steam vegetables.

A WORD ABOUT FIBER

High-fiber foods can create problems for the IBS sufferer (especially those with diarrhea), so never eat them alone or on an empty stomach. In practical terms, this means blend fruit into a smoothie for better digestion. Put veggies into a sauce to eat with pasta, or steam veggies with rice. Peeling chopping, cooking and pureeing fresh fruits, vegetables and beans will help to reduce the impact of insoluble fiber on your GI tract. **Please note: all grains, cereals and tubers have an outer insoluble fiber layer and a soluble fiber interior (the same is true for some fruits and vegetables, such as apples and zucchini). IBS sufferers aren't necessarily allergic to these healthy foods; the problem is that the foods could potentially trigger a reaction if not eaten with soluble fiber foods.

SUPPLEMENTS

There are two supplement protocols given below, one for IBS involving constipation and the other for IBS involving diarrhea. Follow the one that is appropriate for you.

Those with constipation IBS should follow the 30-day herbal detox program in the appendix. This will consist of:

- Two-part 30-day internal cleanse taken morning and night
- Take a fiber supplement that provides a balance of both soluble and insoluble fibers. A flax/borage seed combination is a good choice, particularly one that contains other beneficial

ingredients such as a probiotic blend with fructooligosaccharides (FOS) and herbs like slippery elm bark, marshmallow and fennel seed. Another key ingredient would be L-glutamine, which the intestine uses as fuel to regenerate. This fiber supplement may be added to juices and taken any time of day. When beginning to add dietary fiber to the diet, remember to go slowly, as this can cause some gas if added too quickly.

- Take essential fatty acids (EFA's) to lubricate the digestive tract. A combination of fish and flax (Omega-3) oils with borage oil (Omega-6) is good to reduce inflammation in the gastrointestinal tract. Absorption of the oils may be enhanced with the addition of lipase (a fat-digesting enzyme). Take three to six 1000 mg. capsules twice daily with food.

Select one of the two enzyme formulas described below to take with meals:

- A plant enzyme blend: This supplement should include protease (at least 20,000 H.U.T.), amylase and lipase, as well as papaya and bromelain. Other ingredients in this formula might include soothing herbs like marshmallow and slippery elm. Additionally, a good digestive enzyme formula would contain glutamine (an amino acid) and N-acetyl-glucosamine, which helps soothe an rritated mucosal lining.
- Take HCl/pepsin supplements before meals if stomach acid levels are low. Start with one capsule, and increase by one capsule daily with meals until symptoms are gone. (If you feel a burning sensation, back off to previous dose.) The supplement may contain other soothing ingredients like quercitin, bromelain, gamma oryzanol, L-glutamine and N-acetyl-glucosamine.

If you suffer from constipation IBS, you will also want to:

- Take a probiotic (good bacteria) supplement

with multiple strains as a daily supplement. It should contain a minimum of two to six billion cultures. A prebiotic could be helpful (see appendix).
- Use a liquid calcium/magnesium formula (See Floradix brand in the appendix and Resource Directory.)

*****For cramping and spasms, take a two-part intestinal bowel support formula containing L-glutamine and N-acetyl-glucosamine to support a healthy mucosal lining. Part II consists of a Chinese formula, along with slippery elm and fenugreek, herbs that can soothe cramping (see appendix). Enteric-coated peppermint can also help with cramping and abdominal pain.

****After finishing the 30-day herbal detox program, begin a colon cleanse formula to help with regularity. Look for one containing herbs like cape aloe and rhubarb (that will gently stimulate peristalsis), as well as magnesium oxide to bring water to the bowel. Start with one capsule before bed, and increase by one capsule each night until bowel elimination occurs.

As maintenance, you will want to stay on:

- Enzymes
- Probiotics
- Fiber
- EFA's

A 30-day Liver Detox (see appendix) following the 30-day herbal detox program is also recommended.

FOR IBS DIARRHEA

- Two-part IBS product (see appendix), taken morning and night. This intestinal bowel support formula, containing L-glutamine and N-acetyl-glucosamine, will support a healthy mucosal lining and help with cramping and spasms. Part II of the product consists of a Chinese herbal formula, along with slippery elm and fenugreek, herbs that can soothe cramping (see appendix). For cramping, also try enteric-coated peppermint capsules (see appendix).

- Soluble fiber (see appendix)
- Take essential fatty acids (EFA's) to lubricate the digestive tract. A combination of fish and flax (Omega-3) oils with borage oil (Omega-6) is good to reduce inflammation in the gastrointestinal tract. Absorption of the oils may be enhanced with the addition of lipase (a fat-digesting enzyme). Take three to six 1000 mg. capsules twice daily with food.
- Take a probiotic (good bacteria) supplement with multiple strains as a daily supplement. It should contain a minimum of two to six billion cultures. A prebiotic could be helpful (see appendix).
- Rice bran fiber, mostly insoluble, taken in small amounts and increased gradually as tolerated, can add bulk to stools. Soluble rice fiber is also beneficial in that it is high in antioxidants and natural anti-inflammatories (see appendix).

Select one of the two enzyme formulas described below to take with meals:

- A plant enzyme blend: This supplement should include protease (at least 20,000 H.U.T.), amylase and lipase, as well as papaya and bromelain. Other ingredients in this formula might include soothing herbs like marshmallow and slippery elm. Additionally, a good digestive enzyme formula would contain glutamine (an amino acid) and N-acetyl-glucosamine, which helps soothe an irritated mucosal lining.
- Take HCl/pepsin supplements before meals if stomach acid levels are low. Start with one capsule, and increase by one capsule daily with meals until symptoms are gone. (If you feel a burning sensation, back off to previous dose.) The supplement may contain other soothing ingredients like quercitin, bromelain, gamma oryzanol, L-glutamine and N-acetyl-glucosamine.

- Liquid calcium-magnesium (See Floradix in appendix and Resource Directory.) ** If stool becomes too loose, back off.

LIFESTYLE
- Eat organic foods as much as possible. The GI tract of IBS sufferers is sensitive, so chemicals could have a potentially negative effect.
- Talk to family and friends about your condition, and request their support.
- Start with short walks, then longer ones, through the neighborhood.
- If your social activities have been restricted, start attending a low-key social event.
- When eating in restaurants, call ahead, if necessary, to see what is on the menu. If there isn't time to call, select a steamed vegetable (without fat) and a steamed, broiled or baked protein.
- Drink plenty of water and herbal teas like peppermint, ginger, chamomile and slippery elm.
- Join an IBS support group, if available.

COMPLEMENTARY MIND/BODY THERAPIES
Since stress can be a key trigger for IBS, the following can be very important in the management of this condition:

- Meditation/Prayer
- Massage therapy would be excellent in the management of IBS.
- Acupuncture has stress-reducing effects; ask your practitioner specifically about this.
- Yoga - good not only for exercise but also for stress reduction
- Biofeedback can be helpful in teaching relaxation skills.
- Colon hydrotherapy - If your IBS condition results from an imbalance in the GI tract, (due to such conditions as Candida or parasites), or you have the constipation IBS, colon hydrotherapy could be beneficial.
- Chiropractic
- Music therapy

See appendix for information on the above therapies.

Chapter 4

Dr. Smith's Comments

Research suggests that the stress-related emotional component of IBS releases cortisol from the adrenal glands, which promotes the release of CRF (corticotrophin releasing factor) from the brain (hippocampus, a portion of the limbic system). CRF has been shown to delay gastric emptying and, at the same time, increase colonic motility! In addition, experimentally blocking CRF (with CRF antagonists), relieves depression and anxiety in primates. Thus, stress-released CRF could have the following effects:

- *A factor in IBS - diarrhea predominant*
- *A factor in heartburn, dyspepsia and GERD via delayed gastric-emptying*
- *A factor in anxiety and depression; a treatment for some IBS patients is anti-depressants; hypnosis has been shown to be 88% effective by itself in treating IBS!*

Biofeedback may also be useful. I recommend the Freeze-framer ™ by HeartMath (see appendix).

Physical factors in IBS are becoming more plentiful in the literature (see American Journal of Gastroenterology Vol. 98, issue 2, pp 412-419):

- *Intestinal infections – known as post-infectious IBS – can be a major factor. Many people never had a gut problem until after an episode of gastroenteritis; then IBS-type symptoms become a way of life for many. In the above-mentioned AJG reference, 111 IBS patients had a lactulose hydrogen breath test, and 84% were positive for small bowel overgrowth! One hundred and eleven subjects that were given neomycin experienced a 35% improvement reflected in a composite score, compared with 11.4% placebo (p< 0.05); additionally, patients reported a bowel normalization of 35.3% after neomycin, compared with 13.9% with placebo. The best outcomes were observed if neomycin was successful in normalizing the lactulose breath test. This would implicate bacterial flora in IBS.*
- *Consumption of simple carbohydrates and sugars can feed and increase the population of unfriendly bacteria and yeasts. It has been shown that toxins from Candida yeast can have an effect on the enteric and autonomic nerves of the colon and may help promote constipation-dominant IBS. One would wonder if the immune deficient, carbohydrate-consuming elderly might be a set up for Candida- induced chronic constipation.*

There is a good article in the "Current Opinions" of Gastroenterology [9(4):336-342] entitled: "Inflammatory Bowel Disease and Irritable Bowel Syndrome: Separate or Unified?" The article points out several similarities between the conditions. In reading the article, it becomes clear that intestinal inflammation with increased permeability and immune hyper-responsiveness in the presence of psycho-emotional stress, could constitute a spectrum of physiologic events that occur over time rather than being clear-cut and separate disease entities.

Some interesting findings indicate that IBS is not just a functional (psycho-emotional) disorder with changes in bowel function and abdominal pain. There can be clear-cut physical changes:

- *In the past, IBS bowel biopsy specimens appeared to be normal with routine histology. Now, using immunohistology and closer inspection, increased cytotoxic T cells, natural killer cells, increased numbers of ileal and colonic mast cells with tryptase and increased intra-epithelial lymphocytes are seen. All of these features point to inflammatory changes in the small intestine and colon not unlike the earliest patterns seen in IBD. In fact, some patients with IBS followed for years had biopsy specimens with nerve degeneration in the ganglia of the bowel wall, with infiltration of CD3+ lymphocytes and longitudinal muscle hypertrophy. These are findings that begin to look more like Crohn's disease.*

Interestingly, according to the currently used symptom criteria (Rome criteria), once organic changes (like those above) are made, by definition, a diagnosis of the functional syndrome of IBS can no longer be made! It is easy to see why the process of labeling can lead to oversimplification that could be confusing both to practitioners and patients.

There are at least eight shared pathophysiologic mechanisms in common with IBS and IBD (which includes Crohn's, ulcerative colitis and microscopic colitis):

- Altered mucosal permeability
- Altered interaction of the luminal flora with the mucosal immune system
- Persistent mucosal immune activation
- Altered gut motility
- Sustained severe life stressors
- Histological similarities, especially with regard to inflammatory cells and cytokines
- Positive responses to probiotics, antibiotics and anti-inflammatory agents
- Genetic factors may also play a role in both IBD and IBS. One known factor is a genetic predisposition to enhanced immune reactivity. On chromosome 2, if there is a change from cytosine to thymidine at position 31, there will be increases in IL-1 Beta. This minor change (known as a single nucleotide isolated polymorphism or SNIP) may predispose individuals to chronic inflammatory conditions by increasing COX2 activity and prostaglandin production. In addition, this SNIP can predispose to hypochlorhydria (low stomach acid production) and H. pylori infection. The good news is that these types of small genetic changes (SNIPS) can often be controlled by appropriate |diet and supplementation. If one knew they had this SNIP, it would be important for them to take enzymes, HCl and probiotics and follow the appropriate diet indefinitely.

At this point, I would like to make it clear that I am not saying that IBS will invariably become IBD. I do think in some susceptible individuals the data support that this could be a possibility, particularly if the preventive measures mentioned are not employed. In obtaining histories from IBD patients, it is not uncommon for some of them to report that their earlier symptoms were most similar to IBS.

Since there are many similarities in IBS and IBD (Crohn's and ulcerative colitis), which relate to bacteria, inflammation and stress, there are nutritional options that can be incorporated with benefit as mentioned above: higher fiber (more insoluble), Omega-3 fish oils, probiotics, digestive enzymes, antioxidants, vitamins and minerals. At the same time, minimizing sugar, simple carbohydrates, known food allergens and stress can be most helpful. It is interesting to note that some of the deficiencies found in IBD, namely zinc, folate, iron and vitamin B12, are the very ones that are poorly absorbed in a low-acid environment. It is well known that stomach acid levels decline with age, acid-blocking drugs and genetic susceptibility. Another factor is vitamin D deficiency. The best way to supplement would be 30 minutes of sunshine per day!

I have had patients who were able to implement much of the above and have avoided surgery and continue to be in long-term remission. Unfortunately, with advanced Crohn's or ulcerative colitis, surgery is the only option. Surgery for Crohn's usually involves resection of the severely diseased small bowel, and surgery for ulcerative colitis involves removal of all, or most all, of the colon. If not done correctly, there can be disastrous results. If the surgery is successful, most return to normal lives but can still have recurrent disease! Surgery does not address the cause of these conditions. This is why, with post-surgical patients, I have stressed optional nutritional approaches and lifestyle changes.

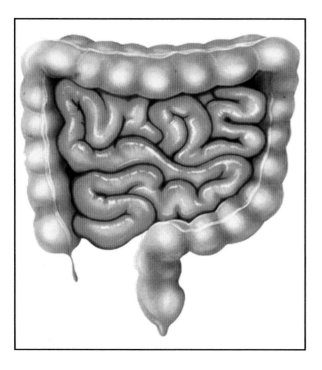

LACTOSE INTOLERANCE
What is it?

Lactose intolerance (also known as lactose malab-sorption or lactase deficiency) is the name given to the condition in which the body in unable to digest lactose (milk sugar). Put another way, the body cannot break down lactose into its component sugars, glucose and galactose. Normally, this splitting is done by the enzyme lactase, which is manufactured in the lining of the small intestine. Lactase, however, is absent or deficient in the intestines of lactose intolerant people, making it difficult for them to handle milk and other dairy products.

Here, it is important to note that lactose intolerance is not the same as a milk allergy. The immune system of the allergic individual launches a response to one or more of the components in the milk, usually a protein. Poor protein digestion is believed to play a role in allergies because the immune response is trig-gered to react to the presence of undigested proteins in the gut lining or in the bloodstream. The person who is allergic to milk products, however, is not necessari-ly lactose intolerant, since lactose intolerance is a function of poor enzyme activity and not an allergic reaction.

What Causes it?

As indicated above, lactose intolerance is due to a deficiency of the lactase enzyme. Failure of the small intestine to produce adequate lactase may be the result of:

- A gastrointestinal disorder that damages the digestive tract, such as celiac disease and Crohn's disease, both of which affect the small intestine.[1] Once intestinal cells are damaged, they are unable to produce enzymes (including lactase) as they once did.
- The aging process; most babies are born with high levels of lactase in their intestines. These levels typically remain high for the first year or two of life, then decline, nearly disappearing in adulthood.[2]
- A rare congenital lactase deficiency (present at birth).
- Injury to the lactase-producing areas of the intestine. Various traumas, such as that from parasites, may cause such damage.[3]

Low lactase levels may also be present in viral and bacterial infections and cystic fibrosis.[4]

Lactose intolerance normally occurs in adults, though it may less frequently affect children. It can occur in infants after a severe bout of gastroenteri-tis, which damages the intestinal lining.[5]

People who are intolerant to the lactose in milk may likewise be sensitive to sugar alcohols such as sorbitol, maltitol and xylitol, and should check labels for presence of these substances so they may be avoided.[6]

When lactose is not thoroughly broken down in the small intestine for any of the reasons discussed, all or some of it enters the colon intact. That por-tion of unsplit lactose that reaches the large intes-tine serves as food for bacteria residing there. As these bacteria feed upon the undigested milk sugar, gases and irritating acids are produced, giving rise to unpleasant symptoms.

Who Gets it?

Lactose intolerance affects up to 75% of the world's population.[7] It is especially prevalent among people of Asian, African, native American, Mexican and Mediterranean ancestry, affecting an estimated 70-90% of people within these groups.[8] Least affected (10-15%) are people of northern

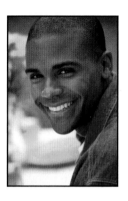

or Western European ancestry.[9,10] Interestingly, most Northern Europeans and their American descendants retain their ability to digest lactose as long as they continue drinking milk.[11] Still, an estimated 50 million Americans are lactose intolerant.[12]

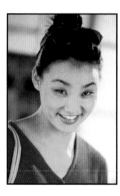

As mentioned, lactose intolerance primarily affects adults. By age six, many people, especially those ethnic groups mentioned above, lose their ability to digest lactose.[13] That ability tends to decline with age, so that most adults, regardless of their heritage, have some degree of lactose intolerance.[14]

People with Crohn's disease (an inflammatory bowel disease) and celiac disease (glucose intolerance) are often lactose intolerant due to damage to the intestinal lining from the disease processes. That damage interferes with lactase production.

What are the Signs and Symptoms?

Within a short time, usually 30 minutes to 2 hours of ingesting milk or dairy products, the lactose intolerant person will develop mild to severe symptoms, which may include:

- Abdominal cramps
- Bloating
- Diarrhea
- Nausea
- Intestinal gas
- Headaches
- Acne

The onset of gastrointestinal symptoms may follow the ingestion of even small amounts of lactose, although individual tolerances to the milk sugar may vary greatly. Some people will be affected by the presence of minute amounts, while others are able to tolerate a glass or two of milk. Some people may have a lactase deficiency and yet be asymptomatic (without symptoms). They would not be considered lactose intolerant.

A severe case of lactose intolerance, if untreated, can lead to generalized intestinal inflammation, which can cause other problems throughout the body.

Although lactose intolerance is rare in infants, when it occurs, the following symptoms may appear: foamy diarrhea with diaper rash, slow weight gain and development and vomiting.[15]

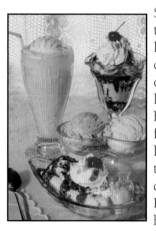

Some dairy products tend to cause more problems than others. Ice cream is often especially difficult for people with lactose intolerance to handle, for some manufacturers add extra lactose to enhance its texture.[16] Hard, aged cheeses, such as Parmesan, on the other hand, are relatively low in lactose and so are generally easier to handle.[17] Fermented dairy products, such as yogurt (with live, active cultures), are usually well tolerated by people with lactose intolerance, as these products have been predigested by bacteria, so that most of

Chapter 4

the lactose has been broken down.[18,19]

How is it Diagnosed?

Anyone suspecting that they may be lactose intolerant may do a simple self-test: Eliminate all sources of dairy products for ten days to see if symptoms disappear. If they do not, then you can rule out lactose intolerance as a cause of the symptoms. If symptoms do subside, it may be as the result of either lactose intolerance or milk allergy. If you are able to tolerate lactose-free or lactose-reduced dairy products or are able to drink milk when lactase enzyme drops are added (or tablets are chewed beforehand), the problem can be narrowed down to lactose intolerance. If a milk allergy is the cause of the problem, there would be no improvement of symptoms expected with the ingestion of lactase.

It may take some detective work to eliminate all dairy products, as these are often hidden in commonly consumed processed foods. Chart 1 lists known and possible sources of dairy products.

Lactose is also used as a filler in some medications, such as Maalox, Premarin, Contact and many types of birth control pills.[20] In fact, it is the base for more than 20% of prescription drugs and about 6% of over-the-counter medications.[21]

There are three diagnostic tools used by the medical profession to identify lactose intolerance: the lactose tolerance test, the hydrogen breath test and the stool acidity test. The last of these is used for infants and small children who may be prone to dehydration, which may result from diarrhea caused by the lactose ingestion required in the first two tests.[22] The test simply measures the amount of acid in the stool, which will be elevated in the lactose intolerant person, as undigested lactose fermented by bacteria in the colon creates lactic acid and other short-chain fatty acids that can be detected in the stool; additionally, glucose may be found in the stool sample as a result of unabsorbed lactose in the colon.[23]

Sources of Dairy Products

- Milk
- Yogurt
- Cheese
- Ice cream
- Creamed soups (canned and powdered)
- Frozen yogurt
- Whipped cream
- Hot dogs
- Lunch meats (unless Kosher)
- Milk chocolate
- Most nondairy creamers
- Pancake, biscuit and cookie mixes
- Protein powder drinks
- Some salad dressings, such as Ranch
- Bread and other baked goods
- Processed breakfast cereals
- Instant potatoes, soups and breakfast drinks
- Margarine
- Candies and other snacks
- Pasta
- Puddings
- Sauces
- Anything that contains:
    Casein
    Lactose
    Caseinate
    Curds
    Milk by-products
    Dry milk solids
    Non-fat dry milk powder
    Whey
    Sodium caseinate

Chart 1

The lactose tolerance test is a blood test that measures blood sugar levels. In preparation for the test, the patient fasts overnight and then drinks a lactose-containing liquid. Blood samples are then taken by a technician to measure blood sugar levels, which should increase significantly after the ingestion of the lactose if the body is properly digesting it. If the lactose is not completely broken down into glucose, the blood sugar level does not rise significantly, and the diagnosis of lactose intolerance is confirmed, especially if symptoms of the disorder are manifesting.[24]

The hydrogen breath test simply measures the amount of hydrogen in the patient's breath. See the appendix for a description of this test.

What is the Standard Medical Treatment?

There is no known cure for lactose intolerance. However, the symptoms may be controlled or eliminated through diet. For the minority of severe cases and for young children,[25] total and complete elimination of all lactose from the diet may be necessary. In this case, special lactose-free dairy products (often available in supermarkets) or dairy substitutes (such as rice milk, nut milk, seed milk, oat milk or goat's milk) may be used. These dairy substitutes may be made at home or purchased in a health food store or in some supermarkets.

The majority of those suffering from lactose intolerance will be able to include some dairy products in their diet, especially if one or more of the following are used:

- Lactose-reduced dairy products (available in supermarkets)
- Lactase enzyme supplements (available in tablet and liquid form without prescription) to be used in conjunction with meals that contain dairy foods
- Fermented dairy products, such as yogurt, kefir, sour cream, acidophilus milk, hard cheeses and buttermilk (available in supermarkets and health food stores)

A few drops of liquid lactase placed in a quart of milk for 24 hours will result in a 70% reduction in the lactose content; a 90% reduction is achieved if the amount of drops used is doubled.[26] Taking 3 to 6 chewable lactase tablets before eating dairy foods will help many with lactose intolerance to consume such products without distress. The more dairy consumed, the greater the number of tablets required. And, it should be noted that these do not work for everyone.

Those who need to strictly avoid all dairy products due to lactose intolerance will want to look to other sources of calcium in their diets. Rich sources would include green vegetables (especially leafy 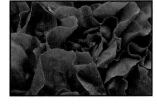 and uncooked), sesame seeds (soak them before eating to deactivate enzyme inhibitors), salmon and sardines.

Lactose Intolerance Facts:

- An estimated 50 million Americans suffer from lactose intolerance, which is an inability to properly digest milk sugar or lactose.
- This condition, which results in a variety of discomforts, such as abdominal cramps and diarrhea, is rarely present at birth, but rather develops over a period of time.
- By age six, many people begin to lose their ability to digest lactose.
- Lactose can be found in dairy products and in some medications.
- Lactose is the base for more than 20% of prescription drugs and about 6% of over-the-counter medications.

Chapter 4

Optional Nutritional Approaches

The following can be used to test for lactose intolerance:

- Lactose-Intolerance Test (see appendix)
- Hydrogen Breath Test (see appendix) measures the amount of hydrogen in the breath.
- Stool Acidity Test for children

Rule out the following:

- Parasites (see appendix for test description) - Parasites can mimic the symptoms of lactose intolerance.

DIET

Follow the Digestive Care Diet in the appendix of this book. Use dairy substitutes listed there. If there is increased inflammation in the digestive tract, a 3-day juice fast (see appendix for recipes) would be helpful before starting the Digestive Care Diet.

Though some people have more tolerance than others to them, the following are relatively low in lactose:

- Hard cheeses like Parmesan
- Yogurt (because most of the lactose has been predigested); homemade is best.

***Note: Eat plenty of foods high in calcium, like black strap molasses, apricots, broccoli, collard greens, kale, spinach, salmon and sardines.

SUPPLEMENTS

- Try a lactose enzyme before eating dairy. Look for a formula with 7,500 A.L.U. of lactase to break down lactose, 600 L.N. to help with fat digestion and 90,000 P. U. of papain for protein digestion. This formula will help digest all components of dairy. (Please note: 3,000 A.L.U. lactase units will break down the lactose in an 8 oz. glass of milk in one hour; 20,000 P.U. of papain will hydrolyze the protein in an 8 oz. glass of milk in one hour.)

- Probiotics/prebiotics (use a non-dairy source) - This helps reestablish the good bacteria and helps with digestion (see appendix). Take a probiotic (good bacteria) supplement with multiple strains as a daily supplement. It should contain a minimum of two to six billion cultures. A prebiotic could be helpful (see appendix).

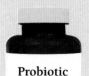

Probiotic

- Take EFAs (essential fatty acids) to lubricate the digestive tract. A combination of fish and flax (Omega-3) with borage oil (Omega-6) is good to reduce inflammation in the gastrointestinal tract. Absorption of the oils may be enhanced with the addition of lipase (a fat-digesting enzyme). Take three to six 1000 mg. capsules twice daily with food.

Essential
Fatty Acids

- Take a fiber supplement that provides a balance of both soluble and insoluble fibers. A flax/borage seed combination is a good choice, particularly one that contains other beneficial ingredients such as a probiotic blend with fructooligosaccharides (FOS) and herbs like slippery elm bark, marshmallow and fennel seed. Another key ingredient would be L-glutamine, which the intestine uses as fuel to regenerate. This fiber supplement may be added to juices and taken any time of day. When beginning to add dietary fiber to the diet, remember to go slowly, as this can cause some gas if added too quickly.

Fiber
Supplement

- Take antioxidant supplements (vitamin C with bioflavonoids - 500 mg. to 3000 mg., vitamin A - 10,000 I.U. daily, Vitamin E – 400 I.U. to 800 I.U. and zinc – 30 mg. to 60 mg. daily) after meals. Other antioxidants may also be taken with these. (See appendix for specification on antioxidants.)

- Multivitamin/mineral supplement (see appendix). Please note: a liquid supplement from your health food store could be extremely beneficial. It should contain vitamin E - 800 I.U., folic acid – 1 mg. to 10 mg., zinc 30 mg. to 60 mg.
- Liquid calcium-magnesium (See Floradix in appendix and Resource Directory.)

***Please note: If there is severe diarrhea, please see the Diarrhea section of this book in Chapter 4.

LIFESTYLES
- Read product labels carefully. Not only are milk and milk solids an issue if your problem is severe, but you must also be aware of processed foods such as breads cakes, cereals and salad dressings.
- Make sure all supplement and medicine labels are marked "no dairy."

COMPLEMENTARY MIND/BODY THERAPIES
- Acupuncture could be helpful during an episode of lactose intolerance.
- Colon hydrotherapy
- Massage
- Yoga
- Meditation/Prayer
- Music therapy
- Chiropractic
- Biofeedback

See appendix for information on the above therapies.

Dr. Smith's Comments
Lactose intolerance increases with age. This may be due to chronic low-grade microbial infection of the small bowel (Candida or bacterial overgrowth). In either case, the brush border enzymes produced by the gut lining will be decreased. Lactase is the enzyme shown to be often the most depleted; it is needed to split the milk sugar lactose. If this does not happen efficiently, symptoms of bloating, diarrhea and malabsorption of calcium may occur.

It is important to note that some patients with osteoporosis may be lactose intolerant. They have increased bone turnover and decreased bone mass, especially in older men and postmenopausal women. Impaired vitamin D status (not enough sunshine) and low calcium absorption have been implicated (AJCN; vol. 22, pp 201-207, 2003). As mentioned previously, low stomach acid, which also occurs with age, may be a significant factor in poor calcium absorption leading to osteoporosis .

Lactose intolerance may be an unexpected factor in IBD or IBS and should routinely be ruled out in these conditions.

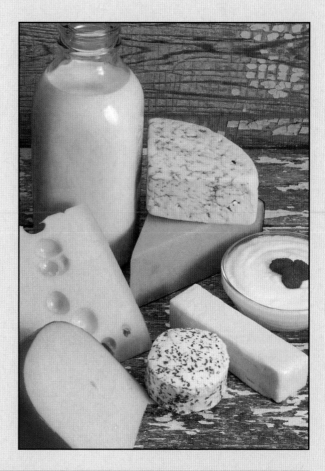

Chapter 4

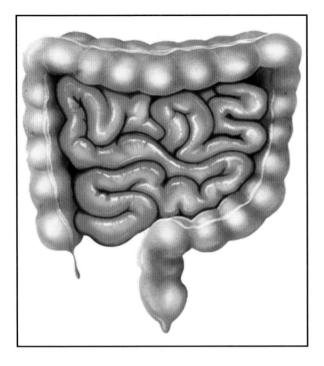

LEAKY GUT SYNDROME
What is it?

When we eat, food passes through the stomach into the small intestine. It is here that nutrient absorption occurs through the semi-permeable mucous lining of the bowel wall. This membrane also shields the bloodstream from unwanted toxins, pathogens and undigested food. In this respect, the gut lining is a vital part of the body's immune system because it limits the volume of potential invaders. Leaky gut syndrome is a condition that develops when the mucous lining of the small intestine becomes too porous, allowing entry of toxins, microorganisms and food particles, as well as pathogens, into the bloodstream. The function of the mucous lining of the small intestine can be compared to that of a window screen, which lets air in but keeps bugs out. It is also like the skin, in that it sloughs off a layer of cells naturally every 3 to 5 days and produces new cells to keep the lining semi-permeable.

What Causes it?

When digestion is impaired by such factors as stress, processed food consumption, inadequate chewing, excessive fluid intake with meals, improper food combining and overeating, it can lead to an excessively permeable (leaky) gut. Here's why: When bacteria present in the intestine act upon undigested food particles, toxic chemicals and gases are produced. These intestinal toxins, known as endotoxins, can damage the mucosal lining, resulting in increased intestinal permeability. As a result of repeated attacks by these toxins, the gut lining erodes over time. This is the basic mechanism by which leaky gut comes into being. It can also be caused or aggravated by a number of other factors, including:

- Alcohol (gut irritant)
- Caffeine (gut irritant)
- Parasites (introduced into the body by contaminated food and water)
- Bacteria (introduced into the body by contaminated food and water)
- Chemical food additives (dyes, preservatives, flavorings, etc.)
- Enzyme deficiencies (as found in celiac disease and lactose intolerance)
- Diet of refined carbohydrates ("junk" food)
- Prescriptive hormones (like birth control pills)
- Mold and fungal mycotoxins (in stored grains, fruit and refined carbohydrates)
- Free radicals (damage chemical compounds present with toxicity)
- Heightened exposure to environmental toxins
- Dental toxins (from restorative materials and invasive procedures)
- Stress

Perhaps the greatest contributors to leaky gut are the drugs listed below:

- NSAIDS (Non-steroidal anti-inflammatory drugs, like aspirin and Motrin)
- Antacids
- Steroids (includes prescription corticosteroids such as prednisone and hydrocortisone)
- Antibiotics (which lead to overgrowth of bad bacteria in the GI tract)

Chapter 4

Digestive Care™

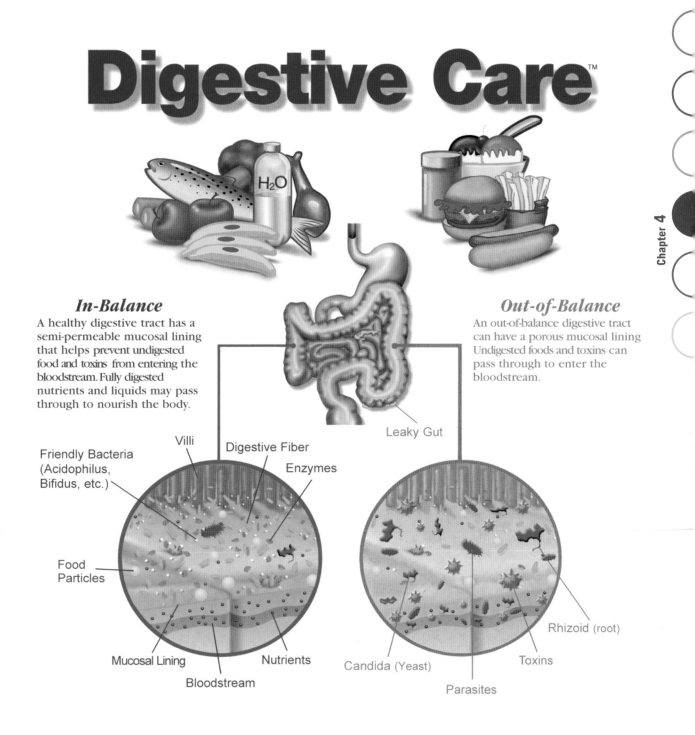

In-Balance

A healthy digestive tract has a semi-permeable mucosal lining that helps prevent undigested food and toxins from entering the bloodstream. Fully digested nutrients and liquids may pass through to nourish the body.

Out-of-Balance

An out-of-balance digestive tract can have a porous mucosal lining Undigested foods and toxins can pass through to enter the bloodstream.

Leaky Gut

Friendly Bacteria
(Acidophilus,
Bifidus, etc.)

Villi

Digestive Fiber

Enzymes

Food
Particles

Mucosal Lining

Bloodstream

Nutrients

Candida (Yeast)

Parasites

Toxins

Rhizoid (root)

H_2O

According to respected author and holistic healer, Elizabeth Lipski, MS, CNN, "NSAIDS can cause irritation and inflammation of the intestinal tract, leading to colitis and relapse of ulcerative colitis … (They) can cause bleeding and ulceration of the large intestine and may contribute to complications of diverticular disease."[1] Prolonged use of NSAIDS blocks the body's natural ability to repair the intestinal lining. Once endotoxins have eroded this membrane, it becomes permeable, rather than semi-permeable. (The "screen" on your "window" gets holes in it.) Now the toxins, pathogens and food particles, which would normally not be permitted to enter the system, literally leak into the bloodstream. The body then becomes confused and attacks these unwanted toxins, developing antibodies to fight them, as if they were foreign substances.

Who Gets it?
People of any age can have leaky gut syndrome. Those who regularly take any of the drugs listed above would very likely suffer from the syndrome, whether they've been diagnosed with it or not.

People with digestive problems (with or without symptoms) will probably have an underlying leaky gut condition, as will people who routinely use large amounts of alcohol and caffeine and those who eat a diet that is high in refined carbohydrates and chemical food additives, which is, unfortunately, the standard American diet.

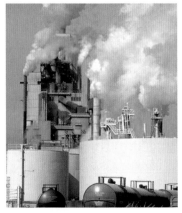

Anyone who has had significant toxic exposure may develop increased intestinal permeability – leaky gut. Gut-damaging toxins may come from pathogens, such as bacteria, parasites and fungi, or from chemicals and heavy metals in the environment (or in the mouth in the form of dental restorations).

Folks who have autoimmune diseases such as those listed below most likely have an underlying gut permeability problem, as well.

What are the Signs and Symptoms?
The net result of the leaky gut is development of autoimmune disease, where the body attacks its own tissues. There are some 80 recognized autoimmune diseases. These include:

- Lupus
- Rheumatoid arthritis
- Multiple sclerosis
- Fibromyalgia
- Sjogren's syndrome
- Thyroiditis
- Crohn's disease
- Urticaria (hives)
- Raynaud's disease
- Alopecia areata
- Polymyalgia rheumatica
- Chronic fatigue syndrome
- Vitiligo
- Vasculitis
- Ulcerative colitis
- Diabetes

Physicians are becoming increasingly aware of the importance of the GI tract in the development of autoimmune diseases, including allergies. In fact, researchers now estimate that more than two-thirds of all immune activity occurs in the gut.[2] Allergies can develop when the body produces antibodies to the undigested proteins derived from previously harmless foods. These antibodies can get into any tissue and trigger an inflammatory reaction when that food is eaten. According to Zoltan P. Rona, MD:

If this inflammation occurs in a joint, autoimmune arthritis (rheumatoid arthritis) develops. If it occurs in the brain, myalgic encephalomyelitis (a.k.a. chronic fatigue syndrome) may be the result. If it occurs in the blood vessels, vasculitis (inflammation of the blood vessels) is the resulting autoimmune problem. If the antibodies end up attacking the lining of the gut itself, the result may be colitis or Crohn's disease. If it occurs in the lungs, asthma is triggered on a delayed basis every time the individual consumes the food that triggered the production of the antibodies in the first place.[3]

Other disorders that are associated with leaky gut include eczema, psoriasis, pancreatic insufficiency, candidiasis and multiple chemical sensitivities. Leaky gut can aggravate existing conditions as well, for it can give rise to such symptoms as fatigue, joint pain, muscle pain, fever, abdominal discomfort, diarrhea, skin rashes, a toxic feeling, memory deficit and shortness of breath, among others.[4]

Leaky gut syndrome can also cause malabsorption and thus deficiencies of many important nutrients – vitamins, minerals and amino acids – due to inflammation and the presence of potent toxins. This malabsorption can also cause gas, bloating and cramps. It can eventually lead to such complaints as fatigue, headaches, memory loss, poor con-

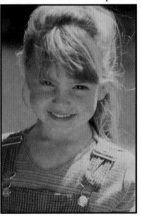

centration and irritability. The set of symptoms known collectively as irritable bowel syndrome (IBS) – bloating and gas after eating and alternating constipation and diarrhea – has also been linked to leaky gut syndrome, as has the more serious inflammatory bowel disease.

Leaky gut has been associated with such cognitive dysfunctions as autism in children. It has been found that some autistic children seem to react to the MMR [measles, mumps, rubella] vaccine with inflammation in the gut lining.[5] It is this inflammation that causes the gut to leak, allowing proteins such as gluten (from most grains) and casein (from milk) to enter the bloodstream, causing an allergic reaction to foods containing those proteins.

Once toxins enter the bloodstream through the leaky gut, their first stop is the liver. When the liver is called upon to work overtime, due to toxic overload, toxins either re-circulate or are deposited in the liver. When they re-circulate to the intestines, they further irritate the lining, increasing its permeability. The recirculation of toxins is medically known as entero-hepatic recirculation: Toxins go from liver to bile to intestines to the bloodstream and then back to the liver to start over. The food allergies that result from leaky gut create inflammation, which causes the gut to leak even more. So, once leaky gut develops, it tends to become progressively worse if measures aren't taken to correct it.

How is it Diagnosed?
The intestinal permeability assessment, which measures levels of mannitol and lactulose (two non-metabolized sugars), is described in the appendix.

What is the Standard Medical Treatment?
Since leaky guy syndrome is not an accepted medical diagnosis, there really is no standard medical treatment. The conventional medical doctor will focus upon treating conditions that arise from leaky gut syndrome – and that treatment will likely be through use of drugs and/or surgery. Those nutritionally oriented physicians familiar with leaky gut will take a different approach, described, at least in part, in the "Optional Nutritional Approaches" section.

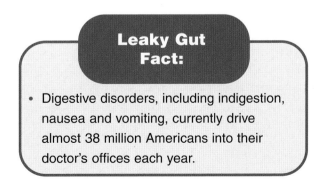

Leaky Gut Fact:

- Digestive disorders, including indigestion, nausea and vomiting, currently drive almost 38 million Americans into their doctor's offices each year.

Chapter 4

Optional Nutritional Approaches

Reducing toxic exposure is of prime importance in preventing and reversing leaky gut syndrome. Some toxins (called exotoxins) enter the body from the outside as the result of exposure to a polluted environment; others (endotoxins) are generated internally. These endotoxins can arise from poor digestion, which allows for adverse bacterial transformation of the undigested food. Digestion can be improved by thorough chewing, avoiding fluid intake with meals, combining foods properly (eat fruit alone, and don't mix protein foods with starchy carbohydrates), reducing stress, eliminating processed foods and eating moderate portions. Maintaining good elimination is also very important. Partially digested food staying in contact with the gut lining and bacteria for long periods of time will exacerbate the problem. Increased exposure will increase the likelihood of creating and delivering immune-reactive substances through the intestinal lining. These immune-reactive substances will be acted upon by the immune tissue in the gut and then sent to the liver for even more immune and detoxification responses that can be harmful.

Leaky gut is associated with a long and growing number of disorders, as stated. It is also the underlying issue in most of the conditions discussed in this section. The following protocols are already listed in most of the conditions in this book. If you have been diagnosed with one of those conditions, then follow that protocol; if not, and you think you have a leaky gut condition, follow the guidelines below:

TEST FOR LEAKY GUT
• Intestinal Permeability Assessment (see appendix)

DIET
Follow the Candida Diet in Chapter 4 (candidiasis) for one month. Then follow the Digestive Care Diet in the appendix.

SUPPLEMENTS
• A plant enzyme blend: This supplement should include protease (at least 20,000 H.U.T.), amylase and lipase, as well as papaya and bromelain. Other ingredients in this formula might include soothing herbs like marshmallow and slippery elm. Additionally, a good digestive enzyme formula would contain glutamine (an amino acid) and N-acetyl-glucosamine, which helps soothe an irritated mucosal lining.
• Take HCl/pepsin supplements before meals if stomach acid levels are low. Start with one capsule, and increase by one capsule daily with meals until symptoms are gone. (If you feel a burning sensation, back off to previous dose.) The supplement may contain other soothing ingredients like quercitin, bromelain, gamma oryzanol, L-glutamine and N-acetyl-glucosamine.

Select one of the two enzyme formulas described above to take with meals.

• Take a probiotic (good bacteria) supplement with multiple strains as a daily supplement. It should contain a minimum of two to six billion cultures. A prebiotic could be helpful (see appendix).
• Take EFAs (essential fatty acids) to lubricate the digestive tract. A combination of fish and flax (Omega-3) with borage oil (Omega-6) is good to reduce inflammation in the gastrointestinal tract. Absorption of the oils may be enhanced with the addition of lipase (a fat-digesting enzyme). Take three to six 1000 mg. capsules twice daily with food. Add extra fish oil capsules, three twice a day.
• Take 10,000 mg. to 20,000 mg. of L-glutamine powder with N-acetyl-glucosamine (NAG) and gamma oryzanol once daily on an empty stomach (see appendix).
• B complex (see appendix)

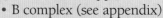

Essential Fatty Acids

Glutamine Powder

- Take antioxidant supplements (vitamin C - 500 mg. to 3000 mg., vitamin A - 5,000 I.U. daily, Vitamin E – 400 I.U. to 800 I.U. and zinc – 30 mg. to 60 mg. daily) after meals. Other antioxidants may also be taken with these. (See appendix for specification on antioxidants and vitamin C protocol.)

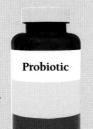

- Take a fiber supplement that provides a balance of both soluble and insoluble fibers. A flax/borage seed combination is a good choice, particularly one that contains other beneficial ingredients such as a probiotic blend with fructooligosaccharides (FOS) and herbs like slippery elm bark, marshmallow and fennel seed. Another key ingredient would be L-glutamine, which the intestine uses as fuel to regenerate. This fiber supplement may be added to juices and taken any time of day. When beginning to add dietary fiber to the diet, remember to go slowly, as this can cause some gas if added too quickly.

****Please note: If you have Candida and parasites, the supplements can be taken simultaneously. For example, you may follow the anti-fungal, anti-parasitic and leaky gut protocols at the same time.

LIFESTYLE
- Avoid or minimize the use of NSAIDS (aspirin, ibuprofen, etc.) and antibiotics.
- Avoid use of antacids.
- Reduce toxic exposure to chemicals. Clean up your environment, and eat organic food as much as possible.

COMPLEMETARY MIND/BODY THERAPIES
- Colon hydrotherapy
- Massage
- Yoga
- Biofeedback
- Music therapy
- Meditation

- Acupuncture
- Chiropractic

See appendix for information on the above therapies.

Dr. Smith's Comments
Increased intestinal permeability, whether it be intermittent or chronic, may be a major contributing factor to most diseases. It has been well established that there are at least four factors that can lead to increased permeability: 1) food allergies 2) malnutrition 3) dysbiosis (abnormal immune response to flora of low virulence or even normal flora) 4) hepatic stress. (Please go to www.mdheal.org by Leo Galland, MD, for further details). Maintaining a well nourished intestinal lining and overlying mucus, with beneficial bacteria from birth throughout life, is of paramount importance in controlling intestinal permeability. There is an excellent review article in the American Journal of Clinical Nutrition, *Oct 2003, pages 675-683. This is a hallmark description of how mucus is made by the intestinal lining, how it is the gel layer of the mucus that allows for bacterial adhesion, how there is cross-talk between the bacteria and intestinal lining and how these vibratory signals profoundly affect what type of immune response is elicited by the intestinal immune system. Suffice it to say that a balance of soluble and insoluble fiber, the right ratio of essential fatty acids, beneficial bacteria, digestive enzymes and supplements for building and maintaining the gut lining would be a very wise dietary choice for everyone to make on a regular basis.*

Chapter 4

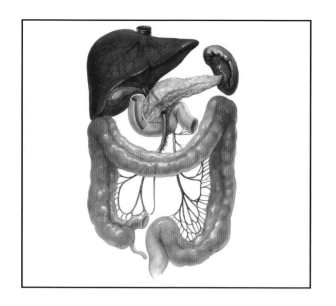

PARASITIC DISEASE
What is it?

A parasite is an organism that lives off another organism. Parasites living inside the human body will feed off our cells, our energy, off the food we eat, even off the supplements we take. Technically, parasites would include bacteria, viruses and fungi, as well as worms and protozoa (single-celled microscopic organisms). For our purposes, however, only worms and protozoa will be considered under the category of parasites. There are over 3,000 varieties of parasite,[1] and they all fall within one of four categories:[2]

- **Tapeworms (Cestoda)** – These large parasites generally reside in the intestinal tract and can grow up to 12 meters in length. The most common varieties are beef and pork tapeworms.
- **Roundworms (Nematoda)** – Also known as threadworms, these parasites range from 0.2 centimeters to 35 centimeters in length. They may reside in the intestinal tract or migrate into lymphatic vessels, the pancreas, heart, lungs, liver or body cavities.
- **Protozoa** – These microscopic single-celled parasites migrate through the bloodstream to all parts of the body.

- **Flukes (Trematoda)** – These parasites range in length from 1 to 2.5 centimeters. They generally travel through the tissues to the liver, kidneys, lungs or intestinal tract.

What Causes it?

Parasites are ubiquitous, which is to say they are everywhere. While precautions can be taken to avoid them, some degree of exposure is probable even when extreme care is taken to prevent parasitic infection. While everyone is exposed to parasites to some degree, not everyone will suffer equally from their ill effects.

What determines whether parasites will set up housekeeping in your body or pass harmlessly through it? While there are doubtlessly many factors at work here, the most important is your general health, specifically your degree of resistance or the strength of your immune system. This, in turn, depends heavily upon your exposure to toxins in the form of chemicals, heavy metals and electromagnetic fields. Some of the damaging chemicals to which we are often exposed include pesticides, personal care products, household cleaners, industrial wastes, solvents, drugs, etc. The threat of heavy metals, especially those used extensively in dentistry, such as mercury and nickel, represents another hidden, yet dangerous exposure to toxins. Finally, environmental toxins in the form of electromagnetic fields from household appliances, video display terminals, electric blankets, waterbed heaters, fluorescent lights, transformers, and numerous others can damage the body's systems. When the body is heavily burdened with these "primary toxins," the table is set for the arrival of the uninvited guest – the parasite, which may be considered a "secondary toxin." If the body is further weakened through poor diet, focal infection (walled-off areas of concentrated toxins and dead and/or infected tissue that can affect remote areas of the body), other disease processes or stress in any form, its resistance to parasitic infestation will be lowered further.

Nutritional deficiency appears to contribute to parasite infestations. Animals kept on diets deficient in protein or vitamins A, B1 and B2, biotin, folic acid or other nutrients have been infested with many types of parasites. When these same parasites have been repeatedly implanted in healthy animals, however, infestations have not occurred, as long as the diet has been adequate.[3] We see then that nutrition affects the internal environment of the body, which in turn plays a key role in determining whether parasites will pass through or set up housekeeping in the body.

Decreased output of enzymes by the pancreas and deficiency of hydrochloric acid (HCl) in the stomach are two factors that can predispose the body to parasitic infection.[4] Stomach acid is one of the body's first defenses against parasites, for in its presence, parasites are destroyed due to the extremely high acidity.

Parasites can enter the body through the mouth, through the nose or through the skin, including through the bottom of the feet. They can also be transmitted via "vectors," or insect carriers. Common sources of parasites include:

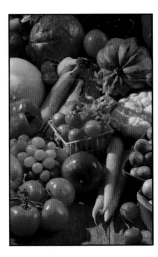

- Contaminated soil
- Contaminated fruits and vegetables
- Raw or rare meat
- Pets
- Mosquitoes
- Contact with feces (such as through day care centers)
- Polluted water/tap water
- Contact with someone who has parasites

Another factor that has contributed significantly to the growing parasite epidemic is the widespread use of drugs that suppress immunity as a side effect. Many of the drugs in common use today are immunosuppressive and therefore increase our susceptibility to parasitic infestation.

Although many external factors contribute to the parasite problem, by far the biggest factor is an internal one: a toxic colon. Colon toxicity is largely the result of an unwholesome lifestyle and resulting bacterial imbalance in the colon. Once the ideal ratio of good to bad bacteria in the colon (80%:20%) is disrupted, the resulting imbalance creates an environment conducive to parasite infestation. Factors that contribute to this imbalance include:

- Antibiotics
- Refined carbohydrates
- Steroid drugs
- Birth control pills
- X-rays/radiation therapy
- Chlorinated water
- Stress
- Low-fiber diet
- Pollution
- Poor digestion and elimination
- Mercury toxicity (often from 'silver' dental fillings)

These factors can also set the stage for overgrowth of the yeast germ Candida albicans. For this reason, Candida and parasites tend to appear together.

Who Gets it?

It's not just third world countries that have parasite problems or Americans who travel extensively, as many people believe. No one is immune from parasite infestation. It is a growing problem in industrialized nations, as recent studies show. Dr. Omar M. Amin of the Parasitology Center in Tempe, Arizona, completed a large parasite study in 2000. His study involved analysis of two fecal specimens from each of 2,896 patients throughout the United States. The type of analysis performed by Dr. Amin (the Proto-fix™– CONSED™ System) employed a new testing protocol, one which resulted in a significantly greater number of positive findings than

Chapter 4

had previously been obtained.[5] Dr. Amin found that 1/3 (32%) of the patients tested positive for parasites, showing one or more of 18 identified species.[6]

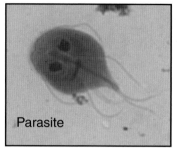

Parasite

While the parasite problem is widespread and growing, it often goes unrecognized. Because parasitic infestation has generally been considered a disease of the tropics, the typical MD is not likely to consider it when making a diagnosis, especially since parasitology is seldom presented in mainstream medical journals or medical schools. There are presently only three nationally reportable parasitic diseases: Cryptosporidiosis, malaria and trichinosis, and apart from the records kept by the Center for Disease Control (CDC) in the United States, there is little tracking for parasites in this country. With lack of information and little training, doctors aren't apt to look for parasites as an underlying cause of illness, which, in fact, they often are. That being the case, accurate statistics are not widely available with regard to parasitic infestation. Nonetheless, a growing number of holistic practitioners are concluding, based on their own clinical observations, that the parasite problem is epidemic in proportions – in developed, as well as in developing nations.

What are the Signs and Symptoms?
Medical texts don't have much to say about parasites other than stating that they can cause diarrhea and malabsorption. It is important to bear in mind, however, that parasites can mimic other disorders and/or produce no noticeable symptoms. When they DO cause symptoms, a wide range can be displayed. These can include:

• Diarrhea or constipation
• Digestive complaints (gas, bloating, cramps)

• Irritability/nervousness
• Persistent skin problems
• Granulomas (tumor-like masses that encase destroyed larva or parasites)
• Overall fatigue
• Disturbed sleep
• Muscle cramps
• Joint pain
• Post nasal drip
• Swollen glands
• Teeth grinding
• Prostatitis
• Sugar cravings
• Ravenous appetite (or loss of appetite)
• Weight loss (or gain)
• Headaches/neck aches/back aches
• Itchy anus or ears
• Dark circles under the eyes
• Light sensitivity
• Elevated eosinophils (white blood cells)
• Low-grade fever
• Nose picking
• Nail biting
• Brain fog
• Pain in the umbilicus
• Bedwetting
• Mucus in stools
• Foul-smelling stools
• Coughing
• Food and environmental sensitivities
• Depressed secretory IgA (an antibody)

Parasites can affect tissue anywhere in the body. Some of the disorders that have been associated with them include arthritis, appendicitis, recurrent yeast infections, allergies, asthma, bronchitis, anemia, irritable bowel syndrome, frequent colds and infections, lactase deficiency, fibromyalgia, gallbladder problems, malnutrition, urinary tract infections, prostatitis, and colitis.[7] Over time, a parasite infection can depress immunity and cause leaky gut syndrome (see previous section), which leads to nutritional absorption problems and has been associated with allergies and other autoimmune diseases.

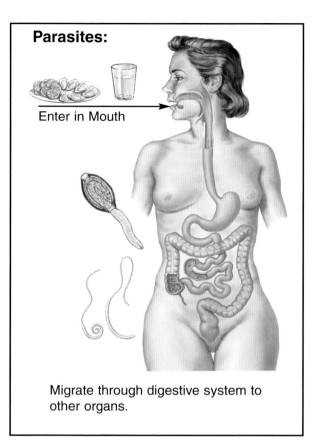

Parasites:

Enter in Mouth

Migrate through digestive system to other organs.

Because they can get into the blood and travel to any organ, parasites can cause problems that are often not recognized as parasite-related. This can result in an incorrect or incomplete diagnosis. For example, chronic infection with Giardia lamblia (giardiasis), considered the most common parasite to affect humans in the US, can be an undetected element or missing diagnosis in chronic fatigue syndrome; giardial infection can be mistaken for irritable bowel syndrome (IBS) or duodenal ulcer;[8] symptoms of the amoeba Entamoeba histolytica can mimic ulcerative colitis or IBS.[9]

Most people don't realize it, but it is not only parasites that can cause damage to the body but also the waste they give off. Giardia lamblia (a.k.a. "Montezuma's Revenge"), for example, invades the upper intestine and gives off toxins that damage enzymes (causing lactose intolerance when the lactase enzyme is damaged). Giardia is often found in mountain streams and in some city water systems, as it is not killed by chlorine. Cryptosporidium is another protozoan that has contaminated some city water supplies. It was the second most prevalent parasite found by Dr. Amin in his 2000 study. The first was Blastocystis hominis.

Interestingly, 1/3 of B. hominis infections were not associated with any symptoms in Dr. Amin's study.[10] Until recently, this disease-causing parasite was considered to be a harmless yeast. In 1967, it was reclassified as a protozoan and deemed a pathogen.[11] It is not unusual for parasites that were once considered harmless to be reclassified as pathogens. Dr. Amin found, in fact, that some protozoa considered as non-pathogenic unexpectedly caused symptoms in 73-100% of the cases studied.[12] This points to a continuing need to reassess the pathogenic potential of parasites.

The waste products from parasites poison the body, forcing the organs of elimination to work overtime and stressing the liver. As the detoxification mechanisms become overwhelmed, nutritional reserves are depleted, and the immune system weakens. The net result is disease development.

How is it Diagnosed?

A stool analysis is usually used to detect parasites. However, they can be difficult to detect since they tend to hide in the lining of the intestine and can live in other organs. If your parasites are in your heart or lungs, they will not show up in your stool regardless of how well it's analyzed. In fact, a single random solid stool sample analyzed in the traditional manner, is unlikely to even reveal the presence of intestinal parasites. Specialized testing (see appendix for laboratory information) is often needed to detect parasites that can be difficult to spot as they go through different stages of their life cycles. Some doctors use purged stool analysis, where the patient is given a laxative beforehand to liquefy the stool and loosen embedded parasites. Then multiple stool samples are submitted for analysis. Another approach is the rectal swab test, designed to detect those parasites that live in the

Chapter 4

mucous membranes that line the intestinal tract.

A "string test" has sometimes been used to detect parasites. Here the patient swallows a capsule that is attached to a string, one end of which is left outside of the mouth. After a few hours, the string is withdrawn and examined microscopically.[13] Another approach, though an invasive one, is to obtain a tissue specimen through a biopsy taken with an endoscope. This lighted, flexible tube is passed into the intestine where a tissue sample is removed through the rectum. Pinworms can be detected in a much more low-tech manner: a piece of tape attached to the anus can pick up these worms or their eggs, which can be detected with microscopic analysis. Blood tests can be used to reveal an elevated eosinophil count, a general indicator for an infection by parasites – except for giardia and amoeba, which rarely cause eosinophilia.[14] A specialized blood test, the ELISA, (see appendix) can be used to diagnose giardia and possibly other parasites. IgG and IgM antibody testing can be done for giardia and Entamoeba histolytica.[15] Other types of blood tests, sputum tests, urine tests and even radiologic tests can be used to detect various types of parasites with varying degrees of success. Analysis of aspirated fluids and the growth of tissue cultures may also be used.[16] Some holistic physicians may rely on various forms of bioenergetic testing to detect parasites.

Parasites have a complex life cycle. Three of the most prevalent parasites found in the United States and worldwide shed at irregular intervals. This means that the parasite might be in the stool two to four days a week but not the rest of the week. If the person is tested for the parasite on a day it is not present, there will be a negative test result. The person would then go untreated. Therefore, it would be best for repeat stool samples (at least two to three) to be taken on non-consecutive days. Also, tests are only available for 40 to 50 types of the 1000+ species of parasites that can live in the body.[17] In view of this situation, a negative lab test is no assurance that a person does not have parasites.

It is best to have parasite testing done by a laboratory, such as Dr. Amin's, that specializes in parasitology. While testing technique is constantly being modified and improved, false negatives still occur. We therefore cannot positively rule out parasites based on even the best lab results. Where we do have positive lab results, they can be very helpful in designing an effective treatment protocol.

What is the Standard Medical Treatment?

Parasites are both under-diagnosed and under-treated in standard medical circles simply because the average medical doctor is not aware of their prevalence. When parasites are detected, they are most often treated with drugs, usually Flagyl (metronidazole), despite its many adverse side effects and the fact that many parasites have become Flagyl-resistant.

Parasite Facts:

- Studies indicate that as much as 85% of the North American population has at least one form of parasite.

- Over time, parasites can be a contributing cause to chronic diseases such as arthritis, multiple sclerosis, asthma, edema, appendicitis and cancer.

- Mainstream medicine tends to overlook parasites as a possible primary cause for many well-known diseases, costing patients many frustrating hours and costing the health care systems many millions of dollars in unnecessary diagnostic tests and ineffective pharmaceutical treatments.

Optional Nutritional Approaches

Because it will not always be possible to identify the type of parasite you have or even to know with certainty that you do have parasites (given the limitations of the testing procedures), it is highly advisable to make a parasite/Candida cleanse a regular part of your natural digestive detoxification program.

Because Candida and parasites tend to travel together, it wise to treat for both simultaneously. This will require strict adherence to an anti-Candida diet, one that emphasizes organic vegetables and meat and excludes refined carbohydrates, sugar in all forms (including fruit) and fermented foods. All starchy carbohydrates, including whole grains, must be limited for a time. You'll want to adhere to this diet for the duration of your parasite cleanse, generally one to three months.

TEST FOR PARASITES
- Complete parasitology (see Proto-fix™ CONSED™ Parasite Test in appendix) -
  If you test positive for parasite, it would be advisable to be retested every year.

DIET
Follow the Candida Diet (chapter 4, candidiasis) for two weeks to one month before going to the Digestive Care Diet in the appendix. Try some of the juicing recipes, adding garlic and pumpkin seeds.

SUPPLEMENTS
The following program can have fewer side effects than prescription medications. Sometimes prescription medication is needed, and it is a good idea to have a health care practitioner's supervision when following the below protocol.

**A 30-day herbal detox would be advisable before starting a parasite program. A possible side effect of eradicating parasites is "die off" or Herxheimer reaction. This can produce an increase in original symptoms or a "flu-like feeling." When parasites are dying in the digestive tract, they give off toxins, and this may create symptoms. A 30-day herbal detox before a parasite program will give the colon and liver some cleansing. This prepares the body for the parasite program. It will also help in eliminating a die-off reaction once you start the parasite program.

The following should be taken for one to two months:

- A two-part cleansing formula that includes capsules and a liquid tincture that would include the following herbs:

- Black walnut (an extract made from the green rind of the hull; it should be in liquid form)
  – Wormwood
  – Garlic
  – Cloves
  – Undecylenic acid
  – Grapefruit seed extract
  – Pumpkin seed
  – Pippli
  – Quassia
  – Rosemary and thyme

Parasite Cleanse

It should be taken three times daily for 15 days, and then a five-day break, followed by another 15 days of use. This can be repeated two to three times. You can start the program at half-strength for the first few days to work into it slowly.

- Make sure you are eliminating from the colon at least one to two times per day. If you experience constipation, add a colon cleanse. Look for one containing herbs like cape aloe and rhubarb (that will gently stimulate peristalsis), as well as magnesium oxide to bring water to the bowel. Start with one capsule before bed, and increase by one capsule each night until bowel elimination occurs.
- Take HCl/pepsin supplements before meals if stomach acid levels are low. Start with one capsule, and increase by one capsule daily with

meals until symptoms are gone. (If you feel a burning sensation, back off to previous dose.) The supplement may contain other soothing ingredients like quercitin, bromelain, gamma oryzanol, L-glutamine and N-acetyl-glucosamine. Inadequate levels of HCl are quite common with parasite infections.

Proteolytic enzymes can also be taken on an empty stomach to help break down the wall of the parasite.

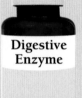

- An enzyme supplement that is high in protease to support the anti-fungal program and help break down the cell wall of the yeast, which is comprised of protein, fat, and chitin, should be taken. A good supplement would contain the following: 300,000 H.U.T. of protease, 112,500 C.U. of cellulase, 45,000 H.C.U. of hemicellulase, 22,500 mcg. lysozyme and 18,000 D.U. of amylase. It should also contain invertase, lactase, malt diatase and lipase. This should be taken before bed on an empty stomach.
- Take a fiber supplement that provides a balance of both soluble and insoluble fibers. A flax/borage seed combination is a good choice, particularly one that contains other beneficial ingredients such as a probiotic blend with fructooligosaccharides (FOS) and herbs like slippery elm bark, marshmallow and fennel seed. Another key ingredient would be L-glutamine, which the intestine uses as fuel to regenerate. This fiber supplement may be added to juices and taken any time of day. When beginning to add dietary fiber to the diet, remember to go slowly, as this can cause some gas if added too quickly.

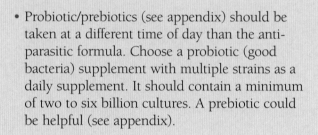

- Take EFAs (essential fatty acids) to lubricate the digestive tract. A combination of fish and flax (Omega-3) with borage oil (Omega-6) is good to reduce inflammation in the gastrointestinal tract. Absorption of the oils may be enhanced with the addition of lipase (a fat-digesting enzyme). Take three 1000 mg. capsules twice daily with food. Add extra fish oil capsules, three twice a day.

- Probiotic/prebiotics (see appendix) should be taken at a different time of day than the anti-parasitic formula. Choose a probiotic (good bacteria) supplement with multiple strains as a daily supplement. It should contain a minimum of two to six billion cultures. A prebiotic could be helpful (see appendix).

When you have finished the anti-parasitic program (one to two months), stay on the digestive enzymes, probiotic, fiber and EFA's from the above protocol, and add the following:

- Take 10,000 mg. to 20,000 mg. of L-glutamine powder with N-acetyl-glucosamine (NAG) and gamma oryzanol once daily on an empty stomach (see appendix).
- Take antioxidant supplements (vitamin C - 500 mg. to 3000 mg., vitamin A - 5,000 I.U. daily and zinc – 30 mg. to 60 mg. daily) after meals. Other antioxidants may also be taken with these (see appendix for specification on antioxidants).
- B complex (see appendix)

***If the anti-parasitic program does not seem to be working, you may need to use antibiotics.

***After finishing the anti-parasitic program, it would be beneficial to do a Liver Detoxification program (see appendix). Stay on the above supplement program while on the Liver Detox program.

LIFESTYLE

- Do not drink untreated tap water (filter or purify before drinking).
- Be careful when eating out at restaurants (avoid salads and other raw foods).
- Have separate cutting boards for meats/fish and fruits/vegetables.
- Have pets tested/treated for parasites.
- Keep pets away from food preparation areas.
- Don't kiss pets or allow them to lick you.
- Don't allow pets to sleep with you or your family – or at least confine them to the bottom of the bed.
- Wash bedding frequently if animals are allowed on the end of the bed.
- Don't allow pets to eat out of your dishes.
- Wear gloves and face mask when changing kitty litter box. Wash hands afterward. If immune-compromised, have someone else do the chore, if possible.
- Wash hands before eating.
- Wash hands after gardening.
- Wear gloves while gardening.
- Make sure meat is thoroughly cooked (no pink showing).
- Wash vegetables and fruits in a diluted hydrogen peroxide/vinegar bath.
- Freeze fish for 48 hours (beef and pork for 24 hours) before preparing. This will kill any parasite larvae.[18]
- Protect children from animal droppings (don't let them use sand boxes where these may be found).
- Wash hands after using the toilet.
- Wash hands after changing a baby's diaper.
- Keep your immune system in good shape (avoid sugar and commercial dairy products).
- Check for parasites regularly.
- Do a parasite cleanse once or twice yearly.
- Don't wipe kitchen counters with rags or sponges. Use disposable paper towels.

- Wash hands after handling raw meat.
- Don't eat raw meat and fish.
- Don't drink unfiltered water in foreign countries (or at home either!)
- Wash hands after touching pets.
- Take herbs, digestive enzymes and probiotics for at least a week prior to foreign travel.

COMPLEMENTARY MIND/BODY THERAPIES

- Colon hydrotherapy
- Acupuncture
- Massage
- Yoga
- Biofeedback
- Meditation/Prayer
- Chiropractic
- Music therapy

See appendix for information on the above therapies.

Chapter 4

General Recommendations For Intestinal Problems

The following is a summary of recommendations that are applicable for all the digestive conditions listed in this chapter

- Clean out your pantry, and restock with healthy foods.
- Learn to read labels.
- Buy and eat organic meats, fruits and vegetables as much as possible.
- Drink plenty of water a day (1/2 your body weight in ounces).
- Replace colas, diet sodas and sugary drinks with herbal teas.
- Drink an 8-ounce glass of water with lemon juice, to taste, each morning and night.
- Replace sugar with lohan or stevia. Never use artificial sweeteners.
- Make sure the oils you use are cold-pressed like olive, safflower, peanut, sesame, grapeseed or coconut. Use butter, not margarine.
- Wash all fruits and vegetables with a vegetable wash (from the health food store) or a 3% hydrogen peroxide solution.
- Soak nuts, seeds and beans overnight for better digestion.
- Chew, chew, chew your foods to mush.
- Reduce portion sizes, and eat smaller, more frequent meals.
- Use Celtic sea salt instead of table salt (see Resource Directory).

Supplements that should be taken on an ongoing basis for maintenance are:

- Digestive enzymes
- EFA's
- Probiotics
- Fiber

The above supplements ensure good digestive health once your digestive tract has healed.

- Do not become constipated. Have at least one bowel movement per day. Two to three is ideal.
- The lifestyle habits that negatively impact your digestive health and ultimately overall health and should be handled are:
  - Smoking
  - Overweight
  - Alcohol abuse
- Exercise frequently, and breathe deeply.
- Try some of the Complementary Mind/Body Therapies in this chapter.

The Health Continuum

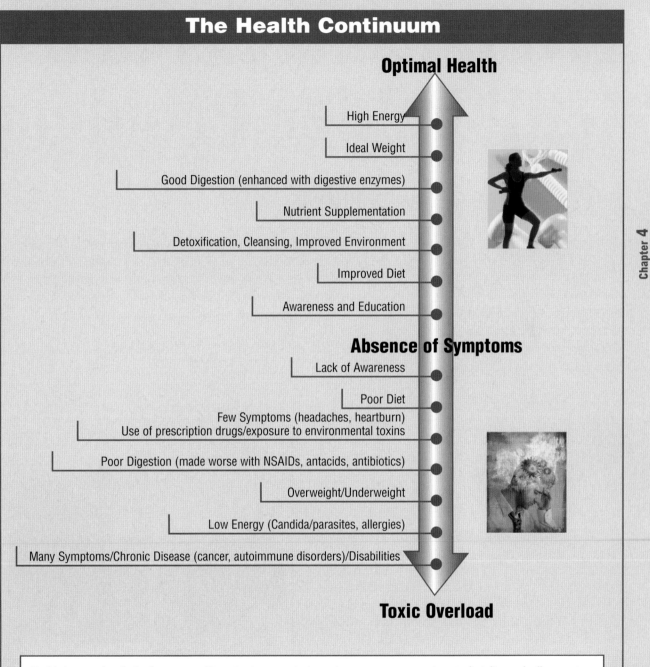

Optimal Health

High Energy

Ideal Weight

Good Digestion (enhanced with digestive enzymes)

Nutrient Supplementation

Detoxification, Cleansing, Improved Environment

Improved Diet

Awareness and Education

Absence of Symptoms

Lack of Awareness

Poor Diet

Few Symptoms (headaches, heartburn)
Use of prescription drugs/exposure to environmental toxins

Poor Digestion (made worse with NSAIDs, antacids, antibiotics)

Overweight/Underweight

Low Energy (Candida/parasites, allergies)

Many Symptoms/Chronic Disease (cancer, autoimmune disorders)/Disabilities

Toxic Overload

Chapter 4

Health is more than lack of symptoms. To maintain or regain it requires awareness, commitment, discipline and adherence to a proactive program emphasizing detoxification and rebuilding through diet and supplementation. The net result will be high levels of energy and a sense of well-being.

The road to chronic disease and disability, on the other hand, begins with lack of awareness, poor diet and symptom suppression through the use of pharmaceutical drugs. Here the stage is set for the development of digestive dysfunction, which increases the body's toxic load and depletes its energy. The net result is development of more and more symptoms, leading ultimately to degenerative disease.

Liver, Pancreas and Gallbladder Problems

The American Liver Foundation reports that more than 25 million people are afflicted with liver and gallbladder disease each year.

CIRRHOSIS
What is it?

Cirrhosis is a degenerative inflammatory disease in which fatty deposits and dense connective tissue build up in the liver causing hardening, drying and scarring of the organ, as well as reduction of blood supply to it. Cirrhosis is considered to be a permanent and irreversible condition.

What Causes it?

For years, alcohol abuse was the most common cause of cirrhosis in the United States. Recently though, hepatitis C (a viral disease) surpassed alcoholism as the major cause of this end-stage liver disease. Hepatitis B and D (also viral) can also lead to cirrhosis. Cirrhosis may result from other chronic diseases, such as congestive heart failure, advanced syphilis, parasitic flatworm infections,[1] cystic fibrosis and the genetic disorders hemochromatosis (excessive iron accumulation) and Wilson's disease (excessive accumulation of copper in the liver). Other inherited diseases that can lead to cirrhosis are alpha-1 antitrypsin deficiency (absence of a serum proteinase inhibitor), galactosemia (galactose metabolism disorder due to an

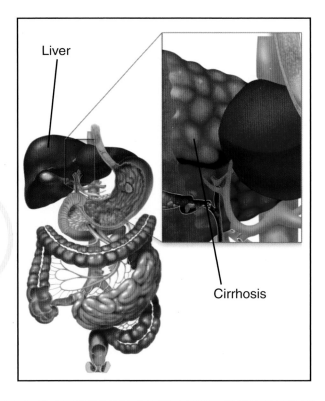

Liver

Cirrhosis

enzyme deficiency) and glycogen storage disease.[2] Toxic overload due to drug abuse (street, over-the-counter or prescription) and environmental chemicals (particularly solvents such as formaldehyde, toluene and trichloroethylene[3]) and ongoing exposure to heavy metals, particularly lead and nickel, can pave the way for cirrhosis.[4] Finally, cirrhosis may be the net result of physical injury to the liver, bile duct obstruction, chronic inflammation or malnutrition.

Drugs that can be particularly damaging to the liver include anti-convulsants, antihypertensive methyldopa, chlorpromazine, drugs used to treat tuberculosis and large amounts of acetamenophen (not toxic if taken as prescribed). These drugs are particularly dangerous if combined with alcohol.[5] Synthetic vitamins A and niacin can also damage the liver if taken in excessive amounts over a prolonged period of time.

A precursor to cirrhosis, steatosis or "fatty liver," characterized by a build up of fat in the liver cells without accompanying symptoms also occurs in association with toxic exposure and alcohol abuse. Diabetes and obesity may additionally contribute to fatty liver, which in turn leads to inflammation, cell death and fibrosis (formation of fibrous tissue).

Who Gets it?

In the year 2000, 26,219 people died in the United States as a result of cirrhosis and chronic liver disease.[6] Among these were people suffering from the disorders mentioned above.

Also at high risk for developing cirrhosis would be people whose exposure to heavy metals and environmental chemicals is high and constant. Those who have an occupational or other chronic exposure to solvents (see chart 1)[7] may be at particular risk for developing cirrhosis, especially if they are also heavy drinkers, because alcohol is also a solvent.

While cirrhosis commonly affects adults, often becoming a life-threatening problem in the fifth or

Sources of Solvents

Trichloroethylene (TCE)
- Photocopy machines
- Correction fluid
- Carpet cleaning solutions
- Floor polishes
- Surgical anesthesia

Toluene
- The food preservative BHT
- Tires
- Furniture wax
- Ink
- Kitty litter
- Guitar string cleaner
- Fragrances in perfumes
- Rug cleaning solutions
- Plastic garbage bags
- Hairspray and hair gel

Formaldehyde
- Paints
- Nail polish
- Pesticides
- Air fresheners
- Cleaning supplies
- Foam insulation
- Glues
- Fuels
- Plywood
- Plastics
- Textiles
- Paper products
- Antiperspirants
- Fertilizers
- Cosmetics
- Mattresses, couches, cushions
- Tobacco smoke
- Carpeting, carpet pads
- Ceiling tile
- Particle board

Chart 1

Chapter 5

sixth decades of life, in rare cases, infants may develop it as a result of biliary atresia, a condition in which the bile ducts are absent or injured.[8] Children can also be affected, frequently as a result of cystic fibrosis or other inherited disorders.

What are the Signs and Symptoms?

As serious as cirrhosis is, the early symptoms may be vague and mild. In fact, a full one-third of people with the disease have no clinical symptoms.[9] The diagnosis of cirrhosis is often made during the course of testing for other conditions or during surgery. Sometimes it's not discovered until an autopsy is done. As the disease progresses, symptoms become more severe. The list below starts off with early signs and symptoms, progressing into those found in late stages of cirrhosis:

- Fatigue
- Loss of appetite
- Nausea or vomiting
- Abdominal swelling
- Upset stomach
- Weakness
- Exhaustion
- Constipation or diarrhea
- Edema (build up of fluid in the legs resulting from the extra load placed on kidneys)
- Light-colored stools
- Indigestion
- Flatulence
- Extreme skin dryness
- Decreased libido
- Ascites (fluid accumulation in the peritoneal cavity)
- Red palms
- Enlarged liver
- Generalized itching (due to bile pigments that are deposited under the skin)
- Bruising (due to bleeding under the skin)
- Abnormal bleeding (due to vitamin K deficiency)
- Decreased albumin (blood protein) levels
- Spider angiomas (raised red dots from which small blood vessels radiate)
- Lowered platelet count
- Varicosities (in stomach, rectum esophagus)
- Jaundice (yellowed skin resulting from elevation of bilirubin, the yellow pigment the liver produces when it recycles worn out blood cells)
- Bright yellow or brown urine
- Anemia
- Gallstones (due to alterations in the bile from the primary condition causing cirrhosis)
- Varices (new blood vessels) in stomach and esophagus (formed when blood from intestines tries to find a way around the blocked liver
- Fever
- Testicular atrophy
- Gynecomastia (enlargement of the male breast)
- Loss of chest and armpit hair
- Psychotic mental changes (such as extreme paranoia) resulting from build up of toxins in the blood
- Facial veins
- Decreased absorption of glucose and vitamins
- Altered hormone production
- Portal hypertension (high blood pressure in the veins connecting the liver with the intestine and spleen)

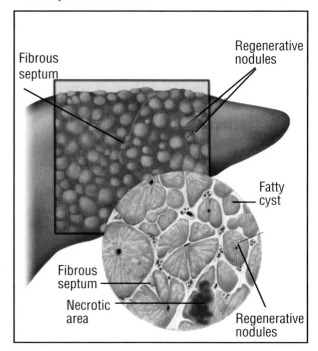

Fibrous septum

Regenerative nodules

Fatty cyst

Fibrous septum

Necrotic area

Regenerative nodules

If left untreated, cirrhosis can lead to such severe complications as gastrointestinal hemorrhage, ammonia toxicity, kidney failure, liver failure, hepatic coma and, ultimately, death.

Serious disorders associated with cirrhosis include insulin resistance, diabetes mellitus, kidney dysfunction, congestive heart failure, osteomalacia and osteoporosis. Those with cirrhosis have a higher incidence of liver and other cancers than those in the general population and are at risk for developing malnutrition, kidney disorders, stomach ulcers, diabetes mellitus and severe drug reactions.

Although cirrhosis is initially a silent disease (no symptoms), eventually symptoms do develop as a result of: (1) loss of functioning liver cells and (2) distortion of the liver by scarring. This scar tissue blocks the flow of blood through the liver. The loss of normal liver tissue slows the processing of nutrients, hormones, drugs and toxins, as well as the production of proteins and other substances by the liver.[10]

As liver cells die, production of the blood protein albumin decreases, leading to edema (water retention in cells or tissues) and ascites (fluid accumulation in the lining of the abdominal cavity), as well as a tendency to bruise and bleed easily (proteins are needed for blood clotting). Cirrhosis can also lead to the creation of varices. Varices are dialated veins that form in the stomach and esophagus when blood from the intestines tries to find a way around the blocked liver. These varices can burst, creating a life-threatening situation.

How is it Diagnosed?

The diagnosis of cirrhosis will entail the use of several diagnostic tests, in addition to a complete physical examination and thorough medical history. Diagnostic work-ups may include such blood tests as a complete blood count, liver enzymes, blood proteins, electrolytes and

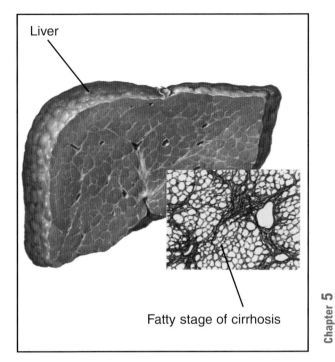

Liver

Fatty stage of cirrhosis

hepatitis B screening. Radiologic procedures could include computerized axial tomography (CAT scan), an ultrasound of the liver, gallbladder and bile ducts and an isotope vein injection study known as a liver/spleen scan. A more invasive study would be vascular imaging of the liver. In this study, a catheter is inserted into the femoral vessels and then passed into the hepatic artery and portal vein where dye is injected to study the alterations in the blood vessels caused by cirrhosis. A laproscopic exam, which involves inserting devices through tiny incisions in the abdomen, may also be done to obtain videos and biopsies of the liver. If esophageal varices are suspected, diagnostic endoscopy (see appendix) may be performed. This test involves inserting a narrow, flexible lighted tube through the mouth into the esophagus and looking for varices (dilated veins) in the esophagus, stomach and duodenum. Diagnosis of cirrhosis is ultimately confirmed through biopsy, which involves obtaining tissue samples by laproscopy or by inserting a needle through the skin into the liver with CAT scan localization of the area of biopsy.

What is the Standard Medical Treatment?

There is no cure for cirrhosis. Medical treatment is aimed at delaying or stopping progression of the disease, minimizing damage to liver cells and reducing complications. Where the cause of the cirrhosis is a known toxin, such as alcohol, removal of that toxin, can usually stop progression of the disease, and in time some degree of liver function may be restored. Where hepatitis is the underlying cause of the cirrhosis, the patient may be treated with steroids or antiviral drugs to reduce injury to liver cells. (See Crohn's disease section for information on the side effects of steroids.) Medications are also typically used to treat such symptoms as itching and water retention (edema and ascites), resulting from portal hypertension. To address the later problem, a salt-restricted diet may be imposed. If unsuccessful, diuretic drugs (like Lasix) may be employed. As a last resort, a shunt, using the patient's own veins, cadaver veins or prosthetic grafts, may be surgically implanted to divert blood flow from the portal vein to another blood vessel in an effort to take some of the pressure off the portal venous system and prevent variceal bleeding.

Reduced salt intake and diuretics may also be used to treat esophageal varices. Other treatment modalities – beta-blocking blood pressure medications and sclerotherapy (injection of a scarring chemical into the vein) may also be used to treat varices.

Elevated blood ammonia can be a serious complication resulting in coma. Lactulose, a synthetic sugar that is not absorbed by the body, has been used in some cirrhosis cases to assist in removal of ammonia from the blood.[11] Neomycin and other antibiotics have been used to decrease intestinal bacteria that produce ammonia.[12] Finally, a restriction of dietary protein may be used to decrease ammonia levels. Such a restriction will result in less toxin formation generally in the digestive tract. Where infections, such as spontaneous bacterial peritonitis develop, antibiotics are used. Immunosuppressive drugs, such as cyclosporine and methotrexate, have been used with cirrhosis patients in an effort to facilitate survival – but at a cost, as these drugs have serious side effects.

A generic drug called colchicine, which is used to treat gout, has also been used to improve liver function and survival in cirrhosis patients since it inhibits collagen (a protein in the body that makes up scar tissue).[13] This drug, however, carries with it serious gastrointestinal side effects. A drug with fewer side effects, which has been used to improve symptoms of cirrhosis, is Ursodiol, a gallstone-dissolving drug.

It is imperative that drugs that are metabolized in the liver (most are) be used with extreme caution in the cirrhosis patient, since detoxification of these drugs is extremely problematic. When the liver stops working, the only treatment option is liver transplant. The encouraging news here is that 80% of those patients receiving liver transplants are still alive five years after the transplant.[14]

Because no "wonder" drugs have been developed to treat cirrhosis and because all drugs can have devastating side effects, all viable natural alternatives should be considered in treatment of the cirrhosis patient, with an emphasis on nutritional supplementation.

Cirrhosis Fact:

- Over 27,000 Americans die from cirrhosis annually, making it the country's third leading cause of death for people between the ages of 25 and 59, and the seventh leading cause of death overall.

Optional Nutritional Approaches

DIET

- Follow the Digestive Care Diet in the appendix of this book. Incorporate as much raw food into your diet as possible. Juicing can be extremely beneficial in this disease. If you do not choose to do a two to three day juice fast, then try to incorporate juice into your daily diet. Green leafy vegetables and beets would be the best choice for juicing.
- You may need to watch protein (especially from animal sources) if ammonia levels are high. If you are having animal protein, limit it to small quantities of poultry and fish. If the liver is too damaged, it may not be able to handle fat-soluble vitamins, namely D, E, A and K except in small amounts Avoid cod liver oil, as well.
- Watch fats, especially fried foods, butter, margarine or hardened fats (such as shortening). Use only the cold-pressed oils listed in the appendix.
- A powdered hypoallergenic vegetable protein with added amino acids, enzymes, vitamins and antioxidants may be beneficial (see Resource Directory).
- Keep sugar, white flour products (such as packaged foods) out of your diet. Carbohydrate consumption should be in the form of vegetables and whole grains (see appendix).
- Do not overeat. Eat small meals more frequently.
- Do not consume alcohol (most important!).

SUPPLEMENTS

Cirrhosis of the liver is a degenerative inflammatory disease. In order to delay the progression of this disease and minimize liver cell damage, supplementation as well as diet (see above) can be very helpful. The recommended supplementation program for someone with cirrhosis can be overwhelming, to say the least, in terms of the number of supplements. See www.renewlife.com for a product that minimizes liver support supplements.

Do not become constipated. A 30-day herbal detox (see appendix) may be helpful. If you need to take something periodically for regularity, try a colon cleanse. Look for one containing herbs like cape aloe and rhubarb (that will gently stimulate peristalsis), as well as magnesium oxide to bring water to the bowel. Start with one capsule before bed, and increase by one capsule each night until bowel elimination occurs.

- Aloe vera, 5 ounces twice a day, could be helpful.
- A liver detox product (see appendix) could be beneficial after the 30-day herbal detox program. A person with cirrhosis could stay on this product indefinitely.

Along with the above program, the following should be added for digestive support:

- A plant enzyme blend: This supplement should include high potency protease (at least 100,000 H.U.T.), amylase and lipase, as well as papaya and bromelain.
- Take HCl/pepsin supplements before meals if stomach acid levels are low. Start with one capsule, and increase by one capsule daily with meals until symptoms are gone. (If you feel a burning sensation, back off to previous dose.) The supplement may contain other soothing ingredients like quercitin, bromelain, gamma oryzanol, L-glutamine and N-acetyl-glucosamine.

Select one of the two enzyme formulas described above, or a formula that includes both; take with meals.

- Take EFAs (essential fatty acids) to lubricate the digestive tract. A combination of fish and flax oils (Omega-3) with borage oil (Omega-6) is good to reduce inflammation in the gastrointestinal tract. Absorption of the oils may be enhanced with the addition of lipase (a fat-digesting enzyme). Take three to six 1000 mg. capsules twice daily with food.
- Take a fiber supplement that provides a balance of both soluble and insoluble fibers. A flax/

borage seed combination is a good choice, particularly one that contains other beneficial ingredients such as a probiotic blend with fructooligosaccharides (FOS) and herbs like slippery elm bark, marshmallow and fennel seed. Another key ingredient would be L-glutamine, which is a primary fuel the intestine uses to regenerate. This fiber supplement may be added to juices and taken any time of day. When beginning to add dietary fiber to the diet, remember to go slowly, as this can cause some gas if added too quickly.

- Take a probiotic (good bacteria) supplement with multiple strains as a daily supplement. It should contain a minimum of two to six billion cultures. A prebiotic could be helpful (see appendix).

The following supplement program includes vitamins, minerals, antioxidants, amino acids, herbs and mushrooms. See www.renewlife.com for specific product information. You may supplement extra if you choose:

Vitamins and minerals
- B complex, to include B1 (thiamine) - 500 mg.
- B2 (riboflavin) – 75 mg.
- B5 (pantothenic acid) – 1500 mg.
- B6 (pyridoxine) 200 mg. (Pyridoxal-5-phoshate, the activated B6, will be easier for the liver to utilize than pyridoxine.)
- B12 (sublingual) 5 mg. 1-2 times daily
- Folic acid - 800 mcg. -1600 mcg. daily
- Choline - 1500 mg. daily
- Vitamin C, at least 2,000 mg. – 3000 mg. daily (or follow protocol in appendix)
- Vitamin E (gamma tocopherol/tocotrienols) – 400 I.U. - 800 I.U. daily
- Selenium - 200 mcg. daily
- Zinc 60 mg. daily
- Trimethylglycine 500 mg. - 1000 mg. daily

Antioxidants
- COQ10 - 60 mg. daily
- NAC (N-acetyl-cysteine) – 600 mg. twice daily

- Phosphatidyl choline (from lecithin) - lecithin granules (1 tbsp three times daily with meals) or capsules 2400 mg. daily with meals
- Alpha lipoic acid – 400 mg. - 800 mg. daily

Amino Acids
- Branched chain amino acids can be helpful - valine –150 mg., isoleucine- 150 mg., leucine – 30 mg. Take 2-4 capsules daily between meals, with juice or before a meal.
- Glutamine, 10,000 mg.- 20,000 mg. daily. Take 10,000 mg. to 20,000 mg. of L-glutamine powder with N-acetyl-glucosamine (NAG) and gamma oryzanol once daily on an empty stomach (see appendix).
- Taurine - 1,000 mg.- 4,000 mg. daily
- L-arginine – 4000 mg. - 8, 000 mg. daily (best taken on empty stomach in divided doses)
- L-methonine 100 mg. - 500 mg. daily

Herbs
- Silymarin (from milk thistle) - 250 mg., up to 4 daily
- Artichoke extract (has properties similar to silymarin) – 300 mg. daily
- Tumeric (from curcumin) – 250 mg., up to 4 daily
- Green tea extract – 100 mg. - 400 mg. daily

Mushrooms
The following mushrooms have been shown to offer powerful immune support and could be beneficial in cirrhosis:

- Cordyceps
- Coriolus
- Maitake
- Reishi
- Shitake

LIFESTYLE
- Drugs (prescription and over-the-counter) can be stressful for the liver. Take with caution.
- Read all labels carefully.
- Try some type of exercise daily.

- Do not become constipated. Use the Life Step™ (see Resource Directory) for proper elimination posture.
- Do not smoke, and avoid second hand smoke.
- Clean up your environment, as all chemicals and toxins can affect liver function.

COMPLEMENTARY MIND/BODY THERAPIES

- Colon hydrotherapy is contraindicated with cirrhosis. Do not use.
- Acupuncture could be helpful in cirrhosis.
- Massage
- Yoga
- Biofeedback
- Meditation
- Music therapy
- Chiropractic

See appendix for information on the above therapies.

Dr. Smith's Comments

Cirrhosis is a process of ongoing deposition of collagen in the liver with resultant fibrosis or hardening of the liver. The serious clinical problems of cirrhosis are:

- *Seriously compromised liver function leading to liver failure and the need for liver transplant*

- *Creation of portal hypertension, which occurs when the fibrous scarring of the liver obstructs the flow of blood to and from the liver; when this happens, the inflowing blood to the liver from the abdominal organs must go through alternative venous routes around the liver in order to get back to the heart. These alternate veins can become dilated and actually rupture. This can be a serious cause of upper gastrointestinal bleeding. These veins are called varices, and they are usually located in the esophagus, stomach and duodenum. To stop the bleeding often requires endoscopy, or at times, surgery. The surgery either involves ligating (tying off) the bleeding veins or doing some type of shunt, which is a venous detour around the liver blockage. With advanced cirrhosis, it is unlikely that nutrition can reverse the situation, but it might slow it down.*

- *Ascites due to cirrhosis; this is the accumulation of a clear fluid in the abdomen, which can cause massive abdominal swelling. Such swelling pushes on the diaphragms and can compromise respiration and even affect blood flow through the kidneys. It is thought to be due to a portion of plasma exuding out of the veins resulting from the backpressure from the cirrhotic liver. It can be controlled sometimes with diuretics, but when severe, it is necessary to drain it with a needle or to surgically shunt it into a neck vein to return it to the heart.*

It is thought that cirrhosis is an ongoing inflammatory process. This inflammation can be due to ongoing viral infection, toxic exposure (often alcohol) and absorption of toxins from the gut, which can also lead to autoimmune liver disease. Whatever the cause, the inflammation creates an oxidative stress environment (excess free radical exposure). The oxidative process is thought to be one of the factors that promotes the deposition of collagen, which is one of the early steps leading to cirrhosis of the liver. Supporting evidence comes from Gastroenterology *[1997; 113: 106973]. This article showed in a small group of hepatitis C patients that vitamin E (d-alpha tocopherol), 1200 I.U. daily, prevented stellate cell activation and hepatic collagen production, both of which are important steps in hepatic fibrosis or cirrhosis.*

A wide variety of supplements may be helpful, including alpha lipoic acid, glutathione, silymarin, N-acetyl-cysteine, glycine, glutamine, selenium, B vitamins and vitamin C.

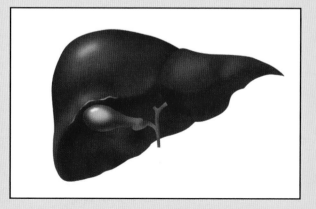

Chapter 5

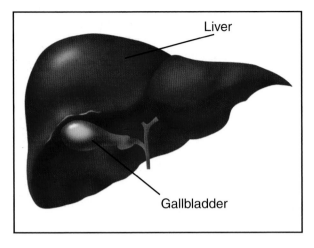

Liver

Gallbladder

GALLSTONES

What is it?

Gallstones are the most common digestive problem associated with the gallbladder. They can be solid, semi-solid or soft masses that are composed of one or more of the following: cholesterol, bile pigment (bilirubin), bile salts, inorganic minerals (usually calcium) and the phospholipid lecithin. Gallstones can range in size from as small as a grain of sand to as large as a golf ball. Very often they are the size of small pebbles. A person can have a single stone, dozens, or even hundreds.

When bile production, circulation or efficacy are compromised, gallstones can occur. The liver produces bile (a yellowish brown or green fluid), excretes toxins into it and then sends it to the gallbladder. It is the job of the gallbladder to hold that bile in storage until food enters the small intestine, at which time the gallbladder should contract, sending bile through the cystic and bile ducts into the duodenum (upper portion of the small intestine). At that time, the fat in the food can be broken down or emulsified. Bile also helps increase peristalsis and retard putrefaction.

There are two major types of stones, cholesterol stones and pigment stones. Cholesterol stones contain more than 70% cholesterol; some are pure cholesterol.[1] Pigment stones are made up of calcium and bilirubin, with a mucous protein core.[2]

What Causes it?

A number of factors appear to contribute to gallstone formation. Primary among them are:[3]

• Inherited body chemistry
• Body weight
• Gallbladder motility (movement)
• Diet

During the normal course of digestion, about 98% of the bile acids that are secreted from the liver and released by the gallbladder are reabsorbed in the ileum. When the ileum is impaired in its ability to reabsorb these bile acids, the bile acid pool is reduced, as is the rate of bile secretion. The net result is an increased risk of developing gallstones.

When the liver produces too much cholesterol or an insufficient quantity of bile salts, then cholesterol crystals can precipitate out of solution and form cholesterol stones.[4] Excess cholesterol in the bile can result from obesity or pregnancy, while a deficiency of bile salts can result from the use of bile salt binding drugs used to treat high cholesterol. A bile salt deficiency is also found in Crohn's disease, a serious gastrointestinal disorder usually affecting the ileum.

The risk of developing gallstones during pregnancy is elevated not just because of the added body weight but also due to increased estrogen levels. Women on birth control pills or hormone replacement therapy would therefore also be at greater risk of developing gallstones than women who were not on these therapies. Increased estrogen levels may increase cholesterol levels in the bile and decrease gallbladder movement.[5] Exposure to some environmental chemicals, such as pesticides, affects the body the same way that excessive estrogen does[6] and so could conceivably play a role in gallstone formation.

Cholesterol stone formation is accelerated if gallbladder contractions are sluggish, as they tend to be when there is too much cholesterol in the bile. This can happen after a person has undergone prolonged fasting or followed a very low-calorie diet. Some cholesterol-lowering drugs can also slow gallbladder contractions, causing incomplete emptying of bile.[7] Delayed emptying of the gallbladder gives cholesterol more opportunity to crystallize into stones.

The bilirubin found in pigment stones is created as part of the body's normal functioning, resulting from the following steps:

- The spleen removes worn out red blood cells from the bloodstream.
- These red blood cells release hemoglobin, a red pigment.
- Hemoglobin is converted to the yellow pigment bilirubin.
- Bilirubin is picked up by the liver and released into the bile.

Pigment stones can form when the body destroys too many red blood cells, a condition called hemolysis, present in hereditary blood disorders such as sickle cell anemia. Pigment stones can also result from alcoholic cirrhosis of the liver. In a cirrhotic liver, the bile cannot adequately dissolve cholesterol; the cholesterol then forms crystals, which settle to the bottom of the gallbladder and eventually become stones.[8] The risk of developing pigment stones is also increased in the patient who has had intestinal surgery.

Diet is less of an influence in pigment stones than in cholesterol stones. It is believed that low-fiber, high cholesterol diets (those high in animal fats) and diets high in starchy foods contribute to formation of cholesterol stones.[9] Over-consumption of fatty and fried foods and refined sugar, as well as inadequate intake of foods containing vitamins E, B and C, are also factors thought to contribute to gallstone formation.[10]

There appears to be a genetic component to gallstones, for they tend to run in families and are more common in some races than others. Parasitic infection can also play a role, for such infection

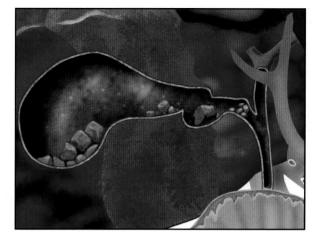

This is an illustration of gallstones.

can lead to a build up of calcium-based stones. Constipation is another condition that can set the stage for development of gallstones. Food allergies also appear to play a role, for allergenic foods may cause swelling of the bile ducts, resulting in impaired bile flow from the gallbladder.[11] Lack of exercise can also contribute to stone formation. In fact, physical activity can reduce the risk of stone formation by 20-40%.[12] Dehydration is another contributing factor. Adequate water intake is necessary to dilute toxins in the body.

The amount of stomach acid produced by the body seems to also play a role in gallstone formation, for stomach acid and fat stimulate the hormones that make the gallbladder contract. A deficiency in hydrochloric acid may impair gallbladder contraction and result in back up of bile.[13]

Once gallstones have formed, they can block the flow of bile from the liver and gallbladder. At times, they can obstruct the pancreas and intestine, as well, creating medical emergencies.

Who Gets it?

As Michael D. Gershon, MD, states, those most prone to biliary problems (problems related to bile and associated structures through which it flows, including gallstones) are people who can be

Chapter 5

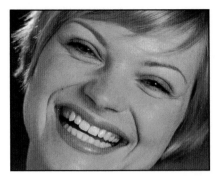

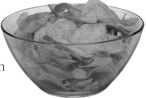

described by the four F's: fair, fat, female and forty.[14] Women are decidedly more prone to gallbladder formation (2 to 4 times more likely to be affected than men),[15] especially when pregnant, taking birth control pills or on hormone replacement therapy.

While gallstones can affect people of any age, the risk for developing them increases with age, especially as middle age approaches. It is believed that the majority of adults over sixty have gallstones,[16] though most will be unaware of it due to lack of symptoms. While more than 20 million Americans have gallstones, about 80% are asymptomatic (without symptoms).[17] Native Americans have the highest prevalence of gallstones in the U.S.; among the Pima Indians of the southwest, 85-90% of the women and 70-80% of the men have gallstones.[18] Mexican-Americans are another high-risk group.

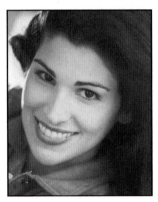

Other people who are at increased risk for developing gallstones are those who have gastrointestinal diseases (especially Crohn's disease and cystic fibrosis), those who are taking cholesterol-lowering drugs, those who eat a high-fat/high-sugar/low-fiber diet, those who have a very low or very high caloric intake and are overweight, those with biliary tract infections, those whose water intake is insufficient, those who lead a sedentary lifestyle, those with food allergies, people with low levels of stomach acid, those who are chronically constipated and those with parasitic infections.

While increased levels of cholesterol in the bile can cause formation of cholesterol gallstones, it is important to know that the level of cholesterol in the bile does not correlate with the total cholesterol in the blood. There does, however, appear to be an association between increased serum triglyceride levels and less soluble bile.[19]

What are the Signs and Symptoms?

Most people who have gallstones never have symptoms.[20] Early symptoms are characterized by incomplete fat digestion. When fat is not completely digested, bacteria in the colon act upon undigested portions of it, resulting in:

• Gas
• Pale stools
• Fatty stools that float
• Foul-smelling stools
• Abdominal distention and bloating
• Chronic belching

Once the stone begins to form, its radius increases at an average rate of 2.6 mm per year, eventually reaching a size of a few millimeters to over a centimeter. Symptoms occur an average of 8 years after formation of the stone begins.[21] The presence of stones creates a possibility that inflammation of the gallbladder (cholecystitis) may develop as a result of stones lodging in the cystic duct (connecting the gallbladder and small intestine), causing a backflow of bile. Serious symptoms may occur when stones become large enough to obstruct bile ducts. These may include:

• Pain in the upper right abdomen (may radiate to the right shoulder, to the back or to the area under the sternum and mimic a heart attack), especially after a fried or fatty meal or ingestion of fat-soluble vitamins – A, D, E and K

- Nausea and vomiting
- Malaise (feeling bad all over)
- Loss of appetite
- Constant itching (the result of bile salts entering the bloodstream)
- Chills, fever (due to infection)
- Jaundice (yellow coloration of skin and whites of the eyes)
- Brown or bright yellow urine
- Light or clay-colored stools
- Shaking
- Food intolerances
- Fatigue
- Headaches
- Anxiety, irritability

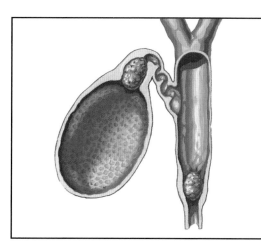

This is an illustration of gallstones in the bile duct.

Attacks of gallbladder pain can last anywhere from 20 minutes to several hours. Pain that occurs when a gallstone blocks the flow of bile from the gallbladder is referred to as biliary colic. Prolonged blockage of bile ducts can cause severe damage to the gallbladder, liver or pancreas and may even be fatal.[22]

How is it Diagnosed?
"Silent" gallstones (those causing no symptoms) are often detected during a diagnostic work up that is done for unrelated reasons. Gallstones may appear on abdominal x-ray, CT scan, MRI scan or abdominal ultrasound. Ultrasound is the diagnostic tool most frequently used to rule out gallstones when they are suspected. Ultrasound (or pulse-echo sonography) is a non-invasive, painless procedure that involves passing a probe externally over the abdomen. Sound waves are introduced into the body through this probe. If gallstones are present, the waves will bounce off of them, revealing their location via an image that appears on a monitor. Ultrasound will also help detect liver cysts, tumor blockage of bile ducts and pancreatic tumors and cysts. A hepatobiliary scan with an intravenous isotope, which is concentrated in the liver and excreted into the bile to be stored in the gallbladder, is an important functional test that can differentiate asymptomatic stones from those

stones blocking the ducts. If the test is positive, the gallbladder will not be seen on the imaging screen, as the isotope will not be able to enter the gallbladder due to cystic duct blockage. This is usually an indication for surgery for gallbladder removal. With a negative test, the gallbladder and bile ducts are well visualized, and the patient's gallstones may not be causing their problem.

Endoscopic ultrasound, where an ultrasound probe is built into the tip of an endoscope (flexible lighted tube inserted into GI tract), can be used to find small stones in the gallbladder and common bile duct that cannot be detected by conventional ultrasound.[23]

Gallstones cannot be diagnosed strictly on the basis of symptoms, for there are other conditions that can cause the same type of abdominal pain, as well as intolerance to fatty food. These can include irritable bowel syndrome (IBS), gastroesophageal reflux disease (GERD) and sphincter of Oddi dysfunction (a tight valve at the junction between the common bile duct and the duodenum).[24] Other conditions that can mimic gallbladder disease include ulcers (usually duodenal), antral gastritis and parasitic disease.[25] When gallbladder disease is suspected, the following should be ruled out: pancreatitis, duodenitis, gastritis and esophagitis[26] – all conditions involving inflammation. In addition, a cardiac evaluation with an ECG and cardiac enzymes may be indicated since heart problems can present as gallbladder disease.

Most conventional doctors are unaware of the role that food allergies or sensitivities can play in gallstone formation. Those who are aware of this relationship may order an ELISA test (see appendix) to detect these.

Those physicians who are aware of the role that low HCl levels may play in gallstones may order a Heidleburg test (see appendix) to measure levels of this important acid. Additionally, physicians usually order a liver function profile since elevation of liver enzymes is commonly an indicator of gallbladder problems.

What is the Standard Medical Treatment?

When stones are silent (causing no symptoms), no treatment is generally recommended, and unfortunately, all too often no lifestyle modifications are recommended to prevent future problems. Those problems can take the form of a gallbladder infection, which invariably will be treated with antibiotics. If the patient does not respond to antibiotic treatment and/or if the bile duct is blocked by gallstones, surgical removal of the gallbladder will most likely be the treatment of choice, due to the drawbacks inherent in other conventional treatments. These treatments include stone removal, widening of the sphincter between the end of the common bile duct and the intestine to allow easier passage of stones and use of drugs and other techniques to break up stones.[27]

Non-surgical approaches to gallstones are generally used for those patients who are unable to tolerate surgery. One such approach involves oral dissolution therapy using bile salts (chenodeoxycholic acid and ursodeoxycholic acid). Here medication that alters the composition of the bile is taken by mouth. The bile salts used in this approach promote increased cholesterol solubility.

While this is a desirable effect, there are drawbacks to oral bile salt therapy: It works only on cholesterol stones; it can have undesirable side effects, including mild diarrhea and possible liver damage; it is extremely slow-working, taking six months or more to dissolve stones; complete disappearance of stones happens only in a minority of cases; there is a tendency of stones to recur after dissolution; full-dose therapy must be continued indefinitely, or stones may re-form when the drug is discontinued.[28]

Contact dissolution is another non-surgical approach to treatment of gallstones. Here a chemical, methyl-tert-butyl ether (MTBE), is injected directly into the gallbladder through a catheter that is passed through the abdominal wall. The downside of this therapy is that the MTBE has an extremely unpleasant odor; it causes pain in the upper abdomen; it may cause nausea and vomiting; it may cause damage to the kidneys if it escapes from the gallbladder; recurrence of stones is possible.[29]

Extracorporeal shock-wave lithotripsy (ESWL) is another non-surgical treatment for gallstones. This is a non-invasive but expensive procedure involving the use of sound waves to break up stones. It only works for small cholesterol stones that are not calcified (less than 10% of the typical gallbladder cases seen in the U.S.), and no more than three stones can be treated at a time. Although this procedure has worked well in combination with bile salt therapy, there have been some associated side effects (biliary pain and some bleeding into the kidney).[30]

The non-surgical approaches described above are, according to the latest edition of the *Merck Manual* (the physician's guide to diagnosis and treatment), " … now largely unavailable owing to greater patient acceptance of laparoscopic cholecystomy."[31] Translation: Patients prefer to have their gallbladders removed!

Removal of the entire gallbladder to cure the gallstone problem may seem extreme, but the thinking is this: Simply removing the stones does no good; the abnormal bile would re-form them.[32] In addition, the damaged lining of the gallbladder tends to allow for recurrent stone formation. Medicine views the gallbladder as a dispensable organ. After all, certain animals (rats, horses, pigeons) get along without a gallbladder, as can most humans. A common temporary side effect can be diarrhea. This usually clears in one to two months as the liver and the intestines begin to compensate for having no gallbladder. About 1% of patients may have chronic diarrhea.

The type of cholecystectomy (gallbladder removal) most commonly done today is the laparoscopic variety introduced in 1988. This "keyhole surgery" involves entering the abdomen through the navel, with three additional small incisions made for the insertion of instruments and small video camera (attached to external monitor), used to guide the surgeon's movements. There are several advantages of laparoscopic over conventional "open" cholecystectomy, which involves a 5" to 8" incision and one week of hospitalization. These advantages include:

• Less pain
• Quicker healing
• Improved cosmetic results
• Fewer complications

The drawback of the laparoscopic method is that the surgeon is unable to explore the common bile duct for stones.

Open surgery is still used today for complex cases and when complications are encountered in the laparoscopic approach. With either surgery, complications are possible. These include:

• Injury to the common bile duct (which connects gallbladder to liver) – This is the most common complication; it can cause leakage of bile and/or infection, and may necessitate corrective surgery. Scarring of any part of the duct may lead to

obstruction, with repeated complex operations. Severe disability and even death can result if the problem is not completely corrected.
• Adhesions – Unnatural connection of body tissues.
• Stones leftover in the bile duct. This usually can be handled with endoscopic removal of the stones via the Ampulla of Vater (opening of the bile duct into the duodenum).
• Bile leakage from the gallbladder bed in the liver, which can cause subhepatic abscess formation requiring either radiologic or surgical drainage.
• A portion of the cystic duct (the "stump") left behind – When this happens, the stump may actually become a "mini-gallbladder" and form stones or contain some undiscovered ones.[33]

Gallstones Facts:

• Gallstones are very common. They occur in one out of five women by age 60, and they are half as common in men.
• Gallstones occur more commonly in older people and in people who are overweight or who lose weight suddenly.
• They also occur more frequently in women who have been exposed to higher amounts of the hormone estrogen over their lifetime by having multiple pregnancies, by taking birth-control pills or by taking hormone replacement after menopause.
• Eighty percent of people with gallstones have no symptoms and do not require treatment.
• Even when gallstone attacks subside on their own, the symptoms will return within a year 50% of the time.

Chapter 5

Optional Nutritional Approaches

Clearly at times there may be no alternative to gallbladder removal, depending on the individual case. In many instances, however, diet and lifestyle modification can play a key role in halting the growth of gallstones and reducing the frequency and severity of gallbladder attacks.

Most nutritionally-oriented physicians are aware that a high-fiber diet featuring whole grains, fruits and vegetables can reduce the amount of cholesterol in bile and the tendency to form stones, and that reduced fat intake (less meat and dairy products) means fewer gallbladder contractions and therefore fewer and less severe attacks. Such doctors would also advocate a low sugar diet based on the fact that several studies have indicated that people who eat a lot of sweets are more likely to develop gallstones.[34] This may be due to the fact that increased sugar entering the liver activates its conversion into triglycerides and then into cholesterol. The liver is the first line of defense against elevated blood sugar from the diet.

When gallstones are suspected, the following should be ruled out:

- Foods sensitivities - ELISA testing (see appendix)
- Low HCl in the stomach - Heidelberg test (see appendix). A simple test of low stomach acid is to take a hydrochloric acid capsule (500 mg. – 650 mg.) before a meal. Then, with each subsequent meal, add another capsule until you feel a burning sensation, then back off to the previous dose (see appendix).
- Parasites - See section on parasites.

Gallbladder disease is easier to prevent than to treat once it has developed.

Diet

Follow the Digestive Care Diet in the appendix of the book. A two to three day juice fast would be beneficial especially in cases of gallbladder inflammation (see appendix). Continue to include fresh juice in your diet daily.

The following could also be helpful:

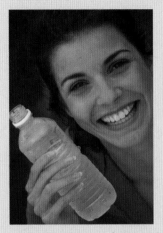

- Decrease coffee intake (coffee can induce gallbladder contractions)
- Reduce intake of sugar and refined carbohydrates, as this has been associated with gallstones.
- Don't skip breakfast (fasting longer than 14 hours elevates gallstone risk).
- Drink plenty of water (about half the body weight in ounces).
- Avoid spicy and fried foods.

Supplements

- A 30-day herbal detox (see appendix) could be helpful twice a year to cleanse the body. You'll want to keep a colon cleanse product on hand to prevent constipation. Look for one containing herbs like cape aloe and rhubarb (that will gently stimulate peristalsis), as well as magnesium oxide to bring water to the bowel. Start with one capsule before bed, and increase by one capsule each night until bowel elimination occurs.

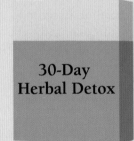

30-Day Herbal Detox

- Follow this up with a Liver Detox (see appendix) for 30 days. This product should contain two parts, one to be taken in the morning and the other at night. It should consist of cholagogues (to stimulate gallbladder contraction and

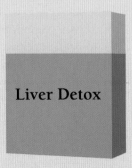

Liver Detox

promote bile flow), such as milk thistle (silymarin), dandelion, artichoke, celadine and curcumin.

Select one of the two digestive enzyme products listed below to take with meals. Choose the HCL formula if you suspect low stomach acid; otherwise, the plant enzyme blend would be a good choice:

• A HCl/protease/pepsin blend: This supplement should include HCL, 500 mg. – 650 mg. and 100,000 H.U.T. units of protease and pepsin 150 mg.
• A plant enzyme blend: This supplement should include high potency protease (at least 100,000 H.U.T.), amylase and lipase, as well as papaya and bromelain.

Other recommended supplements include:

• Take EFAs (essential fatty acids) to lubricate the digestive tract. A combination of fish and flax oils (Omega-3) with borage oil (Omega-6) is good to reduce inflammation in the gastrointestinal tract. Absorption of the oils may be enhanced with the addition of lipase (a fat-digesting enzyme). Take three to six 1000 mg. capsules twice daily with food. Add extra fish oil capsules, three twice a day.
• Fiber is extra important in the gallbladder disease, before or after gallbladder surgery. Take a fiber supplement that provides a balance of both soluble and insoluble fibers. A flax/borage seed combination is a good choice, particularly one that contains other beneficial ingredients such as a probiotic blend with fructooligosaccharides (FOS) and herbs like slippery elm bark, marshmallow and fennel seed. Another key ingredient would be L-glutamine, which the intestine uses as fuel to regenerate. This fiber supplement may be added to juices and taken any time of day. When beginning to add dietary fiber to the diet, remember to go slowly, as this can cause some gas if added too quickly.
• Lecithin (phosphytidyl choline) granules - 1 tablespoon three times daily, before meals, or capsules – 1200 mg. three times daily, before meals, or phosphytidyl choline supplement – 500 mg. daily
• B complex (see appendix) and at least 1,000 mg. of choline daily plus B12 (sublingual form)
• L- methionine - 1,000 mg. daily
• Taurine – 500 mg. to 1,000 mg. 2 to 3 times a day
• Vitamin C – 1,000 mg. to 3,000 mg. per day (or use protocol in appendix)
• Vitamin E – 200 I.U. - 400 I. U. per day
• Enteric-coated peppermint oil has been shown to cleanse the gallbladder. Take one to two capsules 3 times daily between meals.

A LIVER/GALLBLADDER FLUSH can be effective to flush out the liver and gallbladder ****If you have gallbladder disease, it is advisable to have a sonogram first (ultrasound). If there are stones present, and you choose to proceed with a flush, it is imperative that you seek the assistance of a knowledgeable health care practitioner. A practioner will explain the risk to benefit ratio. In addition, be prepared to have surgery or endoscopy if stones become lodged anywhere in the ductal system. This flush is good for liver detoxification, but caution should be used for those with gallbladder disease. The following is one of several versions of the liver/gallbladder flush:

Monday through Friday – Drink as much organic natural apple juice as possible. Eat normally. Continue to take your usual medications and/or supplements.

Saturday – Eat your lunch as usual. At about 3 p.m., drink one tablespoon Epsom salts in 1/4 cup warm water. Follow this with freshly squeezed grapefruit or orange juice to help improve elimination. At 5 p.m., repeat the process – Epsom salts and grapefruit or orange juice afterward, if desired. For dinner, eat citrus fruit or juices (freshly squeezed). Before bed, drink 1/2 cup cold-pressed extra virgin olive oil mixed with 1/2 cup lemon juice. In bed, lie on your right side, with knees pulled close to your chest, for half an hour.

Sunday morning –Upon rising (an hour before breakfast), take one tablespoon Epsom salts in warm water. This will help flush material out of the liver/gallbladder into the intestinal tract.

Please use caution and physician direction for the above flush, which can be done two to three times yearly.

Another effective way to detoxify the liver is through the use of COFFEE ENEMAS. The following are needed to prepare a coffee enema:

• A glass or enamel pot for boiling water
• Two quarts of filtered or purified water
• 4 tablespoons of ORGANIC coffee (ground, not instant)
• Enema bag
• Olive oil to lubricate tip of insertion tube

Prepare the coffee as follows:

• Fill pot with one quart of water.
• Bring water to a boil, and immediately turn off burner.
• Add coffee (4 T.).
• Steep coffee until water is lukewarm (105 to 118 degrees F).
• Pour one tablespoon to 1/2 cup of steeped coffee into enema bag.
• Add one quart of water to the enema bag.
• Save the remaining coffee in a glass container in the refrigerator for use at another time.

To take the enema, follow these steps:

• Hang the enema bag on towel rack, showerhead or shower curtain rod.
• Lubricate the tip of the insertion tube with olive oil.
• Insert tube gently into rectum.
• Lie on your right side.
• Inject and retain the coffee (or as much of it as you can comfortably retain) for 5-20 minutes.
• Sit on the toilet, and dispel contents of the enema.

IMPORTANT NOTE: Coffee enemas, while they may be helpful to the person with gallstones, are not intended to treat any specific condition but rather to assist the body with its natural processes of elimination and detoxification.

LIFESTYLE
• If overweight, lose weight slowly; no crash dieting.
• Avoid synthetic hormones.
• Chew foods to mush for the best digestion.
• Exercise daily to reduce risk of gallstones.

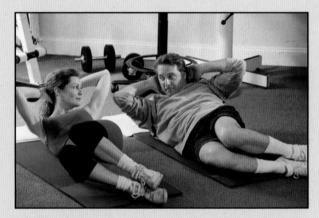

COMPLEMENTARY MIND/BODY THERAPIES
• Colon hydrotherapy could be helpful in cases of constipation and will assist in liver detoxification. Try it with the 30-day herbal detox program, liver detox program or with the liver/gallbladder flush.
• Acupuncture can be beneficial with gallbladder problems.
• Massage
• Yoga
• Biofeedback
• Meditation
• Chiropractic
• Music therapy

See appendix for information on the above therapies.

Dr Smith's Comments

I have seen many patients present with classical signs and symptoms of acute cholecystitis, namely right upper abdominal pain, with radiating pain under the right scapula (shoulder blade), nausea and vomiting, especially after a fatty meal, and yes, commonly with the four Fs: female, fair, fat, and forty and with gall-stones on ultrasound.

However, I would like to point out that there are many other possible presentations ranging from the signs and symptoms of a heart attack, to heartburn, indigestion, ulcers or even small bowel obstruction. In fact, gall-stone ileus is a condition whereby a large gallstone migrates through the wall of an inflamed gallbladder right through the wall of a piece of intestine adherent to the gallbladder. The large stone now in the intestine can cause a bowel obstruction, which often requires surgery unless it is small enough to pass.

Some patients have no symptoms and do not even have gallstones, but can be acutely and deathly ill from what is known as acalculus cholecystitis (without stones and an inflamed gallbladder). This is an extreme example of toxic or infected bile, which can be due to increased intestinal permeability (leaky gut).

Many hospital patients are not eating for various reasons and are on many medications, including antibiotics. This sets the stage for serious malnutrition of the intestinal lining. Most people are not aware that the intestinal lining feeds itself before any food is absorbed into the bloodstream. From the bloodstream and lymphatics, food is then taken to the liver for processing and detoxification if necessary.

In the presence of malnutrition, overgrowth of yeast and/or pathogenic bacteria (often as a result of antibiotics) and stress, there can be a pathologic increase in intestinal permeability. Viral and bacterial particles and toxins and poorly digested food remnants (especially in the colon) that have been sitting there for days can now go to the liver via the circulation.

When the liver is overwhelmed, some substances are detoxified but others get by untouched. In addition, if there is a shortage of sulfur-containing amino acids, the liver itself will take some toxins and convert them into new compounds that are even more toxic!

Thus, there can be highly toxic and/or infected bile that literally burns the liver, bile ducts and gallbladder. When the gallbladder stores this toxic material, it then starts destroying the wall of the gallbladder and is absorbed into the blood, creating a true surgical emergency. If the patient is too sick to be operated upon, radiology can place a drain in the gallbladder as a temporary treatment.

To make matters worse, the toxic bile enters the duodenum and begins a destructive path of inflammatory damage to the duodenum, pancreas and small intestine. This greatly exacerbates the original problem, in that the inflamed pancreas will not deliver needed enzymes, and the inflamed small intestine will be more damaged, allowing more toxins to leak through and creating a dangerous vicious cycle for the body.

The above example is indicative of how the intestine, liver, gallbladder and pancreas are all interconnected, not only in health but in disease as well.

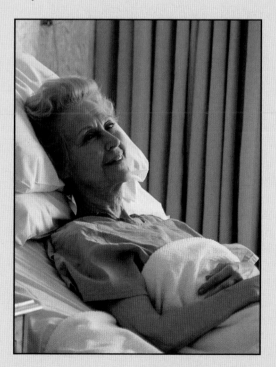

Chapter 5

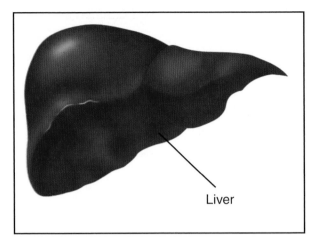

Liver

HEPATITIS

What is it?

Hepatitis is inflammation of the liver. There are many different types of hepatitis; each identified by what causes it. Viral hepatitis is the most prevalent type.

Hepatitis can also be defined in terms of the severity of the case, with three separate categories: acute (inflammation lasting less than six months), chronic (inflammation lasting more than six months) and fulminant – a particularly serious form of acute hepatitis associated with jaundice, coagulopathy (blood clotting dysfunction) and encephalopathy (brain dysfunction).[1]

What Causes it?

Although most cases of hepatitis are thought to be caused by viruses, other factors may also be involved: excessive use of alcohol, street drugs, some medications (both prescription and over-the-counter), injury to the liver and exposure to environmental toxins. Even environmental toxins absorbed through the skin can damage the liver. Chlorinated hydrocarbons and arsenic are examples of agents that are severely toxic to the liver. Obesity may also be a causative factor in hepatitis, for excess weight means excess fat deposited in the liver, causing inflammation (known as fatty liver hepatitis).[2]

One or more of seven specific viruses, listed alpha-

betically as hepatitis A through G, may attack the liver, causing hepatitis. Two other viruses, the transfusion-transmitted virus (TTV) and S.E.N –V (named for the person who isolated it) may also cause the disease. Indeed, other viruses that primarily target organs other than the liver may also attack the liver, causing inflammation. These include such viruses as Epstein-Barr, cytomegalovirus and herpes simplex.

Hepatitis D is a virus that only affects people who have hepatitis B. It is the least common but most serious of the hepatitis viruses. Hepatitis E, rarely found in the U.S., is similar to hepatitis A. Evidence for the existence of hepatitis F is at present only anecdotal. The last hepatitis virus to be discovered (in 1995) was hepatitis G. It does not appear to be a significant cause of acute or chronic hepatitis.[3] Yet another variety of the disease is autoimmune hepatitis, an uncommon liver disease that has the potential to lead to cirrhosis.[4] The cause of autoimmune hepatitis is unknown.

The three most common types of viral hepatitis are hepatitis A, B and C. (HAV, HBV, HCV). These will be the focus of discussion in the paragraphs that follow.

There are over 1,000 drugs and chemicals that can injure the liver, causing drug-induced hepatitis. Some of the major ones are Cimetidine (Tagamet), Cindamycin (Cleocin), Coumadin, Diazapam (Valium), Ibuprofen (Motrin), Metronidazole (Flagyl), Phenytoin (Dilantin), Salicylates (aspirin) and Tamoxifen.[5] Street drugs can also damage the liver, causing inflammation. Both cocaine and the amphetamine Ecstasy can cause acute hepatitis.[6] Use of intravenous and intranasal drugs has long been associated with the transmission of HBV and HCV. Cigarette smoking, while not a direct cause of hepatitis, can increase susceptibility to the liver-toxic effects of some drugs, such as those listed above. Smoking also decreases the liver's detoxification ability.

The only form of hepatitis that has a high rate of

transmission through sexual contact is hepatitis B. The information below shows how the three major hepatitis viruses can be spread:

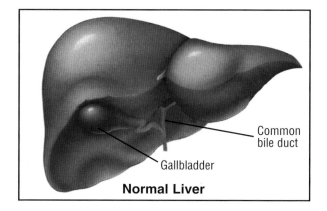

Normal Liver

Common bile duct

Gallbladder

Hepatitis A[7]

HAV is found in the stool of HAV-infected persons. HAV is usually spread from person to person by putting something in the mouth (even though it may be clean) that has been contaminated with the stool of a person with hepatitis A. This can happen when people don't wash their hands after using the toilet and then touch other people's food.

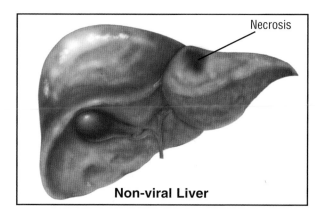

Necrosis

Non-viral Liver

Hepatitis B[7]

HBV is found in blood and certain body fluids. It is spread when blood or body fluid from an infected person enters the body of a person who is not immune. HBV is spread through having sex with an infected person without a condom, sharing needles or "works" when "shooting" drugs, needle-

sticks or sharps exposures on the job, or from an infected mother to her baby during birth. Exposure to blood in ANY situation can be a risk for transmission.

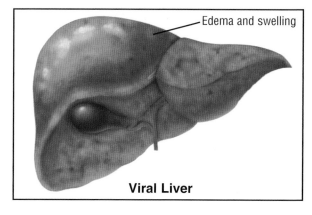

Edema and swelling

Viral Liver

Hepatitis C[7]

HCV is found in blood and certain body fluids. It is spread when blood or body fluids from an infected person enters another person's body. HCV is spread through sharing needles or "works" when "shooting" drugs, through needlesticks or sharps exposures on the job, or sometimes from an infected mother to her baby during birth. It is possible to transmit HCV from sex, but it is uncommon.

Both HCV and HBV (also known as "serum" hepatitis) can be transmitted via transfusion of contaminated blood, though improved screening of donated blood has decreased the incidence of this kind of transmission. HAV (infectious hepatitis), in addition to being transmitted through fecal contamination of food or water, can infect a person who has eaten raw shellfish from polluted waters.[8] Of the three major types of viral hepatitis, HCV is the most serious, since 85% of infections with this slowly progressive but ultimately devastating virus lead to chronic liver disease.[9]

While HBV and HCV can lead to chronic (long term) hepatitis, with HAV, there is no chronic infection, and once you've had the disease, you cannot get it again. Interestingly, low levels of stomach acid (hydrochloric acid – HCl) have been associated with chronic hepatitis.[10]

Chapter 5

Risk Factors Associated with the Three Major Hepatitis Viruses[11]

Hepatitis A

- Household contacts of infected persons
- Sex partners of infected persons
- Persons, especially children, living in regions of the US with consistently elevated rates of HAV during 1987-1997
- Persons traveling to countries where HAV is common (everywhere except Canada, Western Europe, Japan, Australia and New Zealand)
- Injecting and non-injecting drug users
- People eating food or drinking water that is infected with the virus

Hepatitis B

- Persons with more than one sex partner in a six-month period
- Persons diagnosed with a sexually transmitted disease
- Sex partners of infected persons
- Injecting drug users
- Household contacts of infected persons
- Infants born to infected mothers
- Infants/children of immigrants from areas with high HBV rates
- Health care and public safety workers who are exposed to blood
- Hemodialysis patients
- Persons who have hemophilia
- Persons traveling to areas where HBV is common
- Asian and Pacific Islanders (have highest rate of HBV)

Hepatitis C

- Injecting drug users
- Health care and public safety workers
- Recipients of clotting factors made before 1987
- Hemodialysis patients
- Recipients of blood/solid organs before 1992
- People with undiagnosed liver problems
- Infants born to infected mothers
- People having sex with an infected partner (possibly)
- Non-Hispanic African Americans (have highest rate of HCV)
- People who have received a tattoo or body piercing

Who Gets it?

People of any age may develop hepatitis, from birth to old age. The most common age of onset for HBV is between 15 and 24 years, while the HCV virus is generally activated after age 40.

Generally speaking, those at greatest risk for developing any type of hepatitis would be those with a weak immune system and heavy body burden of toxins from any source. Additionally, those with lowered levels of stomach acid would be at increased risk for developing chronic hepatitis. Since HCl levels tend to decline as we age, risk for developing the chronic form of the disease would tend to increase with age as well.

There may well be other, as yet unidentified, risk factors involved for each of the hepatitis viruses.

Vaccines are presently available for HAV and HBV but not for HCV. There is some controversy regarding the safety and efficacy of these vaccines, especially HBV, which is now a routine part of the recommended infant immunization program. The argument prevails that very few infants in the 0 to 1 age group are at risk for this rare blood-transmitted disease (just 0.001 percent in 1996), and yet, in that year, there were 1,080 total reports of adverse reactions to the vaccine in that age group, including 47 deaths.[12]

What are the Signs and Symptoms?

While some people with viral hepatitis have no symptoms, those who do, regardless of virus type, may experience any or all of the following:

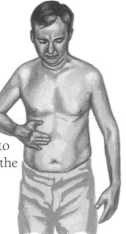

- Fever
- Weakness
- Nausea/vomiting
- Headache
- Muscle aches
- Fatigue
- Dark urine
- Light stools
- Jaundice (yellow pigment to the skin and whites of the eyes)
- Low levels of HCl
- Abdominal discomfort
- Elevated bilirubin (bile pigment) in the blood
- Flu-like symptoms (mild to severe)
- Joint aches/inflammation
- Diarrhea
- Itchy skin lesions
- Personality changes

Unlike HBV and HCV, the onset of HAV symptoms is sudden. Acute forms of HBV and HCV may develop into chronic forms, increasing the risk for liver failure and death from cirrhosis and liver cancer.

It is important to know that hepatitis causes some degree of liver damage, even in the absence of symptoms.

How is it Diagnosed?

Diagnosis of viral hepatitis may be made on the basis of symptoms and confirmed with blood tests that show an elevation of liver enzymes, such as SGPT, GGPT, SGOT and alkaline phosphatase, which leaks out into the blood when liver cells are damaged.[13] Another type of blood test is also used, one which shows the presence of viral antigens (compounds that are foreign to the body, resulting in formation of antibodies against them) or antibodies (chemical bullets) that bind antigens. Viral type (A, B, C, etc.) is identified on the basis of types of viral antigens or specific antibodies in the blood.

In addition to liver enzymes, hepatitis is monitored by counting viral particles. This is done by measuring the RNA of viral particles by a technique known as polymerase chain reaction. In the case of hepatitis C, the higher the level of HCV-RNA, the more aggressive the chronic infection.[14] As patients respond to treatment, their viral particle count measured by PCR drops lower and ideally to zero. A liver biopsy (where a piece of liver tissue is obtained with a needle) can be performed to confirm the diagnosis and identify the type and degree of damage.

What is the Standard Medical Treatment?

There is no cure for hepatitis. Treatment is aimed at protecting the liver and preventing further damage to it.

There is no treatment for hepatitis A beyond rest and fluid replacement and a nourishing diet as recovery progresses. Basically, the disease is left to run its course, giving the body supportive therapies only. Drugs would only tax the liver. Drug therapy is, however, used in treatment of both HBV and HCV in their chronic phase. Alpha-interferon and lamivudine are the two drugs licensed for the treatment of chronic hepatitis B, while interferon, pegylated interferon and ribavirin are licensed for treatment of chronic hepatitis C. Often drug combinations are used for treatment of HCV. Acute HBV and HCV are treated in the same manner as HCV, with rest and fluid replacement.

All hepatitis patients are advised to avoid alcohol. Strenuous exercise should also be avoided, as should liver-toxic drugs and chemicals. Additionally, special care should be taken with hygiene during the contagious phase of the disease (2 to 3 weeks prior to onset of symptoms up through 3 weeks after onset of symptoms). Contact with others should be avoided during this time. It is especially important not to share personal care items that may have blood on them, such as razors, toothbrushes and washcloths.

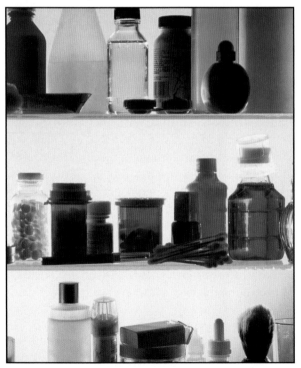

Hepatitis Facts:

- Up to 85% of those with hepatitis C, and a smaller number of those with hepatitis B, develop long-lasting (chronic) hepatitis. Some people with hepatitis B become lifelong "carriers" of the illness and can spread the hepatitis infection to others. Patients with chronic hepatitis C also are infectious, and can spread the virus through blood-to-blood contact.

- About 5% of adults who get hepatitis B will develop a long-lasting form of the disease. The rate is much higher for babies and young children. A small percentage of these patients eventually develop cirrhosis or liver cancer.

- Up to 80% of people infected with hepatitis C will develop chronic infection, and about 20 percent to 30 percent of these patients will develop cirrhosis or liver cancer.

- Since the early 1990s, improved techniques for screening donated blood have greatly reduced the risk of catching hepatitis B or C from blood transfusions. According to the U.S. National Institutes of Health, the current risk of catching Hepatitis C is one in 100,000 units of transfused blood.

- In the United States today, most infectious cases of hepatitis are caused by an infection with one of the hepatitis viruses (A, B, C, D or E).

Optional Nutritional Approaches

It is very important for persons with hepatitis to avoid liver toxicity. This requires the best possible diet, one that is organic and chemical-free. It is also of utmost importance to have bowel elimination daily, for if the bowel is toxic, it puts an extra burden on the liver. All alcohol should be avoided. The reduction of oxidative stress is the most important step, so antioxidant supplementation is suggested. As in all liver disease, it is important that the proper level of iron be maintained, as excess iron is toxic to the liver. Adherence to these principles is very important. Other nutritional suggestions include:

DIET

- Follow the Digestive Care Diet in the appendix of this book. Incorporate as much raw food into your diet as possible. Juicing can be extremely beneficial with any type of hepatitis. A two to three day juice fast is highly recommended, and then try to incorporate juice into your daily diet. Green leafy vegetables and beets would be the best choice for juicing.
- Watch for fats, especially fried foods, butter, margarine or hardened fats (such as shortening) Use only the cold pressed oils listed in the appendix.
- Keep sugar, white flour products (such as packaged foods) out of your diet. Carbohydrate consumption should be in the form of vegetables and whole grains (see appendix).
- Most important: Do not consume alcohol!

SUPPLEMENTS

- Do not become constipated. A 30-day herbal detox (see appendix) may be helpful. If you need to take something periodically for regularity, try a colon cleanse. Look for one containing herbs like cape aloe and rhubarb (that will gently stimulate peristalsis), as well as magnesium oxide to bring water to the bowel. Start with one capsule before bed, and increase by one capsule each night until bowel elimination occurs.

- A 30-day Liver Detox (see appendix) could be beneficial following the 30-day detox program. This Liver Detox product should contain two parts, one to be taken in the morning and the other at night. It should consist of cholagogues (to stimulate gallbladder contraction and promote bile flow), such as milk thistle (silymarin), dandelion, artichoke, celadine and curcumin. A person with hepatitis could stay on this product indefinitely.

As long as anemia is not present, lower iron levels as much as possible. The following will help with this (under physician supervision):

- One to two 100 mg. calcium citrate capsules with iron-containing food
- One 300 mg. capsule of lactoferrin (apolactoferrin form) three times a day.

- Take EFAs (essential fatty acids) to lubricate and nourish the lining of the digestive tract. A combination of fish and flax oils (Omega-3) with borage oil (Omega-6) is good to reduce inflammation in the gastrointestinal tract. Absorption of the oils may be enhanced with the addition of lipase (a fat-digesting enzyme). Take three to six 1000 mg. capsules twice daily with food. Add extra fish oil capsules, three twice a day.
- Take a fiber supplement that provides a balance of both soluble and insoluble fibers. A flax/borage seed combination is a good choice, particularly one that contains other beneficial ingredients such as a probiotic blend with fructooligosaccharides (FOS) and herbs like slippery elm bark, marshmallow and fennel seed. Another key ingredient would be L-glutamine, which the intestine uses as fuel to regenerate. This fiber supplement may be added to juices and taken any time of day. When beginning to add dietary fiber to the diet, remember to go slowly, as this can cause some gas if added too quickly.
- Take a probiotic (good bacteria) supplement

with multiple strains as a daily supplement. It should contain a minimum of two to six billion cultures. A prebiotic could be helpful (see appendix).

For digestive support, take one of the two enzyme products listed below with meals:

- A plant enzyme blend: This supplement should include protease (at least 20,000 H.U.T.), amylase and lipase, as well as papaya and bromelain. Other ingredients in this formula might include soothing herbs like marshmallow and slippery elm. Additionally, a good digestive enzyme formula would contain glutamine (an amino acid) and N-acetyl-glucosamine, which help nourish the gut lining and make the mucus that protects the intestinal lining.
- Take HCl/pepsin supplements before meals if stomach acid levels are low. Start with one capsule, and increase by one capsule daily with meals until symptoms are gone. (If you feel a burning sensation, back off to previous dose.) The supplement may contain other soothing ingredients like quercitin, bromelain, gamma oryzanol, L-glutamine and N-acetyl-glucosamine.

The following supplements support the immune system, help with oxidative stress and help to protect and restore liver function. For information on a product that combines all of the following, go to www.renewlife.com.

- Multivitamin/mineral (see appendix)
- Vitamin C - at least 2,000 mg. to 3000 mg. daily (or follow protocol in appendix)
- Vitamin E (gamma tocopherol/tocotrienols) – one to two daily
- Selenium - 200 mcg. daily
- Zinc - 60 mg. daily
- CoQ10 – 60 mg. daily
- NAC (N-acetyl-cysteine) – 600 mg. twice a day
- Phosphatidyl choline (from lecithin), lecithin granules (1 tbsp. three times daily with meals) or capsules, 2400 mg. daily with meals

- Alpha lipoic acid 400 mg. - 800 mg. daily
- Take 10,000 mg. - 20,000 mg. of L-glutamine powder with N-acetyl-glucosamine (NAG) and gamma oryzanol once daily on an empty stomach (see appendix).
- Taurine - 1,000 mg. to 4,000 mg. daily
- L-arginine – 500 mg. twice daily (best taken on empty stomach)
- L-methonine – 100 mg. to 500 mg. daily

The following herbs can be helpful:

- Garlic – 1000 mg. twice a day.
- Silymarin (from milk thistle) - 250 mg.; up to 4 daily
- Artichoke extract (has properties similar to silymarin) - 300 mg. daily
- Tumeric (from curcumin) – 250 mg.; up to 4 daily
- Green tea leaf - 30 mg. daily

The following mushrooms have been shown to offer powerful immune support and are beneficial to the liver:

- Cordyceps
- Maitake
- Shitake
- Coriolus
- Reishi

For specific product information on the above vitamins, minerals, antioxidants, herbs and mushrooms, see Resource Directory. The digestive supplements are necessary to support good digestion and the integrity of the digestive tract.

LIFESTYLE
- Drugs (prescription and over-the-counter) can be stressful for the liver. Take with caution.
- Read all labels carefully.
- Try some type of exercise daily.
- Do not become constipated - use the Life Step™ (see Resource Directory) for proper positioning during bowel elimination.
- Do not smoke, and avoid second hand smoke.
- Clean up your environment, as all chemical and toxin can affect liver function.

COMPLEMENTARY MIND/BODY THERAPIES

- Colon hydrotherapy - During the 30-day herbal detox it could be beneficial to do colon therapy if constipation occurs. Follow up with a maintenance program as recommended by your colon therapist.
- Acupuncture could be helpful in this condition.
- Massage therapy
- Yoga
- Chiropractic
- Biofeedback
- Meditation/Prayer
- Music therapy

See appendix for information on the above therapies.

Dr. Smith's Comments

As mentioned in the text, hepatitis is inflammation of the liver, which can come from many sources. The major causes of hepatitis are chemical toxicity, alcohol and viral illnesses. Nutritional supplements can be helpful in all of these areas.

I would like to share an example that relates to glutathione levels in white blood cells in hepatitis. There is an article entitled: "Antioxidant status and glutathione metabolism in peripheral blood mononuclear cells from patients with chronic hepatitis C." The investigators wanted to see what role oxidative stress could play in the pathogenesis of hepatitis C virus infection.

They investigated the oxidant/antioxidant status in peripheral blood mononuclear cells from patients with chronic hepatitis C and controls.

Lipid peroxidation products and superoxide dismutase activity in peripheral blood mononuclear cells were higher in chronic hepatitis C patients than in healthy subjects, while glutathione S-transferase activity was reduced in patients as compared to controls. (This is a selenium-dependent enzyme.)

In addition, 35% of patients with chronic hepatitis C, showed lower levels of glutathione and higher levels of oxidized glutathione than normal controls.

Conclusions: Oxidative stress is obs[...] blood mononuclear cells from [...] patients. This process might alter [...] and facilitate the chronicity of th[...]. Hepatology, Vol. 31 (5) (1999) pp. 808-8[...]

The above examples support the need for nutritional support in patients with chronic hepatitis B or C. As one can see looking at the last example, the oxidative stress and resulting glutathione depletion affects not only the liver but also the immune blood cells.

I think a complete nutritional and supplemental program as outlined in the text would certainly benefit the patient while they are receiving anti-viral therapy (Interferon and Ribavirin), and continued support after the viral count is down may help prevent relapse of the infection.

Two good tests to monitor would be the liver detoxification test, and the Comprehensive Digestive Stool Analysis (CDSA done by either Great Smokies Laboratory or Doctor's Data). The liver test demonstrates the liver's ability to detoxify caffeine, tylenol and aspirin (good indicator of overall detoxification capacity), and gives an idea of what nutrients may be needed. The CDSA would be a good indicator of any digestive problems showing up in the stool. This is important since whatever happens in the stool may indicate what is in store for the liver. Many people may not be aware that the liver takes the full burden of whatever is happening in the intestinal tract. Therefore, minimizing toxicity in the liver will help to restore and maintain liver function. This is clearly seen in Primary sclerosing cholangitis where up to 70% of the patients with this disorder have had IBD! It is usually ulcerative colitis, but if it is Crohn's it always involves the colon. This is compelling evidence of the colon and liver connection.

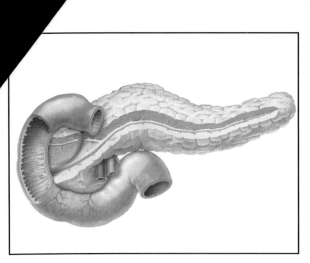

This is an illustration of a healthy pancreas.

PANCREATITIS

What is it?

The pancreas is a large gland located behind the stomach and close to the duodenum (upper portion of the small intestine). Pancreatitis is inflammation of this gland. When functioning properly, the pancreas secretes digestive enzymes (exocrine function) and releases the hormones glucagon and insulin that regulate blood sugar levels (endocrine function). Pancreatitis primarily affects the exocrine pancreas, but in severe chronic cases, the endrocrine pancreas may also be affected.

There are two types of pancreatitis: acute and chronic. The onset of symptoms is sudden in acute pancreatitis and, while the attack may be severe, even life-threatening, recovery is usually complete, without permanent damage to the pancreas. Chronic pancreatitis, on the other hand, involves continuous low-grade persistent inflammation and scarring of the gland, resulting in permanent damage and impaired pancreatic function.

The enzymes produced by the pancreas serve the purpose of breaking down food into its component parts – lipase breaks fat down into fatty acids; amylase breaks starch down into glucose and protease splits proteins into amino acids. These powerful digestive enzymes normally become active only within the opening (lumen) of the bowel, where they are sealed off from the rest of the body.[1] However, in pancreatitis, a process of autodigestion occurs as pancreatic enzymes are activated within the gland itself and leak out into adjacent tissue, causing severe tissue damage.

What Causes it?

Alcoholism, alcohol abuse, gallstones or other gallbladder disease are the major causes of pancreatitis. Gallstones can become lodged in the pancreatic duct, trapping digestive enzymes in the pancreas. The result is inflammation of the gland and leakage of enzymes from it. Over-consumption of alcohol can result in premature activation of pancreatic enzymes. Other causes and factors contributing to pancreatitis may include:

- Viral infection (hepatitis A or D, Epstein-Barr virus, mumps, coxsackie B, mycoplasma pneumonia, campylobacter)
- Hyperparathyroidism (metabolic disorder causing elevated levels of calcium in the blood)
- Hyperlipidemia (metabolic disorder involving high concentrations of fat circulating in the blood)
- Traumatic injury (or surgery) to the abdomen
- Excess iron in the blood[2]
- Hypothermia (accidental exposure to low temperatures)
- Kidney transplants
- Certain medications

Among the medications linked to pancreatitis are thiazide diuretics, antibiotics (sulfonamides, salazopyrine, tetracycline), high dose estrogens, corticosteroids, several immunosuppressive drugs, azathioprine, divalproex and the chemotherapy drug 6-MP.[3,4,5]

In children, pancreatitis may be associated with some of the factors listed above (mumps, abdominal trauma, viral illnesses and medications), as well as cystic fibrosis, hemolytic uremic syndrome, Kawasaki disease and Reye's syndrome.[6]

In some cases of pancreatitis, the cause is unknown.

Who Gets it?
Pancreatitis is most likely to affect alcoholics, people who abuse alcohol and people with gallstones and other gallbladder problems. Those suffering from the conditions listed above or taking the drugs listed above would also be at increased risk for developing the disease. Also at increased risk would be women with a history of several pregnancies and people who go on crash diets.[7]

Pancreatitis affects more men than women, presumably due to the fact that more men abuse alcohol. Onset of symptoms usually occurs between the ages of 30 and 40.[8] In some cases, the disease may be inherited.[9]

Unhealthy Pancreas

What are the Signs and Symptoms?
The most prominent symptom of acute pancreatitis is pain above the naval that may spread across the abdomen and to the back. The pain of acute pancreatitis often comes on suddenly and intensely, but it may be mild in the beginning and gradually increase in severity. It is usually worse when lying down or moving and tends to diminish upon sitting up and leaning forward.

Other symptoms of acute pancreatitis may include:

- Nausea/vomiting

- Fever
- Mild jaundice (yellow tint to skin and whites of the eyes)
- Fatty (clay-colored) stools
- Anxiety
- Chills
- Sweating
- Weakness
- Abdominal swelling/gas
- Increased pulse rate

The symptoms of pancreatitis are similar to those of pancreatic cancer, and indeed pancreatitis can lead to pancreatic cancer.

Symptoms of chronic pancreatitis are much the same as those of the acute variety, except for the fact that some level of pain tends to linger, interspersed with episodes of acute pain. In some rare cases of chronic pancreatitis, pain may be entirely absent. It is possible that pain may disappear as the condition advances and the pancreas loses its ability to make enzymes. Repeated episodes of gallbladder infection and gallstones are often involved in chronic pancreatitis.

Complications of acute pancreatitis may include the following:[10]

- Low blood pressure
- Heart failure
- Kidney failure
- ARDS (adult respiratory distress syndrome)
- Ascites (accumulation of fluid in the abdomen)
- Cysts or abscesses in the pancreas

Complications of chronic pancreatitis may include:[11]

- Obstruction of the small intestine or bile duct
- Pancreatic insufficiency, leading to diabetes (from damage to insulin-producing cells in pancreas)
- Fat malabsorption (and accompanying weight loss)
- Ascites

Chapter 5

- Pancreatic pseudocysts (fluid collections), which may become infected
- Blood clots in the splenic vein

Severe cases of pancreatitis can involve bleeding into the pancreas (leading to shock and sometimes death), dehydration, infection, cysts and serious tissue and organ damage as enzymes and toxins enter the bloodstream.

How is it Diagnosed?

Blood tests may be done to identify abnormal enzyme levels. Blood levels of the carbohydrate-digesting enzyme amylase may be elevated in pancreatitis as a result of leakage of the enzyme into the blood when the gland is inflamed. Blood levels of the fat-digesting enzyme lipase may likewise be elevated, while trypsinogen levels may be low. Pancreas function tests may be ordered to confirm the diagnosis of pancreatitis. Evidence of malabsorption may be found through a test for fecal fat. Changes in blood levels of calcium, magnesium, potassium, sodium and bicarbonate are typically seen with pancreatitis, as are elevated sugar and fat levels in the blood.

Abdominal x-rays, ultrasound or CAT scan may also be performed to provide images of the upper abdomen. These tests may show inflammation and swelling, as well as reveal gallstones and obstruction of bile flow if present.

A special endoscopic procedure called endoscopic retrograde cholangiopancreatography (ERCP) may also be used to put x-ray contrast dye into the bile and pancreas ducts via a long narrow tube, allowing the physician to view the extent of tissue damage in the pancreas and surrounding structures.

What is the Standard Medical Treatment?

An acute attack of pancreatitis will typically last only a few days unless gallstones are blocking ducts, in which case the gallbladder will likely be removed. The patient is typically hospitalized, and, in an effort to rest the pancreas, no food will be given by mouth for a few days in mild cases. Circulation will be supported with intravenous fluids. In severe cases, IV feeding may be necessary for three to six weeks while the pancreas heals.

Analgesics or nerve blocks will likely be used for pain relief rather than risk use of potentially addictive narcotics. High doses of pancreatic enzymes may also help control pain by reducing the secretion of juices from the pancreas. These exogenous enzymes will help rest the pancreas and also correct its underproduction of enzymes, assisting the body in digestion of food once a normal diet is resumed. Pancreatic extract may also be used in the long term. It can help correct greasy stools and weight loss resulting from underproduction of digestive enzymes and malabsorption of fat.

In severe cases, or if complications, such as infection, cysts, bleeding occur, surgical intervention may be necessary. Surgery will be necessary to drain the pancreatic duct or remove part of the pancreas if an obstruction is present. If diabetes has developed, blood sugar levels will be controlled with insulin.

Dietary and lifestyle modifications may be recommended. These would typically include:

- No alcohol
- No smoking
- Reduction of fat in the diet (It stimulates the pancreas.)
- Reduction of sugar in the diet
- Correction of underlying disorders (such as gallbladder disease and metabolic disorders)
- No large meals
- Use of digestive enzyme supplements

By adhering to the above recommendations, most patients with acute pancreatitis will be able to prevent it from becoming chronic. Additional measures, such as supplementation with antioxidant nutrients, may also assist toward this end. This and other alternatives are discussed on the following two pages.

Optional Nutritional Approaches

Pancreatitis can be a severe condition. If you develop symptoms of pancreatitis, consult a physician immediately. Since pancreatic conditions are closely associated with excessive alcohol consumption, abstinence from alcohol would be recommended. Pancreatitis can also be related to gallbladder problems, so refer to the entry on gallbladder in this section for those recommendations.

Diet

- A juice fast (see appendix) can be helpful for most organs under stress. Start with a two to three day juice fast. Begin the Digestive Care Diet in the appendix of this book.
- Stop all alcohol consumption.

Supplements

- If antibiotics have been prescribed, after you have finished taking them, a 30-day herbal detox (see appendix) could be helpful to detoxify the body.

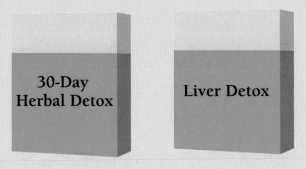

30-Day Herbal Detox   Liver Detox

- Follow up the 30-day herbal detox with a 30-day liver detox program (see appendix).
- Take digestive enzymes with each meal. Select a plant enzyme blend: This supplement should include high potency protease (at least 100,000 H.U.T.), amylase and lipase, as well as papaya and bromelain. Other ingredients in this formula might include soothing herbs like marshmallow and slippery elm. Additionally, a good digestive enzyme formula would contain glutamine (an amino acid) and N-acetyl-glucosamine, which helps soothe an irritated mucosal lining.

- Take EFAs (essential fatty acids) to lubricate the digestive tract. A combination of fish and flax oils (Omega-3) with borage oil (Omega-6) is good to reduce inflammation in the gastrointestinal tract. Absorption of the oils may be enhanced with the addition of lipase (a fat-digesting enzyme). Take three 1000 mg. capsules twice daily with food. Add extra fish oil capsules, three twice a day.
- Take a fiber supplement that provides a balance of both soluble and insoluble fibers. A flax/borage seed combination is a good choice, particularly one that contains other beneficial ingredients such as a probiotic blend with fructooligosaccharides (FOS) and herbs like slippery elm bark, marshmallow and fennel seed. Another key ingredient would be L-glutamine, which the intestine uses as fuel to regenerate. This fiber supplement may be added to juices and taken any time of day. When beginning to add dietary fiber to the diet, remember to go slowly, as this can cause some gas if added too quickly.
- Take a probiotic (good bacteria) supplement with multiple strains as a daily supplement. It should contain a minimum of two to six billion cultures. A prebiotic could be helpful (see appendix)
- Multivitamin and mineral (see appendix).
- Chromium picolinate - 300 mcg. to 600 mcg. daily.
- B complex (see appendix)
- Antioxidant supplement: Take vitamin C - 2,000 mg. to 3,000 mg. or follow protocol (see appendix), vitamin E – 400 I.U. to 800 I.U. daily, zinc – 30 mg. to 60 mg., vitamin A – 500 mg. daily.
- Calcium/magnesium supplement (See Resource Directory.)
- Take 5,000 mg. to 10,000 mg. of L-glutamine powder with N-acetyl-glucosamine (NAG) and gammma oryzanol once to twice daily on an empty stomach (see appendix).

Chapter 5

LIFESTYLE

- If you smoke, try to stop, and avoid second hand smoke.
- Exercise to help with stress.

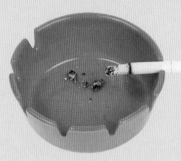

COMPLEMENTARY MIND/BODY THARAPIES

- Colon hydrotherapy could be helpful in eliminating toxins from the colon. Use it with the 30-day herbal detox and the liver detox protocols.
- Acupuncture could be beneficial in this condition when the inflammation has been reduced.
- Yoga
- Massage therapy
- Meditation/Prayer
- Biofeedback
- Chiropractic
- Music therapy

See appendix for information on the above therapies.

Dr. Smith's Comments

I have seen patients occasionally who have severe pancreatitis secondary to small gallstones that affect the flow of pancreatic juice when there is a common connection between the side of the bile duct and the end of the pancreatic duct. Usually patients recover within a few days and have the problem corrected with laporoscopic cholecyctectomy. In some cases, however, the pancreatitis can be severe and even lead to death. This is one reason to consider cholecystectomy if there are multiple small stones.

Some patients are very sensitive to alcohol consumption, which is probably the major cause of pancreatitis. In some of these cases, there are genetic defects that do not allow for the production of inhibitory proteins, which keep the pancreas from prematurely releasing its enzymes. This would be like having too sensitive of a

trigger on a gun. The inappropriate release of the enzymes can cause the pancreas to digest itself, a mild to fatal condition.

Autoimmune chronic pancreatitis has become an important clinical problem and is easily confused with pancreatic cancer. This misdiagnosis can lead to removal of part or the entire pancreas instead of medical treatment with anti-inflammatory steroids. This condition again can be due to auto-antibodies. Such antibodies are produced in response to unrecognized partially digested food or microbial products from leaky gut syndrome. It is these auto-antibodies that cross react with pancreatic tissue (which they view as foreign tissue) and cause major damage to the pancreatic cells and ducts.

Finally, chronic pancreatitis can be due to toxic bile washing into the pancreatic duct causing inflammation. It is easy to see, as mentioned before, that healing the "leaky gut" and liberal use of antioxidants and natural anti-inflammatories could be beneficial.

Pancreatitis Facts:

- The disease affects approximately 50,000 to 80,000 people in the United States each year, and is a common reason for people to be admitted to the hospital.

- In about 30% of cases, no cause can be found.

- Approximately 10% of patients with alcohol-related acute pancreatitis develop chronic pancreatitis.

- Pancreatitis caused by heavy drinking is likely to come back if drinking continues.

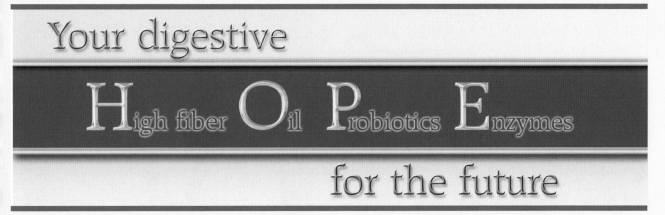

Your digestive

HOPE
High fiber **O**il **P**robiotics **E**nzymes

for the future

Today's health care consumers can be completely overwhelmed with all of the good options that are available to enhance health. So, to simplify the choices, we recommend seven options that are the foundation of nutritional health. HOPE AAA:

High-fiber diet – a balance of soluble and insoluble fiber

Oils – Essential fatty acids, predominantly Omega-3, with some Omega-6 and liberal use of extra virgin cold-pressed olive oil (Omega-9)

Probiotics – Several species of Lactobacilli and Bifidobacteria, several billion organisms per day, along with prebiotics (FOS and inulin) to support the bacteria

Enzymes – Plant-based enzymes to be taken with meals (especially with cooked foods) to assist in digestion of protein, fat and carbohydrates. This is especially important over age 50. Everyone is aware of a decline in his or her physical strength, endurance and libido with age, but many people do not know that their pancreatic, renal, liver and intestinal function declines as well.

Antioxidants - Free radical scavengers, vitamin A, vitamin C, vitamin E, selenium, zinc, glutathione, lipoic acid, to name a few (see appendix for details)

Anti-inflammatory compounds – Many herbs like Boswellia, curcumin, silymarin, dandelion, marshmallow, slippery elm and aloe have the ability to lower inflammation in the GI tract (as well as in the entire body).

Alkaline diet – At least 80% of everyone's diet should include vegetables, fruits, seeds, nuts and sprouted grains and legumes to create an alkaline mineral reserve in the body. If the first morning urine pH is lower than 6.5, it is a general indication that the body may be too acidic. This occurs with inadequate fluid intake and excess stress, as well as with a diet high in protein, animal fats, simple carbohydrates and excess sugars and sodas.

There is tremendous synergy when all seven of the above options are combined together to promote gastrointestinal health and thereby total body health. It is interesting to note that HOPE-AAA, through the consumption of organic, whole, raw, fermented and sprouted foods from vegetables, fruits, seeds, nuts, grains and legumes, has been the mainstay of the human diet since the beginning of recorded history. With the passage of time and processing of food, human taste preferences have changed, especially in industrial countries. Only a small percentage of the world's population is willing to choose raw, whole foods as the mainstay of their daily diet. Availability, sanitation, use of chemicals in farming and the prevalence of food preservatives, are important issues that now face us. This is due to the tremendous demand by society to have clean, convenient foods always available. As recently as 100 years ago, 90% of America's population produced most of their own food from gardens or small farms. Today, this number is under 10%.

Since our high-speed technological society does not appear to be interested in returning to a more individual-based agricultural society, supplementation has become a fact of life. Thus, fibers, oils, probiotics, digestive enzymes, antioxidants, and anti-inflammatories, all of which are critical for optimum health (especially with aging) can now be safely supplemented into our diets. But most important, is to choose a diet of whole organic foods whenever possible as mentioned above.

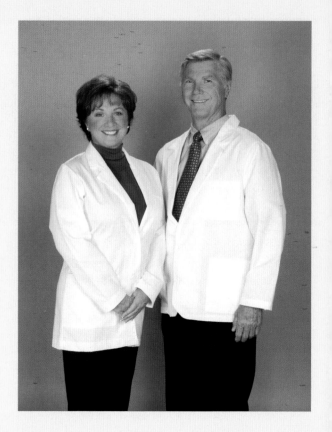

We have had the honor of working with many people with life-threatening illnesses who have chosen the road less traveled. They combined the organic whole food diet with the appropriate supplements and are still alive, and often are doing better than before they became ill! We call them health athletes. Many of them are now spending their lives helping others with similar problems.

One may wonder, why do we become sick? Illness is a wake up call! Usually it is the body's attempt to respond to problems that are out of balance due to improper nourishment of the body, mind and soul. To a large extent, this can be the case with all illnesses. Our concern should be to help the body by meeting its needs as presented in this book. Unfortunately, too many people spend their energy worrying about what is "out there" ready to jump on them, be it infection, arthritis or cancer. Today we have ready access to knowledge and products to help us make the necessary changes. Remember: health is a choice, not a God-given right. We hope we can continue to inspire you to make healthy choices for your life.

Sincerely,

Dr. Leonard Smith, M.D.
Brenda Watson, N.D.

Appendix

THE DIGESTIVE CARE DIET

BASELINE PRINCIPLES
The following dietary guidelines will greatly assist anyone, especially those who cannot tolerate wheat (gluten), dairy (casein), foods with high mold count, or those with Candida or an overgrowth of other fungi in the body, those with ulcerative conditions, gastritis or other digestive upsets. There are certain rules of thumb that should be followed and other factors to understand concerning the digestibility of certain foods, food combining and timing principles and what foods to consume as a standard fare, as well as what to eat when dining out.

Food Combining Principles – Basic food combining principles require the separation of protein foods from carbohydrate foods and the consumption of raw fruits by themselves. There are more strict rules of food combining, but these are the major problem combinations facing people in food choices. These rules can be easily followed without too many restrictions. But first it is vital to understand what proteins are and what carbohydrates are. Generally speaking, proteins are primarily foods that build body tissues, and carbohydrates are primarily involved in energy production.

Generally, proteins come from animals, and carbohydrates come from plants. So animal proteins are all flesh foods from beef to fish, eggs, fowl and dairy products, and plant proteins come from soy products, grass juices, plankton (spirulina and chlorella and other blue-green algae), nuts, seeds, sprouts and beans that are sprouted and cooked at low temperatures. Complex carbohydrates come from vegetables and grains. Wheat, oats, barley, rye, quinoa, amaranth, corn and rice are the most common grains. Processed grain products made from refined grains are considered simple carbohydrates; these include breads, pasta, bagels, cookies, muffins, cakes, tortillas, cereal, granola, etc. These and other simple carbohydrates (like fruit and sugar) are considered a health hazard when taken in excess due to their effect of raising blood sugar, triglycerides, cholesterol and insulin levels. Fruits are an important source of antioxidants, enzymes and minerals. If eaten in moderation, generally they do not raise blood sugar and insulin levels. The only reason to avoid fruits is in the case of intestinal dysbiosis or yeast overgrowth.

The reason these two food groups (proteins and carbohydrates) do not mix well is that their digestive enzymes require opposite pH ranges for digestion and tend to cancel each other out when mixed together. Usually our digestive systems can handle small amounts of these foods together, but not at the ratios and volumes of food that are often consumed. These indigestive bouts can create fermentation and putrefaction of undigested foods. Protein-digesting enzymes of the stomach (namely pepsin) require an acidic stomach environment in

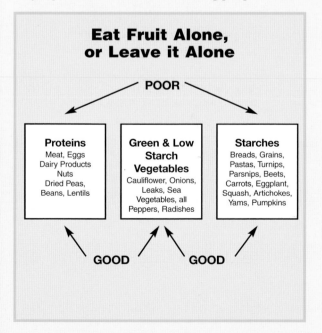

Eat Fruit Alone, or Leave it Alone

POOR

Proteins	Green & Low Starch Vegetables	Starches
Meat, Eggs Dairy Products Nuts Dried Peas, Beans, Lentils	Cauliflower, Onions, Leaks, Sea Vegetables, all Peppers, Radishes	Breads, Grains, Pastas, Turnips, Parsnips, Beets, Carrots, Eggplant, Squash, Artichokes, Yams, Pumpkins

GOOD   GOOD

order to function properly. Carbohydrate-digesting enzymes require more of an alkaline medium to function. But both groups are more easily digested when eaten with vegetables, especially raw. Raw vegetables provide both enzymes to help the whole process along, as well as much needed fiber.

FOOD TIMING PRINCIPLES

The digestive system can best digest a heavy meal, one of proteins and fats (with low-starch vegetables), early in the day, optimally between 7 a.m. and 2 p.m., while it does much better with lighter carbohydrate and vegetable meals later in the day from 2 p.m. 'till around 7 p.m. This allows the body plenty of time to do its digesting early and have the digestive tract clear to allow a restful sleep. Also, proteins are more acidic, and their stimulatory effect is more appropriate early in the day, for breakfast and lunch, whereas consuming more alkaline meals later prepares the body for sleep. Recall how you feel after a heavy starch/carbohydrate meal; you get sleepy. This alkaline reaction is following the body's natural chemistry, as the brain's chemistry of sleep requires a more alkaline body pH. And, as the body cleanses itself through the night, it naturally becomes more acidic by morning, and you wake up! Thus the cycle continues. But when we disrupt it through faulty food combinations and wrong food timing, we alter its natural digestive cycles. For example, when we eat fruit for breakfast we become too alkaline too early in the day, and this will usually trigger sleepiness too early, thus giving rise to sugar or caffeine cravings to stimulate us. Conversely, when we eat a heavy protein meal late, we become too acidic for that part of the body's circadian rhythm, and we do not get a restful sleep. On the other hand, food timing may not be critical if small food portions are eaten and differences in digestion are considered.

The 80% Rule – This is where you can occasionally eat a small amount of protein with a carbohydrate meal and vice versa, depending on the integrity of the digestive system. When you are experiencing symptoms, it is best to be stricter, and when stronger, give yourself a little leeway. For example, you could eat a whole small piece of sprouted grain toast with a morning vegetable omelet, or grate a small amount of Parmesan cheese on your pasta (providing you are okay with dairy and wheat) along with a garden salad. As long as the carbohydrate amount is under 20% of the meal, your body can compensate for these small amounts of improperly combined foods periodically. If you listen to your body, you will know what works best for you.

About Beans – Usually slightly challenging to digestion, as they are gassy, beans are best consumed one type at a time with as few other foods as possible to eliminate excess indigestion. Also, taking digestive enzymes high in amylase helps in their digestion. Soaking and washing beans before cooking eliminates enzyme inhibitors in the coat and makes for easier digestion. Sprouted beans similarly are much easier to digest.

About Gluten – This is the protein part of certain grains and is the problematic portion to certain individuals. It is found in wheat, rye, barley and oats. But it is definitely wheat that creates most of the problems for people's digestive tracts. This is partly because of the recent hybridization of wheat that has increased the gluten content of the grain at the expense of the more nutritive germ and fibrous vitamin B-rich bran layers. Gluten is responsible for making nice high-rising breads, gluey bagels and soft pancakes or pie crusts. This is the active sticky ingredient in wallpaper paste! It is also responsible for a host of digestive problems, mainly an immune over reaction in the small intestines. Gluten is found in many prepared foods, so read all labels, and watch out for burger substitutes (garden burgers, fake hotdogs and lunchmeats), as well as prepared soup bases.

About Soy – Another digestive challenge, soy, is not all that the current marketing campaigns would have you believe. Uncultured soy products are difficult to digest! These include texturized vegetable protein, isolated soy protein, soy protein isolates, soy flour, soy nuts, soy milk and the edamame bean. Soy that has been fermented or broken down by beneficial bacteria (similar to how cabbage becomes sauerkraut, or milk becomes yogurt) is the least challenging to people's digestion. These forms include tempeh, miso and, natto. Tofu is not cultured, but is precipitated into a curd from soymilk and is a more concentrated protein than other forms of soybean preparations; it can be better digested if eaten with vegetables, or eaten in soup broth.

About Dairy – Much depends on if you are lactose intolerant, your blood type (type B's and AB's usually do the best with dairy products) and if the dairy is cultured, as in yogurt, or if the product is raw or pasteurized, since pasteurization makes dairy products more difficult to digest. This applies to milk and cheese. It is almost impossible to buy raw milk, unless you know someone who raises goats or cows. Raw cheese, however, is available in health food stores. Usually people can digest feta, cottage and Ricotta cheeses better than other cheeses. But again, much depends on the other factors mentioned.

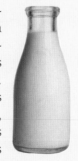

Gas-Producing Foods – Several vegetables, including mushrooms, broccoli, cabbage, cauliflower, Brussels sprouts, and other members of the Brassica family, along with certain fruits, (cherries and grapes) and beans, contain raffinose (long-chained polysaccharide molecules). When raffinose ferments in the digestive tract, it can cause

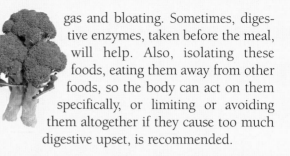

gas and bloating. Sometimes, digestive enzymes, taken before the meal, will help. Also, isolating these foods, eating them away from other foods, so the body can act on them specifically, or limiting or avoiding them altogether if they cause too much digestive upset, is recommended.

Necessary Fats – Eating fats and oils early in the day with protein meals is easier and more efficient than having them too late in the day or evening. Sautéing vegetables in olive oil or having oil in a salad dressing for dinner is OK, but heavy fatty meats or meals are better for breakfast and lunch. Also, make sure you avoid oils in clear bottles, and buy ones that are expeller or cold-pressed in opaque bottles to protect them from photon decay from ultraviolet light. Extra-virgin olive oil and coconut oil are two of the safest, most available oils in stores. Also Omega-3-containing oils, like flax, evening primrose, borage, pumpkin seed and hemp seed oils, as well as cold-water fish oils, are an important part of the optimum diet.

Slippery-wet Foods vs. Dry, dehydrated, fiberless foods – Avoid excessively cooked foods where much of the water is cooked out, and the fiber is broken down by the heat. Eat raw, fiber-rich foods as much as possible, and eat foods that are wet versus dry; for example, chips and toast are dry, where whole grains and vegetables are wet foods. Oatmeal is a better choice than dry cereal, and slippery flax seeds (when soaked in water), okra and aloe vera are all examples of slippery wet foods that assist in a healthy gut and good bowel movements.

For those with significant health challenges, food sensitivity testing should be a major consideration before beginning any diet. The simplest and least expensive diet would be one that consists only of vegetables, fish, chicken, turkey and olive oil. The following diet is a general guideline and is broader and more easily tolerated.

ONE WEEK MENU

Day 1

Breakfast

- Vegetable omelet (2-3 eggs – organic eggs are best – and 2-4 vegetables of choice, cooked in real butter, extra virgin olive oil, grape seed oil or coconut oil.
- 6 oz. organic yogurt or 2-4 oz. cottage cheese with 2-3 teaspoons flaxseed oil stirred in
- Sliced tomatoes or celery sticks or sweet red pepper slices

Lunch

- Poached, grilled or broiled salmon, mahi mahi, cod, haddock, grouper or tuna steak
- Garden salad with mixed greens (no or little iceberg lettuce), carrots, beets, celery, radish…
- Olive oil-based salad dressing with balsamic or apple cider vinegar, lemon juice, herbs…

Dinner

- Minestrone or vegetable soup
- 1-2 slices of sprouted bread* with organic butter
- Spinach salad with grated carrot, beets or tomato, toasted pine nuts, pan- or oven-roasted pineapple and olive oil and lemon. (Put pineapple in a hot skillet, and sear both sides for several minutes, or place in toasted oven to sear. This will make the fruit more compatible with the other foods in the meal.)

*If sensitive to wheat, use millet or rice bread.

Snack

- Rice ice-cream banana split (1 small banana, sliced; top with Rice Dream ice-cream substitute, a drizzle of raw honey, if desired, or rice syrup; sprinkle with a few carob or organic chocolate chips).

Day 2

Breakfast

- 2-3 poached or soft-boiled eggs
- 1/2-1 piece of sprouted grain toast (sprouted bread* is good) with
- Organic butter or almond butter
- 2-4 radishes or celery sticks with almond or peanut butter or cucumber slices

*If sensitive to wheat, use millet or rice bread.

Lunch

- Grilled or broiled chicken or turkey or a variety of vegetables (carrots, zucchini, yellow squash, beets, onions, cauliflower, mushrooms) Brush the tops with olive oil and lemon, if desired, and sprinkle with herbs like oregano, tarragon, thyme or basil, garlic or onion flakes.
- Coleslaw, mixed with grapeseed oil Vegannaise (available in the refrigerated section of health food stores), or use olive oil and cider vinegar or lemon juice, Celtic sea salt and pepper.
- Steamed vegetables (green beans, asparagus, zucchini, broccoli…) with butter, salt…
- Small bowl of onion or vegetable-based soup if desired

Dinner

- Stir-fry with brown rice or quinoa and 5 vegetables and 2 shrimps or scallops, if desired, (see "soaking and cooking grains"). Sauté onions, garlic and several vegetables together in sesame or olive oil while cooking rice. Broccoli, summer squash, carrots, bok choy, Chinese cabbage and ginger root are all good choices. Vegetables should be warmed through but not overcooked. Season with tamari soy sauce (available in health food stores).
- Cucumber-seaweed salad: Soak 1 small handful of arame seaweed in a bowl of water for 10 minutes. Meanwhile, slice one cup of cucumbers and squeeze out excess water. Drain arame and place arame and cucumbers in a bowl, and sprinkle with rice vinegar (1-3 tablespoons) and a few drops of toasted sesame oil (about 1-3 teaspoon).

Snack

- Sliced pineapple, mango or papaya, sprinkled with coconut flakes

ONE WEEK MENU (CONT.)

Day 3

Breakfast

- Scrambled tempeh – (Sauté 1/4 small onion, 1 rib celery in 1-3 T. olive oil; add 1/4 to 1/3 package of tempeh, crumbled over vegetables. Add 1/2 c. or more vegetables of choice: zucchini, Daikon radish, kale, tomato, grated carrots, mushrooms…Sauté a few minutes, stirring all. Add 1/4 c. water, 1-2 T. tamari soy sauce and 1/2 tsp. granulated garlic). Serve with:
- Sliced tomatoes, sweet red bell peppers or celery sticks with almond or peanut butter.
- 1/4 to 1/2 c. cottage cheese with 1-3 tsp. flax seed oil, or 16 oz. container organic yogurt.

Lunch

- Split pea or lentil soup
- Large garden salad with mixed greens and several vegetables; non-dairy dressing
- 1-2 pieces of manna bread,* plain or with organic butter, almond or cashew butter
*Avoid if wheat-sensitive.

Dinner

- Vegetarian chili - prepared or homemade. (Sauté 1/4 onion, 2 cloves garlic, 1-2 ribs celery and 1/2 bell pepper, in 2-3 T. olive oil for several minutes. While sautéing, add 1/2 tsp. cumin powder, 1 tsp. chili powder, 1/2 tsp. granulated garlic and pinch of salt. Then add 1 can pre-cooked kidney or black beans and 1 whole, fresh chopped tomato. Add a little water if too dry. Season to taste with Celtic sea salt and hot peppers, if you like.) Serve with brown rice or with organic corn chips.
- Dinner salad with Romaine lettuce and some of all the vegetables you added to the chili.

Snack

- Brown rice crackers and salsa

Day 4

Breakfast

- Scrambled eggs with sautéed onion, mushrooms, bell peppers and/or Swiss chard and grated raw milk cheese (substitute soy cheese if sensitive to dairy) on top just before serving. (Cheddar, jack or Swiss)
- 1/4 c. soaked flax seeds added to organic yogurt or kefir. (Soak 2-3 tablespoons flax seed overnight in 1/3 c. or so of water.)

Lunch

- Tuna nicoise salad – (Steam or lightly pan-sauté a fresh piece of tuna. Break into bite-sized pieces, and place on a bed of greens with olives, cucumbers, chopped parsley and scallions. Top with sliced tomatoes and dress with olive oil, lemon juice and Celtic sea salt.) Or make a simple tuna salad with a dolphin-safe canned tuna. Add chopped celery, onion, and tomato and either Vegannaise mayonnaise or olive oil and vinegar, salt and pepper.

Dinner

- Rice pasta or semolina pasta with vegetables. (Sauté several vegetables, onion, kale, garlic, zucchini in 2-3 T. olive oil; add several pinches of basil, oregano, Celtic sea salt and fresh lemon, lime or orange juice, to taste, or several chopped sun-dried tomatoes and a few pan-roasted pumpkin seeds or pine nuts. Also add a dollop of Vegannaise or sour cream for a creamier version. Optional: sprinkle with rice Parmesan cheese or a tiny bit of fresh grated Parmesan or asiago cheese.)
- Caesar salad: Crush a clove or two of garlic in the bottom of a salad bowl; add a pinch of sea salt, and crush well. Add a couple tablespoons of olive oil and stir. Then add fresh lemon juice (about 1/4 of a lemon), about 1/2 tsp. honey and 1 tsp. Vegannaise (for a creamy dressing - optional). Stir together, and add chopped Romaine and other vegetables of choice. Toss, and add rice Parmesan or a tiny bit of fresh-grated Parmesan or asiago cheese and black pepper, if desired.

Snack

- Fresh seasonal fruit or oatmeal with raisins and walnuts

ONE WEEK MENU (CONT.)

Day 5

Breakfast

- Scrambled tofu: Sauté together onion, celery or bok choy and mushrooms, bell pepper and kale in 2-3 T. olive oil or sesame oil with a pinch of sea salt. Then add 1/4 pound firm tofu, squished, 1 T. tamari soy sauce and 1-2 T. nutritional yeast. Warm through for 3-5 minutes.
- Sliced tomatoes or sweet red bell pepper or celery or bok choy with almond, cashew, hazelnut or peanut butter.

Lunch

- Large Greek-type salad without the potato salad, but with feta cheese on top. Substitute Romaine for the iceberg lettuce; olive oil and vinegar dressing with oregano.
- Sliced turkey breast on salad or 1-2 hard boiled eggs or baked tofu or tempeh strips (slice tofu or tempeh into finger-sized slices, and sprinkle with olive oil, tamari soy sauce, and drizzle with honey, or use a pre-pared Teriyaki sauce, Szechuan sauce, BBQ sauce or a Thai-peanut sauce to coat the fingers. Bake in toaster or regular oven 12-15 minutes. You can pre-make these for several days, and use several different sauces for variety.)
- Clear-based soup, chowder or stew

Dinner

- Mexican tortillas, tacos or burritos - black or pinto beans (canned or home-cooked), shredded Romaine lettuce, shredded cabbage, chopped fresh tomatoes, onions, avocado, and grated raw milk cheese, if desired (small amount). Warm shells if using tortilla or taco shells, according to directions, to crisp. Warm burrito wrappers, and place filling ingredients on each; top with fresh or favorite salsa.

Snack

- Sprouted bread or millet or rice bread with organic fruit juice-sweetened jam

Day 6

Breakfast

- Power shake – 12 oz. almond milk or fresh vegetable juice. Place in blender; add 1 organic egg (raw), 1-2 T. flaxseed oil or flax oil blend, or take several flaxseed oil perles, 2-3 T. favorite greens powder, 1-2 .T flax powder, 1 scoop of a glutamine-rich intestinal lining builder (see Resource Directory) (**Optional: 1 T. organic coconut oil (to help with Candida), 1/2 tsp. vanilla, almond or peppermint extract, 2-4 oz. organic yogurt or kefir, 1-2 T. whey. Blend, and enjoy.

Lunch

- Baked chicken or turkey breast or favorite fish and vegetables – Place in a bread pan or casserole dish with water or stock, olive oil, herbs, spices, sea salt, covered, until done. Add chopped veggies of choice – cauliflower, broccoli, string beans, celery – to baking dish.
- Coleslaw – shredded red, green or Chinese cabbage, carrot mixed with Vegannaise mayonnaise, 1/2 tsp. or so apple cider vinegar, Celtic sea salt and powdered cayenne, if desired.

Dinner

- Baked potato or yam with organic butter, olive oil, sour cream, chives, salt and vegetables; after potato is baked, add butter or oil and chopped broccoli, onion, chives, mushrooms…)
- Fresh garden salad with olive oil-based dressing or a honey/mustard…

Snack

- Seasonal fresh fruit

ONE WEEK MENU (CONT.)

Day 7

Breakfast

- Poached egg with Hollandaise sauce or grated raw cheese on sprouted grain tortilla (or wheat-free substitute)
- Sliced tomato, sweet red bell pepper or Daikon slices.

Lunch

- Veggie sticks with dips – carrots, celery and jicama sticks, radishes, broccoli, cauliflower...
- Hummus – store-bought or homemade (chick pea dip: Blend together 1 can cooked chick peas, juice of 1/2+ lemon, 1 clove garlic, 2-3 T. tahini (sesame butter), salt to taste and water to blend)
- Avocado dip – 1-2 mashed ripe avocados. 1-2 T. diced onion, if desired, juice of 1/2 lemon, sea salt and hot pepper (if desired), to taste.

Dinner

- Broiled or pan-sautéed Portabello mushroom sandwich (brush mushroom with olive oil, and sprinkle with tamari soy sauce, then pan sauté, bake a few minutes or broil lightly.) Serve as a sandwich on sprouted grain bread or in a sprouted tortilla (or wheat-free substitute) as a roll-up, along with Vegannaise, lettuce, onion, shredded carrot, cabbage or sun-dried or fresh tomato, leftover rice...; or stuffed with cooked rice and covered with a gravy or sauce or just butter, salt and pepper.
- Garden salad with lots of seasonal vegetables and a tasty dressing

Snack

- Fresh popped corn, topped with sea salt, nutritional yeast or veggie-herb condiment.

Notes

- For a snack or meal replacement in the Digestive Care Diet, use Living Fuel™, a hypoallergenic protein powder with vitamins, antioxidants, minerals, fiber, enzymes and probiotics. See Resource Directory.
- Use organic foods as much as possible, as the nutritional value is 10-15 times higher than non-organic, and they are grown without pesticides.
- Soak all grains, beans, seeds and nuts in water 6-8 hours at room temperature before using or cooking to eliminate phytates and enzyme inhibitors. This makes them more digestible. Canned products will probably not be soaked (sprouting grains and beans enhances their digestibility).
- Vegannaise is a mayonnaise found in health food stores made with healthy ingredients, found in the refrigerator. Buy the grapeseed oil variety, not the canola one.
- Avoid hydrogenated or partially hydrogenated oils in prepared foods; also avoid oils that are in clear containers, as they easily become rancid.
- If using yogurt, select those without fruit, as fruit-protein combinations can cause indigestion. You can either get lemon, vanilla, coffee, or maple-flavored, or just don't eat the fruit with the yogurt. Save it for later, or freeze it, and use it in a fruit smoothie.
- Rice milk, almond milk and oat milk can substitute for cow or soy milk.
- Substitute suggested vegetables, spices and dressings for ones that you like, and switch around items and ingredients to suit your tastes.
- Lunches will usually have to be prepared or gathered ahead of time, if you go to work.
- Most of these menus can be ordered and created when going out to eat. Most restaurants have a protein and salad combination that can be ordered for lunch or a carbohydrate/starch meal that can be adapted for dinner. Example: If seafood and pasta are ordered for dinner, the pasta can be eaten with vegetables and the seafood taken home and used for the next day's lunch. Or, if steak and potato is served for lunch, the steak can be eaten with a salad, and the potato can be taken home for dinner.

Juicing—Fresh vegetable juices are very important to help restore nutrition and to heal the gut. As juicing removes fiber, it concentrates a tremendous amount of nutrition and allows the digestive system to rest. Although fiber is essential, it requires work on behalf of the entire digestive system, and to get this superior nutrition without the work is of great benefit to a worn out, sick digestive system. Basically, any juicer will do in a pinch, but there are some that are much better than others: 1) The quality of the juice is superior. 2) There is less oxidation of the juice. 3) They are easy to use and clean. The slow-speed, masticating types, such as the Sampson, Omega twin gear, Green Star and Green Life, are the best. The Champion is a good all-around one, but does not process greens very well, and the spinner-types are the least desirable, especially the ones that don't eject the pulp, where you have to stop and clean the basket out often. There is also a manual hydraulic press, called the Welles Press, available to squeeze out remaining juice from the pulp.

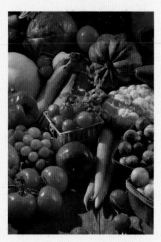

JUICE COMBINATIONS

Carrot combinations are sweeter and carry other vegetables well. People usually like 30-60% carrot and varying amounts of the other vegetables. Fruits do not mix well with vegetables, except apples. 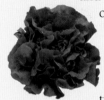 Greens include beet greens, spinach, kale, turnip, collard, lettuces (except iceberg), sprouts, Swiss chard and celery and are especially good for the stomach and to thin heavy, sluggish bile. Try these combinations:

- Carrot-Beet-Spinach
- Carrot-Beet-Greens-Red Bell pepper
- Carrot-Beet-Celery
- Carrot-Celery
- Carrot-Apple
- Carrot-Celery-Apple

 Non-carrot-based combinations are better for type-0 blood types, people with Candida or those who have blood sugar imbalances. Use a watery vegetable, like cucumber, celery or tomato, to take the place of carrot. Cabbage and ginger are great to heal the gut, especially cabbage because of its vitamin K and U that help heal the intestinal lining. Use varying amounts to your liking, and add a clove or two of garlic or a hot pepper, if desired. Hot peppers promote healing, but go easy, as a little goes a long way. And when using ginger root, start with a thumb-sized amount per 8-10 oz. glass. Try these combinations:

- Celery-Cabbage-Cucumber-Red bell pepper
- Celery-Cabbage-Cucumber-Ginger

- Celery-Cabbage-Spinach-Ginger
- Spinach-Kale-Sprout-Chard-Cucumber-Ginger
- Tomato-Celery-Daikon radish (or red radishes)
- Tomato-Celery-Cabbage
- Tomato-Spinach-Celery-Swiss chard
- Tomato-Beet-Cucumber

STORING JUICE

It is always best to make and drink juices fresh, but most can be stored for 24 hours and still retain a lot of their benefits. Store in a small glass jar, where you fill to the very top, eliminating any air space that would oxidize the juice. Top off with water, if necessary. Juices can also be frozen, but freezing and thawing will destroy certain vitamins; this, however, is better than not juicing at all, as is day-old juice. These flexible guidelines usually make juicing more workable to people.

Amounts

You really cannot drink too much juice, as it is very good for the body to have all of this nutrition. People usually consume from 8 to 64 ounces per day. If you are drinking a lot of carrot-based juice and turn orange, it is due to the liver-cleansing effect, not from carotene.

OVERVIEW OF STANDARD MEDICAL DIAGNOSTICS

X-RAYS

CT Scan (Computerized Tomography) – imaging anatomical information from a cross-sectional plane of the body; each image is generated by a computer synthesis of x-ray transmission data obtained in many different directions in a given plane (*Stedman's Concise Medical Dictionary*)

Lower GI Series (Barium Enema) – Administration of barium, a radiopaque contrast medium, for radiographic and fluoroscopic study of the lower intestinal tract. This test, performed by a certified radiologist, involves introduction of barium into the colon through the anus for the purpose of detecting ulcers, diverticuli, polyps and other abnormalities in the colon and rectum. Since the colon must be completely empty, the patient must adhere to a very restricted diet for a day or two before the test. Laxatives or enemas may alternatively be used to cleanse the bowel. No solid food is to be consumed for 8-10 hours before the test begins. The process takes 1-2 hours and may involve some discomfort from the pressure of the barium, followed later by constipation.

Upper GI Series (Barium Swallow) – A fluoroscopic-radiographic examination of the esophagus, stomach and duodenum; a contrast medium, usually barium sulfate, is introduced. During this test, the radiologist is actually watching your digestive system function. Since an empty stomach is necessary, 4-8 hours of pre-test fasting is required. The barium, which is swallowed, coats the lining of the upper GI organs, allowing the radiologist to see such abnormalities as growths, ulcers, scarring or hiatal hernias. He or she can also see blockages and any problems with muscle contractions that may be present. The test typically takes 1-2 hours and may result in constipation as the barium moves through the GI tract. Discomfort is minimal and risks limited. Pregnant women should avoid this test, as well as any other involving radiation.

SCOPES

Colonoscopy – involves visual examination of the inner surface of the entire colon through an elongated endoscope (colonoscope), usually fiberoptic. This test is performed only by gastroenterologists (specialists in GI disorders) in a hospital setting. Strict dietary restrictions must be adhered to prior to testing and enemas or laxatives administered beforehand, as a clean, empty colon is necessary. Sedatives and pain medication are administered. The procedure takes approximately 30-60 minutes. Colonoscopy has become the gold standard for complete evaluation of the colon. Even though a barium enema is effective in detecting a problem in the colon, it is usually necessary to follow with colonscopy to actually see and biopsy the area of concern. Some choose colonscopy to avoid the radiation associated with barium enemas.

Sigmoidoscopy – Inspection, through a rigid or flexible endoscope, of the interior of the sigmoid colon (the lower left portion of the colon). This procedure is often recommended for patients who have chronic constipation, diarrhea or pain. It is also used as a screening tool for colorectal cancer. The sigmoidoscopic exam may detect suspicious growths, ulcers, bleeding, inflamed tissues or muscle spasms. Using the endoscope, which is inserted into the anus, the physician can snip off a tissue sample with a tiny instrument in the scope and send it to the lab for further analysis. The diet is restricted to clear liquids for a day or so prior to sigmoidoscopic examination, which is usually done in a doctor's office and typically takes no more than 10-20 minutes. To more thoroughly cleanse the bowel, enemas or laxatives may be given. Slight cramping and pressure may be experienced as air is introduced into the colon to improve visibility. Some bleeding may occur afterwards. Serious complications, such as perforation, are rare. The limitation of both the flexible and rigid sigmoidoscopes is that they show only the rectum (rigid scope) or rectum and sigmoid (flexible scope). Neither of these scopes should be considered a complete evaluation to rule out any condition of the colon. They have largely been replaced by colonoscopy. The main advantage of sigmoidoscopes are they are easier to use, cost less, and they can be used in an office setting without anesthesia. In addition, in the absence of available colonoscopy, they can be about 70% effective in screening for colorectal cancer. This can be increased to near 100% if combined with a barium enema.

Upper Endoscopy – Use of an endoscope (an instrument for the examination of the interior of a tubular or hollow organ) to visually examine the organs of the upper GI tract: the esophagus, stomach and duodenum. The endoscope is a flexible tube that contains a light and a tiny video camera that relays an image to an external monitor. This test may be ordered if you have persistent nausea or vomiting, stomach pain or bleeding, suspected ulcers, celiac disease or swallowing problems. Eight to ten hours of fasting prior to the test is required. You may be given a sedative to help relax you, and a local anesthetic will be applied to your mouth and throat (via spray or gargle) before the endoscope is inserted through your mouth. The entire test usually takes only 15-20 minutes and is not painful. Complications, such as bleeding and perforation, are rare. You may have a sore throat or some bloating following the procedure, but these effects should disappear within 24 hours. You will not be permitted to leave the facility until the effects of the sedative have worn off (1-2 hours) and may not be allowed to drive yourself home.

Virtual Colonoscopy – a new FDA-approved colon screening technique that allows the visualization of 100% of the colon surface (as opposed to the 70-80% that is visible using conventional colonoscopy). In this procedure, a spiral CT scan is taken of the gastrointestinal area. Semi-transparent, three-dimensional images of the patient's colon are then computer-generated and examined by a radiologist. In preparation for virtual colonoscopy, the patient must take a gentle laxative the night prior to testing. A minor period of fasting is also required. The test itself involves introducing a small amount of air into the colon to distend it. Virtual colonoscopy eliminates the use of the long tube (and the barium), as well as the anesthesia, used in conventional colonoscopy. It is therefore considered to be a safer, less invasive procedure. Some data are now showing that this test may not be as accurate as was originally thought. Thus, it may be a good screening test, but still not as definitive as a barium enema.

SONOGRAPHY

Ultrasonongraphy (Ultrasound) – the location, measurement or delineation of deep structures by measuring the reflection of transmission of high frequency (> 30,000 hz.) or ultrasonic waves. Computer calculation of the distance to the sound-reflecting or absorbing surface plus the known orientation of the sound beam gives a two-dimensional image (*Stedman's Concise Medical Dictionary*). Ultrasound is an effective diagnostic view of the contents of the abdomen. It is painless and requires no preparation. It is especially helpful in looking for gallstones and biliary duct dilation. It is cheaper, quicker and may be more effective than CT scan for bililary tract conditions. Ultrasound is possibly more effective than CT scan in evaluating the ovaries and fallopian tubes.

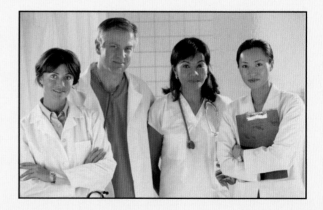

TESTS

Adrenal Hormone Saliva Test – Elevated levels of the stress hormone cortisol, along with depressed levels of another adrenal hormone, DHEA, can profoundly affect GI functioning. These stress hormones can be measured through saliva testing. The test is done at home (upon doctor's orders). Four samples of saliva are taken at designated times over a 16-hour period and sent to a lab for analysis. For the hour preceding the saliva sample, none of the following should be used: caffeine, food, chewing gum, alcohol, nicotine, dental floss and toothpaste. The Pharmacon Adrenal Saliva Test is available to physicians through Great Smokies Diagnostic Laboratory and Metametrix Clinical Laboratory.

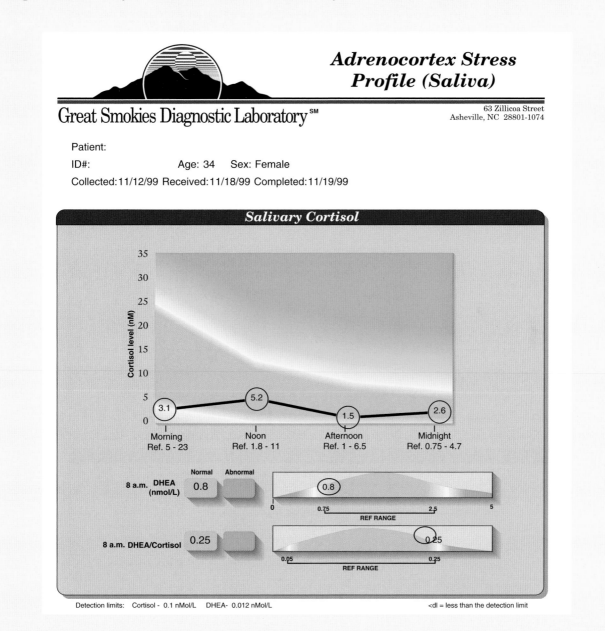

Comprehensive Detoxification Profile – analyzes saliva and urine after challenge doses of caffeine, aspirin and acetaminophen in order to assess the Phase I and Phase II functional capacity of the liver to convert and clear toxic substances from the body.[1] This profile includes markers for oxidative stress and important antioxidants. This test is provided to physicians by Great Smokies Diagnostic Laboratory.

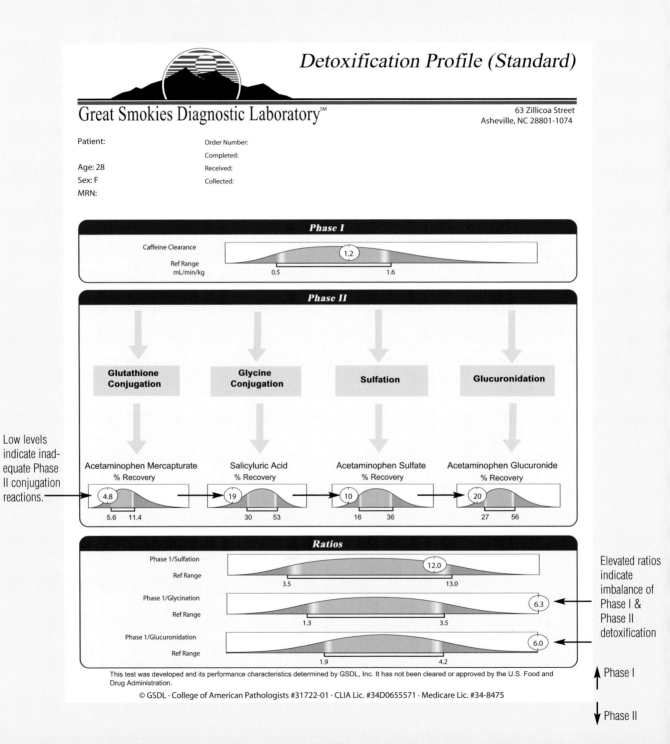

Comprehensive Digestive Stool Analysis (CDSA) – evaluates stool for presence of parasites and levels of beneficial flora, imbalanced flora, pathogenic bacteria and yeast. In addition, it screens for malabsorption and production of short-chain fatty acids. This test is indicated for patients with abdominal pain, chronic diarrhea and other GI-related symptoms. It is available through physicians who may obtain it from Great Smokies Lab and Doctors Data.

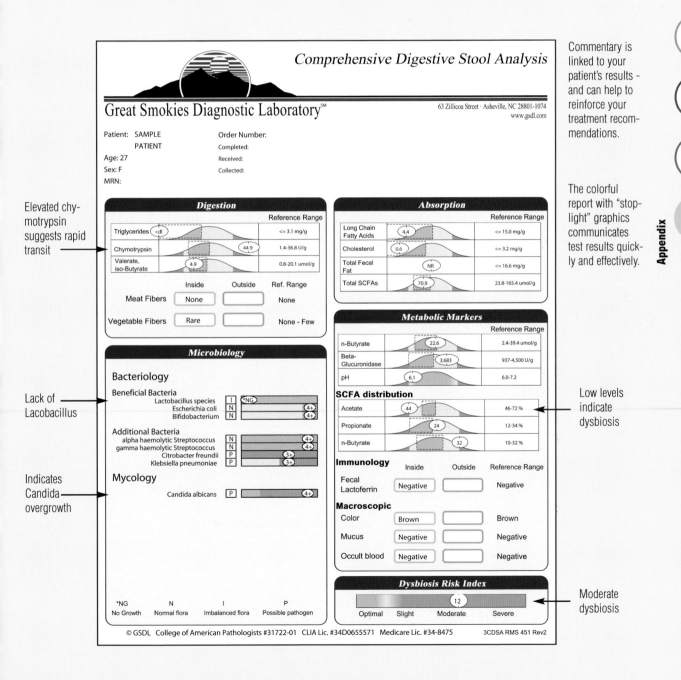

Commentary is linked to your patient's results - and can help to reinforce your treatment recommendations.

The colorful report with "stoplight" graphics communicates test results quickly and effectively.

Elevated chymotrypsin suggests rapid transit

Lack of Lacobacillus

Indicates Candida overgrowth

Low levels indicate dysbiosis

Moderate dysbiosis

ELISA (Enzyme-Linked Immunosorbent Assay) – a blood test that measures IgE, IgG, IgG4 and IgA antibodies and thus is able to identify both immediate and delayed allergic reactions (sensitivities). Food sensitivity tests are available through Immunolabs, Metametrix, Great Smokies and Elisa/Act LRA Biotechnology.

Gluten Sensitivity Test – Individuals with celiac disease have abnormal levels of specific antibodies (antigliadin) in their blood. Analysis of blood or stool for this antibody can help diagnose gluten sensitivity. If the antigliadin antibody test is positive, then a tissue transglutaminase blood test will confirm the diagnosis of celiac disease. This test can be obtained as a part of the food sensitivity ELISA mentioned above. The diagnosis of celiac disease can also be made on the basis of biopsy of tissue from the small intestine obtained during endoscopy.

HCl Challenge – This test may be done at home without the supervision of a doctor. To perform it, take one tablespoon of apple cider vinegar with a meal. If pain or warmth is felt in the stomach, this is an indication that sufficient HCl is being produced and no additional is needed. If no symptoms are noticed, take two tablespoons of apple cider vinegar with the next meal. If no warmth or pain is noted, continue to add one tablespoon at each meal until a warm sensation in the stomach is experienced, then decrease the amount of vinegar by one tablespoon. The same test can be done using HCl tablets to help establish the optimal dose.

Heidelberg Capsule – consists of a tiny pH sensor and a radio transmitter compressed into a large capsule. This test is used to determine the amount of stomach acid present. When swallowed by the patient, the sensors in the capsule measure the pH of the stomach contents and relay the findings by radio signal to a receiver located outside the body. The receiver is connected to a computer and printer, which record a continuous record of gastric pH for as long as the capsule remains in the stomach. The capsule is tethered to a long thread, allowing easy removal upon completion of the test. (Heidelberg capsules without tethers are sometimes used to evaluate the entire GI tract.) Typically, the patient ingests a solution of baking soda after swallowing the Heidelberg capsule. The baking soda alkalizes the gastric juice, which gradually returns to an acidic level. The rate at which the pH changes from alkaline back to acid provides an accurate measurement of the stomach's ability to produce HCl.[2]

Helicobacter Pylori Stool Antigen Test – This is a non-invasive, FDA-approved test that measures H. pylori antigens shed directly into the stool. It is useful for detecting the major causal bacterium associated with peptic ulcers, chronic gastritis and increased risk of gastric cancer. It is also useful for monitoring success of therapy with regard to eradication of H. pylori. This test is available to doctors through Great Smokies Lab.

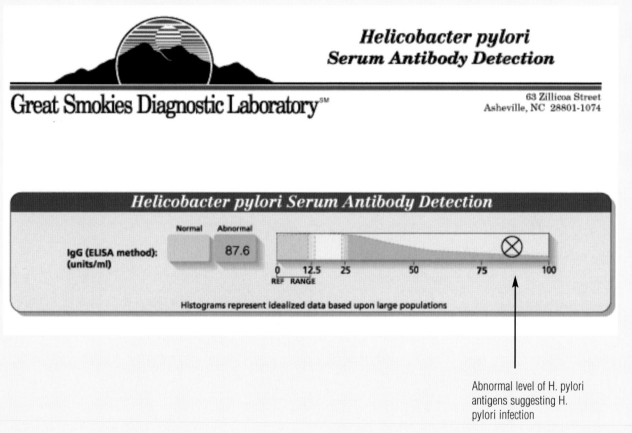

Abnormal level of H. pylori antigens suggesting H. pylori infection

Hormone Profile (female) –This profile from the Great Smokies' Lab analyzes eleven saliva samples over a 28-day period for the levels of key hormones, providing clues about menstrual irregularities, infertility, endometriosis, breast cancer and osteoporosis. The comprehensive profile includes the Adrenocortex Stress Profile and the Comprehensive Melatonin Profile to reveal how the sex hormones are influenced by cortisol, DHEA and melatonin.

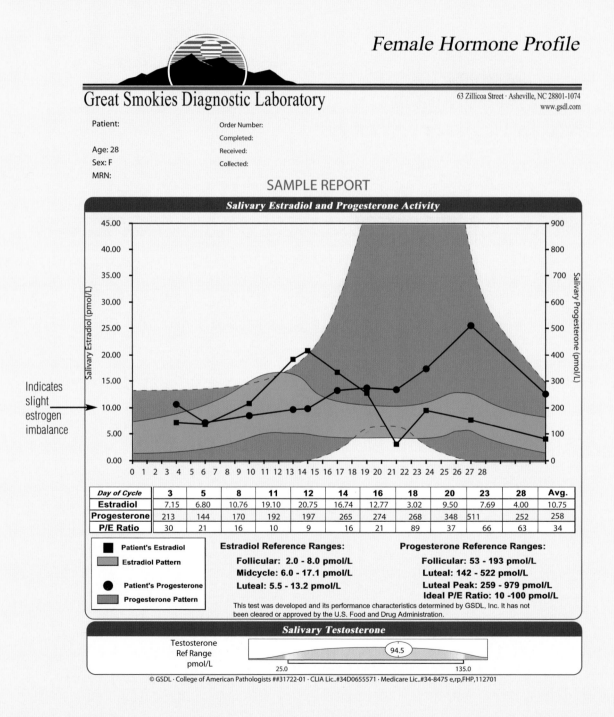

Female Hormone Profile

Great Smokies Diagnostic Laboratory

63 Zillicoa Street · Asheville, NC 28801-1074
www.gsdl.com

Patient:

Age: 28
Sex: F
MRN:

Order Number:
Completed:
Received:
Collected:

SAMPLE REPORT

Salivary Estradiol and Progesterone Activity

Indicates slight estrogen imbalance

Day of Cycle	3	5	8	11	12	14	16	18	20	23	28	Avg.
Estradiol	7.15	6.80	10.76	19.10	20.75	16.74	12.77	3.02	9.50	7.69	4.00	10.75
Progesterone	213	144	170	192	197	265	274	268	348	511	252	258
P/E Ratio	30	21	16	10	9	16	21	89	37	66	63	34

- ■ Patient's Estradiol
- Estradiol Pattern
- ● Patient's Progesterone
- Progesterone Pattern

Estradiol Reference Ranges:
Follicular: 2.0 - 8.0 pmol/L
Midcycle: 6.0 - 17.1 pmol/L
Luteal: 5.5 - 13.2 pmol/L

Progesterone Reference Ranges:
Follicular: 53 - 193 pmol/L
Luteal: 142 - 522 pmol/L
Luteal Peak: 259 - 979 pmol/L
Ideal P/E Ratio: 10 -100 pmol/L

This test was developed and its performance characteristics determined by GSDL, Inc. It has not been cleared or approved by the U.S. Food and Drug Administration.

Salivary Testosterone

Testosterone
Ref Range
pmol/L

94.5

25.0   135.0

© GSDL · College of American Pathologists ##31722-01 · CLIA Lic..#34D0655571 · Medicare Lic..#34-8475 e,rp,FHP,112701

Hormone Profile (male) – This profile from Great Smokies' Lab analyzes four saliva samples over a 24-hour period for levels of testosterone. Elevated levels suggest androgen resistance, while decreased levels can result from such causes as hypogonadism, hepatic cirrhosis, lipid abnormalities and aging. The comprehensive profile includes the Adrenocortex Stress Profile and the Comprehensive Melatonin Profile to reveal how testosterone is influenced by cortisol, DHEA and melatonin.

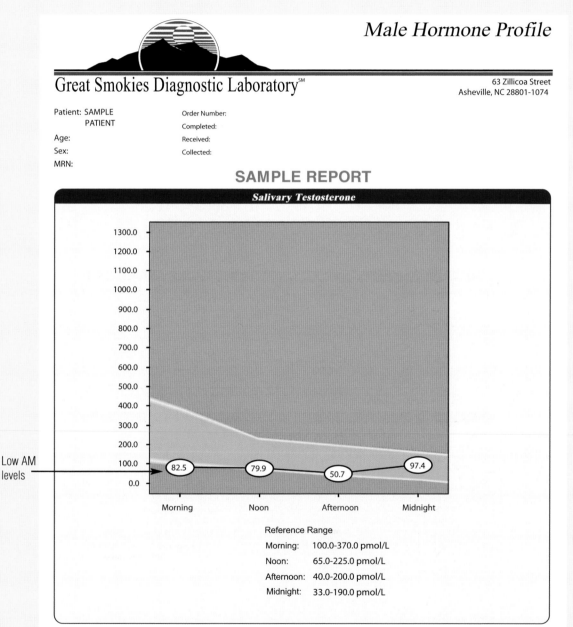

Male Hormone Profile

Great Smokies Diagnostic Laboratory℠

63 Zillicoa Street
Asheville, NC 28801-1074

Patient: SAMPLE PATIENT

Order Number:
Completed:

Age:
Received:

Sex:
Collected:

MRN:

SAMPLE REPORT

Salivary Testosterone

Low AM levels

Morning	Noon	Afternoon	Midnight
82.5	79.9	50.7	97.4

Reference Range

Morning:	100.0-370.0 pmol/L
Noon:	65.0-225.0 pmol/L
Afternoon:	40.0-200.0 pmol/L
Midnight:	33.0-190.0 pmol/L

This test has been developed and its performance characteristics determined by GSDL, Inc. It has not been cleared or approved by the U.S. Food and Drug Administration.

© GSDL · College of American Pathologists #31722-01 · CLIA Lic. #34D0655571 · Medicare Lic. #34-8475

Appendix

Intestinal Permeability Assessment – analyzes urine for the clearance of two non-metabolized sugars, lactulose and mannitol; identifies leaky gut syndrome and malabsorption. This test is available through physicians connected to Great Smokies Lab. Although the body cannot metabolize or use the sugars mannitol and lactulose, if digestion is functioning properly, mannitol, because it is a small molecule, will readily be absorbed across the gut wall, while lactulose will be poorly absorbed due to the fact that it is a large molecule. In the mannitol/lactulose test, the patient collects a random urine sample and then ingests a liquid containing a mixture of the two sugars. Urine is again collected over the next six hours and submitted for laboratory analysis. If the urine shows high levels of mannitol and low levels of lactulose, it is an indicator that food is being properly absorbed. When levels of both sugars are high, leaky gut syndrome is diagnosed. (Low levels of both sugars would be indicative of general malabsorption of nutrients, while low mannitol, along with high lactulose, has been found in people with inflammatory bowel disease and celiac disease.[3])

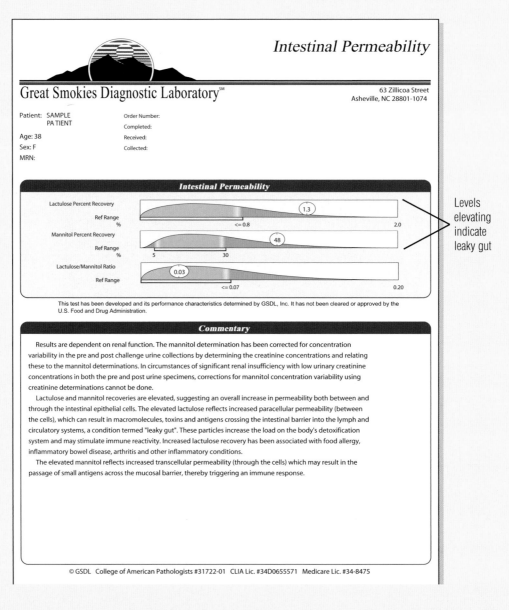

Lactose Intolerance Breath Test – a simple, noninvasive test that detects lactose intolerance by measuring the amount of hydrogen in the patient's expired air. Excess gas (including hydrogen) is typically produced in the colon of the lactose intolerant person when bacteria ferment undigested lactose. The hydrogen is absorbed from the intestine, carried via the bloodstream to the lungs and exhaled. In the test, the patient ingests a lactose-containing beverage; a small tube is then placed in his or her nostril for the purpose of extracting exhaled air. The breath is then analyzed for excess hydrogen using gas chromatography. It should be noted that certain foods, medicines and cigarettes can alter the outcome of this test, and so their use should be avoided beforehand. This test is available through Great Smokies Lab.

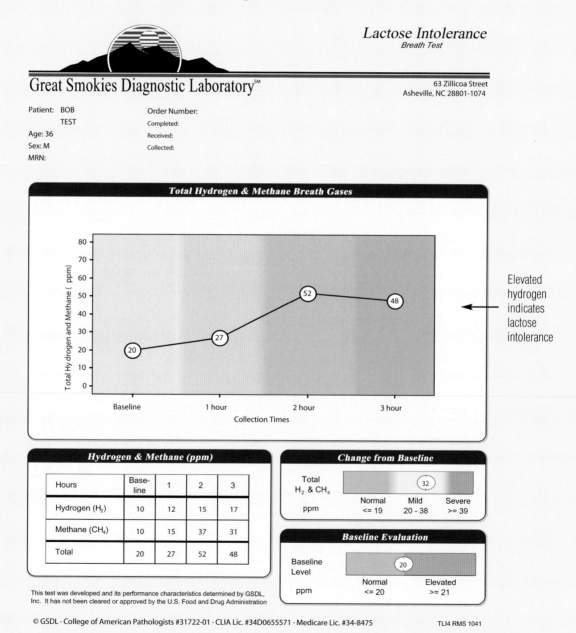

This test was developed and its performance characteristics determined by GSDL, Inc. It has not been cleared or approved by the U.S. Food and Drug Administration

© GSDL · College of American Pathologists #31722-01 · CLIA Lic. #34D0655571 · Medicare Lic. #34-8475   TLI4 RMS 1041

Appendix

Proto-fix™ CONSED™ Parasite Test – "involves filtering of fixed specimens, mixing with CONSED™ and ethyl acetate, vortexing, centrifugation, decanting all but the fecal plug, and mixing with CONSED™ diluting reagent. The plug is then transferred to and mounted on a slide for examination."[4] This test kit, obtained from a physician, contains materials and instructions for the patient, so that he or she may provide, prepare and submit the needed stool specimens for analysis. The test checks for all categories of parasites, as well as fungi spores, common yeast and other pathogens. It test is available through the Parasitology Center, Inc. in Tempe, AZ.

Self Basal Temperature Test – Check Thyroid Activity

There is considerable evidence showing that the current blood tests for the diagnosis of mild sub-clinical hypothyroidism can be misleading. In his book, *Hypothyroidism, an Unsuspected Illness*, Broda Barnes, MD and Endocrinologist, explains that detecting low thyroid function is as simple as checking basal (baseline upon awakening) temperature.

Instructions:
Place a thermometer (preferably digital) within easy reach on the bedside. If possible, avoid using a mercury thermometer to eliminate the possibility of accidental breakage and the potential mercury toxicity. If you use a mercury thermometer, take measures to prevent breakage.

Put the thermometer in your armpit for five minutes. Do this before you've gotten out of bed, had coffee or food or done anything significantly physical. Dr. Barnes suggests using the axillary (armpit) temperature, rather than the mouth, because so many people have low-grade unsuspected sinus infections. These infections generate heat only in the oral cavity, thereby falsely raising the oral temperature. If you do not have infections, you may take your oral temperature. For young children or the disabled, you may use the rectal temperature. Record your temperature each morning for five days.

For women, additional consideration is needed during ovulation, since ovulation somewhat elevates temperature. Because of this, women who menstruate should start recording their temperature on the second or third day of menstruation.

Normal axillary (arm pit) or oral temperature is in the range of 97.8 – 98.2 degrees F. Normal rectal temperature is 98.8 – 99.2 degrees F. Data on your daily basal temperatures will assist in assessing your cellular thyroid hormone activity. Dr. Barnes estimates that greater than 40% of the adult population has hypothyroidism, hypertension, obesity, depression, as well as constipation and many other ailments.

Dr Smith's Comments

One major cause of decreased basal body temperature is low conversion of thyroid hormone T4 (tetraiodothryronine) to the more active form, T3 (tri-iodothyronine), which occurs throughout all the cells of the body. This is highly significant since the thyroid hormone T3 enters the nuclei of the cells and starts the process that upregulates the production on mitochondrial protein, which thereby makes more mitochondria. More healthy mitochondria make more ATP, which is the energy currency of the body. Low ATP equals low energy and low basal body temperature. The failure of the body to convert T4 to T3 is often due to decreased activity of the converting enzyme 5'dioidinase. This enzymatic insufficiency can be due to decreased intracellular selenium levels.

Supplementing with 200 micrograms of selenium may be helpful if there are persistent low basal temperatures. Also, research (J. Clin. Endocr. and Metab, Vol. 87,1687,2002), has shown that there is an improvement in Hashimoto's auto-immune thyroiditis (with a decrease in thyroid peroxidase auto-antibodies) in response to selenium supplementation. Finally, there is published prospective research that supports that 200 micrograms of selenium per day decreased some cancers (colon, prostate and lung) by up to 50%! (JAMA, 276:1957-63,1996).

Another common problem is elevated cortisol (from chronic stress). Cortisol blocks the entry of T3 into the nucleus (which begins mitochondrial reproduction). Here again, uncontrolled chronic relentless stress with elevated cortisol levels (especially in the evening) will lead to lower ATP production, chronic fatigue and low basal temperatures. Stress management may be the single most significant strategy one could employ to improve their health and energy. (See biofeedback and meditation in Optional Nutritional Approaches sections.)

OVERVIEW OF SUPPLEMENTS FOR DIGESTIVE CARE (AS DESCRIBED IN THE OPTIONAL NUTRITIONAL APPROACHES SECTIONS)

Aloe Juice or Aloe Syrup

Aloe has been used for its medicinal properties for many years. In the Optional Nutritional Approaches sections of this book, we recommend aloe for its' soothing properties in gastrointestinal distress. The following is a list of some of the properties of aloe:

- It has enzymes, not found in any other plant, that the body can use.
- It is the only plant source of vitamin B12.
- It is the most potent source of the largest immune-enhancing polysaccharides.

The best quality aloe supplement is one that is organic and uncooked. Cooking aloe at high temperatures denatures the enzymes and compromises quality. Aloe's potency and effectiveness depend on the number of nutrients and their biological availability to the cells of the body. Herbs that might be found in a good aloe product would be marshmallow, chamomile, burdock or echinacea. For added intestinal support, the product should contain the amino acid L-glutamine.

Antioxidants

An antioxidant is an electron donor that provides electrons to neutralize free radicals. A free radical is usually an atom or molecule that is missing an electron in its outer shell (or boundary). It will "steal" electrons from the outer layer of cell membranes and create damage, which can be relatively minor, but if allowed to continue, can lead to serious illness. It is important to understand that all free radical activity is not bad; it is necessary for many chemical reactions to occur and for the immune system to fight infections. Many of the immune cells produce and release free radical molecules to kill pathogenic organisms. The problem comes when there is an excess of free radicals that comes from stress, environment, diet or from an overactive immune system. Free radical excess burdens the body with cellular dysfunction and inflammation, which can lead to a multitude of symptoms ranging from fatigue, low energy, poor digestive and mental function, generalized aches and pains to heart attacks and cancer.

In fact, there are many blood and urine tests now available to determine whether your body has reached a critical level of free radical activity. These tests can easily be done by your health care practitioner: malondialdehyde, lipid peroxide, 4-hydroxy and 9-hydroxy nonenal and 8 hydroxy deoxyguanosine (8OHDG). Since inflammation can be closely linked to decreased antioxidant levels, another screening test called hsCRP (highly sensitive C-reactive protein) is especially helpful. An article in the *NEJM*, (Oct. 23, 2003, 349:1595-1604) states that a hyperimmune marker in the blood called myeloperoxidase (an enzyme released from white blood cells) may be the best indicator of an impending heart attack.

One of the common causes of inflammation, with decreased antioxidants, is low-grade infection. Low-grade infections do not present with elevated blood counts, fevers and localized problems like urine infections and pneumonia; instead, they present with the symptoms mentioned above, fatigue and low energy, etc. The causative pathogens can be H. pylori, Chylamidia pneumoniae, herpes viruses, Cytomegalovirus, Epsein-Barr virus, hepatitis virus, as well as many others. These pathogens in very small numbers cause the immune system to over-react and release free radicals in excess of what is needed, thereby promoting ongoing inflammation and increasing the body's need for antioxidants. These low-grade infections can be successfully treated with antibiotics, natural immune stimulants (some herbs and mushrooms), anti-inflammatory agents and

antioxidants. In many cases, if there is a dental source (usually gingivitis), it can be corrected with appropriate dentistry.

It may not be commonly known that antioxidants come in many sizes and shapes, ranging from vitamins to minerals and enzymes to food.

- Vitamins - vitamin C, vitamin E, vitamin A and the various carotenoids: beta carotene, alpha carotene, zeaxanthin, cryptoxanthin and lutein
- Minerals – zinc and selenium - critically important in hundreds of enzyme reactions; some of these enzymes are directly related in antioxidant production, while other enzymes, by not working correctly, allow for increased free radical activity, thereby indirectly affecting antioxidant status.
- Enzymes – Glutathione reductase, superoxide dismutase and catalase are well known enzymes with antioxidant effects in the body.
- Miscellaneous antioxidants include: alpha lipoic acid (very potent and a recharger of the many other antioxidants), glutathione, amino acids N-acetyl cysteine, glycine and glutamine (These three combine to make glutathione.) Glutathione binds heavy metals like mercury and thereby slows down oxidative stress (free radical activity).
- Herbs – Pycnogenol (pine bark extract), OPCs (grape seed extract) and milk thistle extract (silymarin) help enhance liver function.
- Foods – Blueberry, raspberry, cranberry, bilberry, strawberry and blackberry are just a few of the deep-colored foods that are high in antioxidants as measured by the ORAC (oxidation-reduction antioxidant capacity). At the other end of the food spectrum, there is rice bran soluble fraction, with at least 70 different measurable antioxidants!

It is easy to see that this is a very broad and variable topic but one that is very important to human health. Understanding your antioxidant status and replenishing the supply when needed with a wide variety of foods and supplements can have a significant impact on most any health condition.

Amino Acids
Amino acids are the building blocks that join together and create proteins, which are an integral part of every cell in the body.

- Arginine - L-arginine has also been shown to support the immune system, as well as maintain a positive nitrogen balance and reduce protein catabolism. It enhances wound healing and promotes healing of the mucosal lining of the gastrointestinal tract. Antioxidants should always be taken with L-arginine to prevent excess oxidation from nitric oxide (which is produced from L-arginine).

- Branched-Chain Amino Acids - The three branched-chain amino acids (BCAAs) are leucine, isoleucine and valine. These are essential amino acids (meaning that the body cannot make them). They are needed for maintenance of muscle tissue and preserving muscle glycogen stores. BCAAs also increase protein synthesis in the liver and muscles and help to restore liver function. A study published in the *American Journal of Clinical Nutrition* (vol. 56, 158-63, 1992) showed that children on BCAA supplementation who were waiting for liver transplant had improved height, weight, total body potassium and arm circumference as compared to controls.

- L-glutamine – is a conditionally essential amino acid that is critical in helping to eliminate excess acid in the body through the liver and then via renal handling of ammonia. In addition, it is an important fuel for the cells lining the entire gastrointestinal tract and other rapidly overturning cells. This includes lymphocytes (immunity), fibroblasts (connective tissue) and reticulocytes (bone marrow). The recommended dosage ranges from 3,000 mg. to 20,000 mg. per day based on the severity of the condition. Glutamine results in improvement of GI func-

tion, reverses muscle atrophy, decreases rate of infection and length of hospital stay in ICU patients, and, in high doses, even was shown to reduce mortality in serious illnesses (see review article from Harvard Medical School in the *American Journal of Clinical Nutrition*, Vol. 75, No. 5, 789-808, May 2002).

- – L-glutamine Powder – with N-aceytl-glucosamine (NAG) and gamma oryzanol. The amino acid L-glutamine is the primary fuel for the cells of the intestinal tract. It is essential in the repair of the intestinal lining (leaky gut). N-aceytl-glucosamine (NAG) is the "glue" that forms the mucosal layer. This mucosal layer acts to protect the underlying intestinal tissue from exposure to enzymes, acid and bacterial assault, while providing a selectively absorptive surface. L-glutamine converts to N-acetyl-glucosamine, thus rebuilding the mucous lining of the digestive tract. Clinical studies show gamma oryzanol orally administered is effective as an anti-inflammatory. It is effective in a broad range of gastrointestinal disorders, such as gastric and duodenal ulcers, gastritis and irritable bowel syndrome. In double blind studies in Japan, it was reported to be 90.8% effective in gastrointestinal disorders. It is derived from rice bran oil. In summary, a product that combines L-glutamine, N-aceytl-glucosamine (NAG) and gamma oryzanol, as well as herbs like cranesbill, marshmallow, and ginger, could be highly effective in reducing inflammation at the digestive tract.

- – L-glutamine Poultice – Take L-glutamine powder, and add enough water to make a paste. Apply topically for rectal conditions.

- Methionine – is an amino acid precursor to S-adenosyl-methionine (SAM-e). This is an important methyl donor that helps in many cellular functions. Methionine is necessary for the manufacture of choline, and it is the precursor for cysteine, which is essential in glutathione production. Deficiencies of these nutrients are noted in those with alcohol-induced fatty livers. With excessive alcohol consumption, hepatic (liver) metabolism is extremely impaired, often resulting in cirrhosis. By increasing methionine, choline and glutathione also increase, which may prevent ethanol-induced fatty livers. Methionine supplementation may also be beneficial to those with other liver abnormalities, including Gilbert's syndrome. Those who consume high levels of alcohol may benefit from methionine supplements (1 to 2 grams daily). If supplementing with methionine, it is essential to supplement with riboflavin, vitamins B6 and B12, as well as trimethylglycine, to prevent homocysteine buildup.

• Taurine – An important amino acid in liver detoxification, taurine increases cellular uptake of potassium and magnesium. Taurine levels can be depleted by chronic Candida infections of the intestinal tract.

Essential Omega-3 Oils (Essential Fatty Acids)

Mounting research suggests that getting the right amount of essential fatty acids is as important as getting your daily vitamins. Essential fatty acids are necessary to support the body's cellular processes and fight disease. Essential fatty acids are polyunsaturated fats that are required for the proper structure and function of every cell in your body, and they are critical for optimal health.

These fats are not made by the body and must be obtained through supplementation. EFA's increase the absorption of vitamins and minerals; nourish the skin, hair and nails; promote proper nerve functioning; help produce hormones and support gastrointestinal health. We have recommended flax, borage and fish oils in the "Optional Nutritional Approaches" sections of this book. These essential fatty acids provide a balance of Omega-3, -6 and -9 for optimal health and good overall gastrointestinal health. Additionally, a balance of EPA and DHA (eicosapentaenoic acid

and docosapentaenoic acid found in fish oils) has been shown to be helpful in managing inflammation of the intestinal tract, especially inflammatory bowel disease (Crohn's and ulcerative colitis). The Omega-3 oils have also been shown to be of value in heart disease, immune kidney disease and rheumatoid arthritis.

In addition to flax, fish and borage oils, recommended maintenance doses of fish oil are around 1000 mg. EPA and 500 mg. DHA when treating major inflammatory conditions. The high percentage of remission with Crohn's (59%) (reported in the *New England Journal of Medicine*, 1996; vol 334:1557-60) was revealed in a study that used enteric-coated fish oil, which was thought to be more effective since it could not be affected by stomach acid.

Fiber

Fiber is critical for optimum function of the GI tract. The daily amount varies from 20-60 grams per day. Fiber maintains normal colon function. Along with friendly bacteria (Lactobacilli and Bifidobacteria), it creates short-chain fatty acids that enhance colon function and help prevent colon cancer. We recommend 3 types of fiber:

1. Borage fiber - According to the US Department of Agriculture, borage seeds contain the nutrients listed below. Other than fat and oils, which have been removed, most of the following ingredients would be present in the borage fiber:

   • Macronutrients (carbohydrates, protein, fats), fiber, glucose, galactose and gamma-linolenic acid (an essential fatty acid)
   • Vitamins, such as ascorbic acid (vitamin C), beta carotene (pro-vitamin A) and choline, niacin, riboflavin and thiamine (elements of the B complex)
   • Minerals, including calcium, cobalt, iron, magnesium, phosphorus, potassium, sodium and zinc

- Other plant compounds, including allantoin, lactic acid, malic acid, mucilage, rosmarinic acid, and tannin (Warkinton 2002)

2. Flax fiber – contains generous quantities of both soluble and insoluble fiber. Soluble fiber is well known to be an effective cholesterol-lowering agent. Insoluble fiber is needed for regular bowel movements and prevention of constipation. Lignans, another component of flax fiber, contain plant-based estrogens. These estrogens (enterodiol and enterolactone) protect estrogen receptors in both men and women from xenoestrogens (toxic and dangerous artificial estrogens). Flax seeds are an outstanding source of many other essential nutrients, including folate, vitamin B-6, pantothenic acid, magnesium, potassium, iron, thiamine, copper, zinc, calcium and phosphorus. Flax meal also appears to have anti-inflammatory properties. As an added bonus, flax seeds contain all 8 of the "essential" amino acids.

3. Rice fiber – Soluble fiber contains water-soluble vitamins, hypoallergenic protein, inositol, minerals and unique carbohydrates. These carbohydrates consist of short- and medium-chain complex carbohydrates that are chloride ion blockers, which help control diarrhea. The insoluble fiber provides excellent bulk to the stool. The stabilized rice bran-fine has over 70 antioxidants, including tocopherols, tocotrienols and gamma oryzanol. A combination of these three fractions constitutes a good multi-dimensional approach to a hypoallergenic fiber.

Herbs
The use of herbs dates back to the ancient Sumerians who described their medicinal use some 5,000 years ago. Most ancient cultures relied on herbs as their only medicine. The effects of herbs on the body are well known and documented. *The Herbal PDR* (Physicians Desk Reference), *The German Monograph E* (a resource for physicians), and the National Institute of Health (NIH) website, www.nih.org, all provide extensive information on the use of many herbs.

IBS Supplement
IBS Formula (for cramping and diarrhea)

– **Part 1** (Intestinal Lining Support) contains L-glutamine, N-acetyl-glucosamine, gamma oryzanol and other ingredients the body needs to build and maintain a healthy mucosal lining in the intestine.

– **Part 2** (Bowel Support) contains a formulation of Western and Chinese herbs that have been traditionally used to support proper bowel health and function.

Minerals
See the multivitamin/mineral complex below.

Probiotics and Prebiotics
Probiotics literally means "for life," which may be a good name for the beneficial bacteria since they: help digest food, crowd out pathogenic (disease-producing) bacteria, make many of our vitamins (especially B vitamins and vitamin K), produce antibiotics to kill pathogenic bacteria, make short-chain fatty acids to help promote good colon function, increase fecal bulking, promote mineral absorption and prevent colon cancer. [See *American Journal of Clinical Nutrition*, Feb. 2001, vol 73, number 2(S), an excellent review supplement of prebiotics and probiotics).] All of the above are obviously "life promoting" events.

The definition of "prebiotic" was introduced by Gibson and Roberfroid. They defined prebiotics as "non-digestable food ingredients that beneficially affect the host by selectively stimulating the growth and /or activity of one or a limited number of bacteria in the colon." This definition overlaps with the definition of dietary fiber, with one important exception: selectivity for certain species. This selectivity was shown for Bifidobacteria, which may be promoted by the ingestion of substances, such as fructooligosaccharides and inulin, transgalactosylated oligosaccharides and soybean oligosaccharides (*American Journal of Clinical Nutrition*, Feb. 2001, vol 73, pp363S).

Prebiotic carbohydrates (known as oligosaccharides) are found in many fruits and vegetables: Jerusalem artichoke, onions, chicory, garlic, asparagus, tomatoes and bananas. It certainly is wise to add these foods to the diet. However, concentrated prebiotics of short-chain fructooligosaccharides (FOS) and inulin can be obtained in one gram (quarter- to half-teaspoon) amounts and are even more effective. Most of the probiotic benefits above are improved significantly by merely adding prebiotics.

Symbiotics is a newer term describing the administration of prebiotics and probiotics together or as a single product. This seems to produce better results than doing either alone. Possibly this is due to the FOS supporting the Bifidobacteria and Lactobacilli through the stomach and intestines on the way to the colon. Upon reaching the colon, the probiotics then are better supported and probably more functional.

Generally, it is believed that combinations of 2-4 strains of each, Lactobacilli and Bifidobacteria, may be more beneficial than one strain of each, but this has not been clearly proven. The number of viable organisms does appear to have a direct effect on the concentrations of beneficial bacteria in the colon. This number ranges from 2-10 or more than a billion bacteria per capsule. There are other strains of bacteria, such as certain E. coli and Streptococci, as well as others, that may also be considered probiotic bacteria.

The concept of modulating gut microbial populations for therapeutic benefit and ecological balance now also applies to yeasts. Saccharomyces boulardii (S. boulardii) is a beneficial yeast that has been shown to help correct overgrowth of Candida and diarrhea associated with overuse of antibiotics. A particularly virulent form of AAD (antibiotic associated diarrhea) comes from Clostridium difficile bacteria. It has been shown that S. boulardii liberates a proteolytic enzyme that chops up the two toxins (Toxin A and Toxin B) liberated by C. diffficile that causes much of the problem [American Society for Microbiology, Infection and Immunity, 1999 Jan;(1): 302-307].

We are rapidly approaching the time when conventional medicine will embrace gut ecology as a major part of health. Management of intestinal microflora balance may supplant the indiscriminate and often inappropriate overuse of antibiotics.

VITAMINS/MINERALS

A good multivitamin, antioxidant mineral complex would include the following: vitamin A (acetate) 10,000 I.U. (international units); pure ascorbic acid, 1,000 mg.; vitamin D3, 200 I.U.; d-alpha tocopherol succinate (vitamin E), 400 I.U.; thiamine HCl (B1,) 100 mg.; riboflavin HCl (B2), 25 mg.; riboflavin 5' phosphate (activated B2); niacinamide, 100 mg.; inositol hexaniacinate (no flush niacin); pyridoxine HCl (B6); pyridoxal 5' phosphate (activated B6), folic acid, 800 mcg. (micrograms); hydroxycobalamin (activated B12), 1,000 mcg.; biotin, 800 mcg.; pantothenic acid (calcium pantothenate, B5); calcium (citrate), 300 mg.; magnesium (citrate), 200 mg.; zinc (picolinate), 25 mg.; selenium (selenomethionine), 200 mcg.; manganese (asparate), 20 mg., chromium (picolinate), 200 mcg.; molybdenum (asparate), 100 mcg.; boron (glycinate), 2 mg.; di-potassium (aspartate), 99 mg.; mixed carotenoids, 15,000 I.U., vanadium (aspartate), 200 mcg., and extra antioxidant and liver protection can be added with N-acetyl-cysteine, up to 1,000 mg.

This type of product provides a good baseline, since it lacks added iron, copper and iodine, minerals that should be supplemented on an individual basis. The addition of the activated form of B vitamins is important since patients with toxicity problems may not convert their B2, B6 and B12 to the usable forms. In order to get this many nutrients in a capsule form, it would require about 8 capsules. Ideally, a hypo-allergenic product with no hidden excipients, binders, fillers, shellacs, artificial colors or fragrance should be selected. In addition, the product should not contain dairy, wheat, yeast, gluten, corn, sugar, starch or preservatives of hydrogenated oils.

Health care practitioners can order this type product for their patients through Pure Encapsulations, Douglas Labs or Vitamin Research Products. A good choice in the health food stores would be Source Naturals.

VITAMIN C FLUSH –
How to do an Ascorbate (Vitamin C) Calibration Protocol ("C Flush") to Determine Your Functional Ascorbate Need

Which Ascorbate is Best to Use?
It is preferable to use a 100% L-ascorbate, fully reduced, buffered mineral ascorbate form of vitamin C that contains a proper balance of the major essential buffering minerals: 1) potassium, 2) magnesium, 3) calcium and 4) zinc. No DL-ascorbate or D-ascorbate should be used, as humans do not absorb the D-ascorbate form. People take up only the L-ascorbate. Per gram of ascorbate, we find best outcomes, patient compliance, and satisfaction from a balanced mineral content of potassium (66 mg.), calcium (27 mg.), magnesium (11 mg.) and zinc (400 mcg.).

This means that if you were taking a half-teaspoon of buffered ascorbate that has no masking or "inert" agents in it, you would have 1.5 grams of ascorbate containing potassium, 99 mg.; calcium, 40 mg.; magnesium, 16 mg.; and zinc, 600 mcg. If there is less than 1.5 grams per half-teaspoon,

there is likely to be a hidden or masking agent that may cause digestive or immune problems.

How to do your Ascorbate Calibration "C Flush"
When possible, it is best to start (especially the first use of this protocol) on an empty stomach, first thing in the morning. Allow yourself that day to finish the "flush." Most people saturate their ascorbate need within a few hours. Occasionally, the need is much greater, and it may take a number of hours to complete the initial calibration "flush."

Dissolve each half-teaspoon (1.5 grams) of fully reduced, buffered mineral L-ascorbate powder in 2 or more ounces of water or diluted juice (juice diluted 1:1 with water). Plan to count and record each dosage. After dissolving the L-ascorbate and allowing any effervescence to abate (typically dissolves within two minutes), drink the beverage. The amount of L-ascorbate needed depends on how quickly your body uses it. Below are suggestions for how to best determine your needs based on your level of health.

- A healthy person begins with a level half-teaspoon dissolved in 1-2 ounces of water or diluted juice every 15 minutes.
- A moderately healthy person begins with 1 teaspoon every 15 minutes.
- A person in ill health begins with 2 teaspoons every 15 minutes.
- If, after four doses, there is no gurgling or rumbling in the gut, you should double the initial dosage and continue every 15 minutes.

Continue taking the ascorbate every 15 minutes until you attain a watery stool or an enema-like evacuation of liquid from the rectum (your 'flush'). This is as if a quart or so of liquid is expressed from the rectum.

Caution: Do not stop at loose stool. You want to energize the body to "flush out" toxins and reduce the risk that they may re-circulate and induce problems. At this time, stop consuming the buffered ascorbate for the day. However, if your calibration dosage is more than 50 grams of vitamin C, you should consume a dosage of vitamin C of at least 10% of the total L-ascorbate needed to induce the L-ascorbate calibration "flush" in the later afternoon or evening. Many people find that preparing a "batch" of ascorbate allows for easier, more timely consumptions of the beverage, rather than making up a new batch at each interval. Example: 30 grams (10 teaspoons) may be dissolved in 10-20 ounces of liquid. If this method is chosen, we recommend using a capped, dark bottle to avoid air or light (photo-) oxidation of the ascorbate. Dissolved ascorbate is stable for a day if kept cool or cold and tightly sealed.

Helpful Hints and Insights

1. Most people find that the flush is easy to do. Since the amount of time can vary quite a bit, it is best to do your first ascorbate calibration on a day when you can stay home for most of the day. Once you have done an ascorbate calibration/flush, you will have a better idea of how much time is needed.

2. For most people, it takes somewhere between 3-8 teaspoons of ascorbate to flush. It could differ for others: 15 grams, 20 grams or more than 50 grams, depending on your health status and how quickly your body uses up ascorbate.

3. Sometimes people remain bloated for the rest of the day of calibration. Occasionally, people have loose stools for a day or so after doing the ascorbate flush. This usually means a block to needed magnesium uptake, a lack of healthy probiotic organisms, or a lack of L-glutamine/PKA (PERQUE Endura Guard) for intestinal cell energy.

4. Some people have reported hot stools that seem to burn the anus after several evacuations. If you have this experience, you can use a natural salve, such as calendula ointment, to soothe the area. This tends to cease after the first few times you do the calibration.

5. People with hemorrhoids, irritable bowel disease or inflammatory bowel disease may find that the ascorbate activates their tissues in the healing process. Use PERQUE Pain Guard (soluble quercetin dihydrate and soluble OPC) and active probiotics for two weeks prior to your flush to strengthen tissues, if needed, prior to your ascorbate calibration. Sometimes it is better to increase ascorbate and bioflavonoids slowly over time before doing an ascorbate calibration.

6. Usually, people find that they feel better than they have in a very long time after the first ascorbate flush. Some report a greater sense of well-being after the second or third flush. The overall consensus is that, as time goes on, doing these calibrations helps people feel increasingly better.

For additional information, questions, and inquiries on this Ascorbate Calibration protocol, please contact:

PERQUE LLC
Client Services Department
14 Pidgeon Hill Drive, Suite 180
Sterling, VA 20165
Tel: 800-525-7372   Fax: 703-450-2995
Email: clientservices@perque.com

ALTERNATIVE THERAPIES

Acupuncture

Acupuncture, along with Traditional Chinese Medicine, is part of an ancient system of treatment techniques for enhancing energy flow through the body. It involves the stimulation of specific acupuncture points along the energy pathways (called meridians). That stimulation is accomplished through insertion of needles, application of heat, massage, laser, electricity or a combination of these.

Biofeedback

Biofeedback is a treatment technique involving attempts to consciously control bodily functions believed to be involuntary, such as blood pressure or heart rate, through use of equipment that monitors the function and signals changes in it.

It has been shown that stress can have profound effects on the gastrointestinal tract, including increasing the intestinal permeability and altering motility. When this happens, there is increased uptake of undigested food, microbes, as well as microbial and other toxins that are in the food or GI tract at any given time. The undigested food and various toxins cause an upregulation of the immune system, which can lead to cellular dysfunction, inflammation and auto-immunity. Therefore, learning to recognize and minimize chronic stress can be valuable in healing and maintaining intestinal health, as well as overall health. Meditation or biofeedback can be very helpful in modifying and reducing the body's response to stress. For many people, biofeedback adds an additional feature of allowing one to see (via some type of monitor), the baseline response to stress. During the course of a session, one can then feel the changes in the body and correlate them with what they see changing on the monitor.

One of the more widely used, and effective biofeedback devices is called Freeze-Framer™ by HeartMath. This device employs software that is loaded on a computer and a pulse-sensing device that is placed on a finger. Information from the user's pulse beat is converted into a mathematical formula known as Heart Rate Variability (HRV). HRV is a special way of looking at the minute variations in the time between heartbeats. Generally, having a higher HRV indicates a healthier heart that is more capable of adapting to change on demand. Medical literature has abundant research on the value of monitoring HRV to help determine

cardiac health. HeartMath found a particular range of HRV that could be achieved by slow abdominal breathing while holding positive, loving thoughts in mind or having an "attitude of gratitude." The results are remarkable. The monitor shows a distinct change in the pattern of baseline HRV, to one of larger and deeper wave fluctuations. The physiologic result is an autonomic balancing of the heart, which manifests as:

- Boost in immune system, with increased secretory IgA levels
- Decrease in cortisol (stress hormone)
- Increase in DHEA (anti-stress hormone)
- Lowered blood pressure
- Improved overall physiologic and psychological well being
- Neutralization of the effects of stress on the body

It is recommended to practice with this device for about 20 minutes twice daily for optimum results. The developers of this program have a nice way of stating what happens, "A change in heart changes everything." This statement is supported by the fact that the heart creates the largest electromagnetic field of the body. The body entrains (responds) to the dominant frequency generated by the heart. When the heart is in balance (from an autonomic nervous system perspective), the other body organs tend to come into balance, as well.

Castor Oil Packs

A warm castor oil pack over the abdominal area may be used in cases of constipation and abdominal discomfort. To make one, gather the following items: castor oil, a piece of wool or cotton flannel cloth large enough to cover the abdomen when folded, a piece of plastic the same size as the flannel or larger, a heating pad or hot water bottle and a large towel. Make the pack by thoroughly saturating the flannel with castor oil and wringing it so it is not dripping. Lie down, and apply the pack to the lower abdominal area. Cover the flannel with plastic to protect your clothing and bedding. Then cover the plastic with the towel. Place the heating pad or hot water bottle over the towel, and leave in place for one hour (longer if desired, three hours maximum), while relaxing. Repeat the procedure three times per week or more for a period of three months. Thereafter, the pack may be applied weekly. Following completion of an application, wash the abdomen with a solution of two teaspoons of baking soda dissolved in one quart of water. Your flannel pack may be stored in a plastic bag in the refrigerator when not in use. Add more castor oil to it for subsequent uses.

Colon Hydrotherapy

Colon hydrotherapy is a safe, effective method of removing waste from the large intestine, without the use of drugs. By introducing pure, filtered and temperature-regulated water into the colon, human waste is softened and loosened, resulting in evacuation through natural peristalsis.

Massage

Massage therapy is a hands-on treatment of the muscular structure of the body that involves use of stroking, rubbing, kneading, tapping and/or vibrating motions for the purpose of improving circulation and muscle tone and relaxing the mind and body.

Meditation

This practice involves focused contemplation for the purpose of quieting the busy mind and relaxing the body. Typically, the focus is upon a sound, a word, an image, a thought or upon one's breath.

Music Therapy

This is an established health care profession that integrates music and music activities into treatment programs to promote and maintain wellness or to address the physical, emotional, social and intellectual challenges faced by patients.

Sauna

Application of dry or wet heat (steam) in an enclosed room or structure for the purpose of inducing sweating. The effect of such "hyperthermic therapy" is to release toxins through the skin, relax muscles and ease aches and pains. A hot tub bath can also have a therapeutic effect.

CLEANSING PROTOCOLS

Liver Cleanse

Liver formulas are usually designed to support liver detoxification mechanisms, while reducing the amount of detoxification stress.

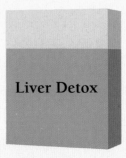

A complete liver detox program would support phase I and phase II detoxification pathways, which are overworked when liver toxicity is present. This support is best achieved with antioxidants and herbs. A complete liver detox program would ideally include three separate supplements:

- A 2-part detox system of herbs and antioxidants
- A flax fiber supplement
- Essential oils (flax, fish and borage)

The 2-part liver detox program would be followed for 30 days. Part I would include a combination of the following antioxidants and herbs:

- NAC (N-aceytl-cysteine)
- Alpha lipoic acid
- Selenium
- Vitamin C and E
- Taurine and methionine (amino acids)
- Phosphatidylcholine choline
- Milk thistle, dandelion, green tea and turmeric

This antioxidant liver formula (part I) should be accompanied by a nighttime formula (Part II) that would include herbs to increase bile flow. Ayurvedic medicine (from India) uses some wonderful herbs that have been quite successful in liver detoxification. They include:

- Belleric myrobalan fruit (Terminalia bellerica)
- Boerhavia diffusa root and herb
- Eclipta alba root and herb
- Tinospora conrdifolia stem
- Andrographis paniculata leaf
- Picrohiza Kurroa root

This combination of antioxidants and herbs (parts I and II) creates a total liver detox formula, which can be followed continuously while adhering to dietary guidelines. A good flax fiber supplement added to this program will help absorb the toxins that are being eliminated from the liver.

Nutrient supplementation might include multi-vitamin/mineral support and/or the addition of super foods (such as green drinks), with emphasis on B vitamins.

After completing this detox program, many people feel rejuvenated and have noticeably more energy. Those who are in good health need this type of detox to stay on that path. Those with chronic health problems (especially those with liver damage), need this type of detox as part of their recovery process. The 30-day program may be repeated for optimal results.

Thirty-Day Detox Protocol

Since most of us in today's world lead busy, stressful lives, it is of utmost importance to keep the cleansing program as simple as possible. There are two areas to address in beginning a cleanse: The first focuses on the cleansing of the colon, while the second targets the remaining channels of elimination – liver, blood, lymph, skin, kidneys and lungs – supporting them with herbs. This is whole body detoxification.

When the liver is overburdened with toxins, the load is passed on through blood and lymph circulation to other organs of elimination: liver, colon,

kidneys, lungs and skin. It is therefore wise to begin a general cleanse that is designed to support all of these organs simultaneously, with special emphasis on the liver. General cleanse kits are easy to use and constitute a 30-day cleansing program. Such kits should include herbs that provide support for all organs and systems of elimination. Included in an effective herbal cleansing formula would be:

- **Milk thistle** – stimulates bile secretion, acts as an antioxidant, and strengthens the cells of the liver to protect them.

- **Dandelion** – stimulates bile and acts as a gentle laxative.

- **Beet** – helps reduce damaging fats in the liver.

- **Artichoke leaf** – stimulates secretion of bile and protects cells of the liver.

- **Mullein, an expectorant** – helps expel mucus from the lungs.

- **Burdock** – helps purge toxins that cause skin conditions.

- **Corn silk** – a diuretic to flush the kidneys

- **Red clover** – a blood purifier and expectorant

- **Larch gum** – helps the lymphatic system.

The formula should also include herbs to support the heart (hawthorne berry) and the adrenal glands (ashwaganda). It must also address colon detoxification. Among other colon cleansing herbs, it would contain aloe, rhubarb and triphala to stimulate peristalsis and magnesium hydroxide to regulate water in the bowel. It is very important that the colon function properly or it will not be capable of eliminating toxins from the liver. These toxins will then recirculate, creating more of a problem. Formulas like this should be taken in the evening before retiring. Kits containing these herbs that address both colon and whole body cleansing make your cleanse very easy to perform.

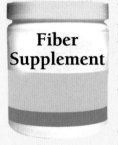

Fiber is also important in a preventive or beginning detox program. Cleansing stimulates the liver to release toxins into the bile, which is then secreted back into the digestive tract (via the gallbladder). It is necessary to ingest extra fiber for these toxins to be absorbed and removed in the bowel elimination. One of the best fiber supplements is flax, as it is about 50% soluble and 50% insoluble fiber. Soluble fiber absorbs the toxins, and insoluble fiber sweeps the colon. Flax is also available in organic (pesticide-free) form, which is a plus. Never do a cleansing program without adding fiber for support to pick up and eliminate the toxins.

A final component in your complete body detox program would be daily intake of essential fatty acids from good quality oils. Essential fatty acids (EFAs) are fats the body cannot make from other materials and therefore must obtain from outside food sources. EFAs lubricate and soothe the colon. They are also crucial in virtually every vital function of the body, including heart health and immunity. While there are several good sources of essential fatty acids, some of the best are:

• Fish oils – high in Omega-3
• Flax – high in vegetable Omega-3
• Borage – high in Omega-9

These essential oils are important in the digestive tract. A good product has the digestive enzyme lipase in the gel cap. Lipase is the enzyme that breaks down fat. It is a great way to enhance a detox program, for consuming oils without lipase puts a strain on the digestive organs.

Healing Crisis

While the net result of a cleanse will be elimination of toxins from the body, improved health and more energy, it is quite common to feel worse before feeling better. As herbal cleansing formulas kill disease-causing microorganisms such as Candida and parasites, toxins are released into the system. If they are released faster than the body can eliminate them, you may experience such symptoms as fever, fatigue, diarrhea, cramps, headache, increased thirst, loss of appetite, flu-like conditions, skin eruptions or irritations. These symptoms are due to a 'die-off' reaction known as the Herxheimer Reaction or healing crisis. It is sometimes difficult to distinguish between such a reaction and an actual illness. A natural health care practitioner can be of assistance in this regard. Generally speaking, the healing crisis is short-lived (a day or two, but usually no longer than a week). Symptoms may range from mild to severe, depending upon the rate of cleansing. The following steps will help to avoid, reduce or eliminate a severe healing crisis.

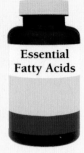

• Start at very low doses of your herbal cleansing formula – half the recommended dose (or less, if necessary), and then gradually increase to the recommended level during a 30-day period.
• If liver support herbs are not present in your cleansing formula or you have a history of liver problems, support the liver with an appropriate herbal formula.
• Initiate the necessary dietary modification two weeks before starting the herbal cleanse.
• Get colon hydrotherapy sessions.
• Increase your water intake.
• Always take a fiber supplement.

A healing crisis, while uncomfortable to experience, is actually a sign of healing in progress. So, if the symptoms are mild and tolerable, there is no need to adjust the dosage of your herbal cleansing product. Try to resist the temptation to suppress symptoms with drugs: it will only increase the body's toxic load and halt the cleansing process.

When you start a detox (cleansing) program, especially as a first-time cleanser, it is important to keep it simple. A realistic commitment is required to stay excited about creating long-term optimal health. Some detox options may not be available to you, or you may not be able to fit them into your schedule. The whole body herbal cleansing program is not a one-time affair. It is best incorporated into a prevention program at least twice a year. It is the first step toward complete detoxification. For people who have many health problems, it may be necessary to seek the services of a natural health care practitioner or physician who can design a custom program. Regardless of whether you choose this option or elect to use a pre-formulated cleanse, this is your first step in the detoxification process, the cornerstone of good health. Whichever option is chosen, clean the digestive system, and support the organs of elimination before moving on to more advanced cleanses, like those that address Candida, parasites, heavy metals or liver detoxification.

To summarize, a simplified 30-day whole-body cleanse would look like this:

1. Maintain a 'clean,' healthy diet, one which excludes refined starches and includes the following:

   - Plenty of fresh organic fruits and vegetables
   - Organic meat, (2 1/2 ounces per meal for women, 3 1/2–4 ounces per meal for men)
   - Ezekiel bread (sprouted whole grain)
   - Herbal teas
   - Purified water (with minerals added back) – 7 to 10 glasses daily
   - Fresh juices (optional)
   - Cold-pressed (unrefined) olive oil
   - Real butter

2. Take an herbal detox formula (which contains herbs discussed in this chapter) morning and night for 30 days. To help support the body in the cleansing process during this time, also add:

   - Essential oils after breakfast and dinner (one to two capsules)
   - A balanced flax fiber supplement before bed
   - Vitamins, minerals after meals
   - Super foods such as green drinks
   - Plant enzymes (containing HCl, if necessary) with meals.

3. Skin brush.

4. Take a hot therapeutic bath, steam bath or sauna three times a week.

5. Try colon hydrotherapy at least three times or more during the 30–day detox.

6. Exercise for 30 minutes: walking, yoga or rebounder.

Resource Directory

CALCIUM/MAGNESIUM SUPPLEMENTS

Floradix Calcium Magnesium with Zinc and Vitamin D
Flora, Inc.
P. O. Box 73
805 E. Badger Road
Lynden, WA 98264
1-800-446-2110
Web Site: www.florahealth.com

CANDIDA INFORMATION

Web Site: www.candida-yeast.com

CELTIC SEA SALT

The Grain and Salt Society
273 Fairway Drive
Asheville, NC 28805
1-800-TOP-SALT (867-7258)
Web Site: www.celtic-seasalt.com

COMPLEMENTARY MIND/BODY THERAPIES (ORGANIZATIONS)

Acupuncture

American Academy of Medical Acupuncture
4929 Wilshire Boulevard
Suite 428
Los Angeles, CA 90010
323-937-5514
Web Site: www.medicalacupuncture.org

Biofeedback

Heart Math
14700 West Park Avenue
Boulder Creek, CA 95006
800-372-3100
fax: 831-338-9861
Web Site: www.heartmath.com

Chiropractic

American Chiropractic Association
1701 Clarendon Blvd.
Arlington, VA 22209
800-986-4636
Web Site: www.amerchiro.org

Colon Hydrotherapy

I-ACT (International Association of Colon Therapists)
P.O. Box 461285
San Antonio, TX 78246-1285
210-366-2888
Web Site: www.i-act.org

Masssage Therapy

American Massage Therapy Association
820 Davis Street, Suite 100
Evanston, IL 60201-4444
847-864-1178
Web Site: www.amtamassage.org

Meditation

Web Site: www.meditationsociety.com

Music Therapy

American Music Therapy Association, Inc.
8455 Colesville Road, Suite 1000
Silver Spring, MD 20910
301-589-3300
Web Site: www.musictherapy.org

Yoga

Yoga Research and Education Center
P.O. Box 426
Manton, CA 96059
530-474-5700
Web Site: www.yrec.org

COMPOUNDING PHARMACIES

International Academy of Compounding Pharmacists
1-800-927-4227, ext. 30
(To find a compounding pharmacist in your area, call the
above number and leave a message.)
Web Site: www.pofsupport.org/linkpharmacies. htm

DENTAL INFORMATION (HOLISTIC)

DAMS (Dental Amalgam Mercury Syndrome)
3226 17th Ave. South, #1
Minneapolis, MN 55407
1-800-311-6265

DIAGNOSTIC TESTING LABS

(Can Only be Used by Licensed Physicians)
Great Smokies Diagnostic Laboratory
63 Zillicoa St.
Asheville, NC 28801-1074
800-522-4762
Web Site: www.gsdl.com

Doctor's Data
P.O. Box 111
West Chicago, IL 60185
1-800-323-2784 or 630-231-9190
Web Site: www.doctorsdata.com

Mead Labs, LLC (Pharmacon Adrenal Saliva Test)
1211 N.W. Glisan St., Ste. 202
Portland, OR 97209
1-888-509-8500
Web Site: www.meadlabs.com

Meta Metrix
4855 Peachtree Ind. Blvd.
Norcross, GA 30092
1-800-221-4640

Parasitology Center, Inc.
903 S. Rural Road, #101-318
Tempe, AZ 85281
480-767-2522
fax: 480-767-5855
Web Site: www.parasitetesting.com

DIGESTIVE DISEASE ORGANIZATIONS FOR PATIENTS

American Celiac Society
59 Crystal Ave.
West Orange, NJ 07052
973-325-8837
E-mail: AmerCeliacSoc@netscape.nt

American Liver Foundation
75 Maiden Lane
New York, NY 10038
800-465-4837 or 888-443-7872
Web Site: www.liverfoundation.org

Celiac Disease Foundation
13251 Ventura Blvd., #1
Studio City, CA 91604-1838
818-990-2354
Web Site: www.celiac.org

Celiac Sprue Association/USA, Inc.
P.O. Box 31700
Omaha, NE 68131-0700
402-558-0600
Web Site: www.csaceliacs.org

Center for Ulcer Research and Education Foundation
1161 San Vincente Blvd., Ste. 304
Los Angeles, CA 90049
213-825-5091

Crohn's & Colitis Foundation of America, Inc.
386 Park Ave. South, 17th Floor
New York, NY 10016-8804
800-932-2423 or 212-685-3440
Web Site: www.ccfa.org

Digestive Disease National Coalition
711 2nd Street N.E., Ste. 200
Washington, DC 20002
202-544-7497
Web Site: www.ddnc.org

Food Allergy Network
10400 Eaton Place, Ste. 107
Fairfax, VA 22030-2208
800-929-4040 or 703-691-3179
Web Site: www.foodallergy.org

Gluten Intolerance Group of North America
15110 10th Ave., S.W., Ste. A
Seattle, WA 98166-1820
206-246-6652
Web Site: www.gluen.net

Hepatitis Foundation International
504 Blick Dr.
Silver Spring, MD 20904-2901
800-891-0707 or 301-622-4200
Web Site: www.hepfi.org

International Foundation for Functional Gastrointestinal Disorders
P.O. Box 170864
Milwaukee, WI 53217-8076
414-964-1799
Web Site: www.iffgd.org

Intestinal Disease Foundation, Inc.
Landmarks Building, Ste. 525
One Station Square
Pittsburgh, PA 15219
412-261-5888 or 877-587-9606
Web Site: www.intestinalfoundation.org

National Digestive Diseases Information Clearinghouse
Two Information Way
Bethesda, MD 20892-3570
301-654-3810
Web Site: http://digestive.niddk.nih.gov

Pediatric Crohn's & Colitis Association, Inc.
P.O. Box 188
Newton, MA 02168
617-244-6678

United Ostomy Association, Inc.
19772 MacArthur Blvd., Ste. 200
Irvine, CA 92612-2405
800-826-0826 or 714-660-8624
Web Site: www.uoa.org

HEMORRHOIDS

Pilex®
25675 Meadowview Ct.
Salinas, CA 93908-9396
831-484-7820 or 800-745-3995 (10 to 8 EST)
fax: 831-484-2203
Web Site: www.pilex.com

HERBAL CLEANSING/DIGESTIVE PRODUCTS

Renew Life Formulas, Inc.
2076 Sunnydale Blvd.
Clearwater, FL 33765
800-830-4778
Web Site: www.renewlife.com

HOLISTIC PHYSICIANS

American Academy of Environmental Medicine
7701 E. Kellogg St., Ste. 625
Wichita, KS 67207-1705
316-684-5500
Web Site: www.aaem.com

American Association of Naturopathic Physicians
2366 Eastlake Ave. E.
Seattle, WA 98102
206-323-7610
Web Site: www.naturopathic.org

American College for Advancement in Medicine
23121 Verdugo Dr., Ste. 204
Laguna Hills, CA 92653
949-583-7666
fax: 949-455-9679
Web Site: www.acam.org

American Holistic Medical Association
4101 Lake Boone Trail, Ste. 201
Raleigh, NC 27607
919-787-5146

Institute for Functional Medicine
4411 Pt. Fosdick Dr., N.W., Ste. 305
Gig Harbor, WA 98335
800-228-0622
Web Site: www.functionalmedicine.org

National Institute of Environmental Health Sciences
P.O. Box 12233
Research Triangle Park, NC 27709
919-541-3345
Web Site: www.niehs.nih.gov

IBS SUPPORT GROUP

Web Site: www.ibsgroup.org

IRON SUPPLEMENTS

Floradix Iron & Herbs
Flora, Inc.
P. O. Box 73
805 E. Badger Road
Lynden, WA 98264
1-800-446-2110
Web Site: www.florahealth.com

LIFESTEP™

Renew Life Formulas, Inc.
2076 Sunnydale Blvd.
Clearwater, FL 33765
800-830-4778
Web Site: www.renewlife.com

MAGAZINE

Sully's Living Without – A Lifestyle Guide for People with Food & Chemical Sensitivities
P.O. Box 2126
Northbrook, IL 60065
Web Site: www.LivingWithout.com

MEAL REPLACEMENT

Living Fuel Rx (see www.livingfuel.com) is a hypoallergenic, complete, functional alkaline food that is suitable for food-sensitive individuals. It is an organic, wild-crafted, all natural, raw, plant-based, optimized meal replacement powder. In addition, it is a foundational food for all blood types and all metabolic types. Living Fuel Rx provides complete building blocks and fuel for the body, brain and every cell in a nutri-ent-dense restricted calorie format. Most people, including professional athletes, find that they can thrive on one serving for 3-4 hours. The product is also being successfully used with infants, pregnant women and senior citizens. The protein source for Living Fuel Rx is entirely plant-derived, with added amino acids (glutamine, taurine, lysine and N-acetyl-cysteine) to create a complex similar in composition to egg protein.

Each serving of Living Fuel Rx has more calcium than milk, more potassium than bananas, more fiber than oatmeal, more friendly bacteria (probiotics) than yogurt, more protein than a half dozen egg whites and more greens or berries, cofactors, vitamins, minerals, antioxidants and other phy-tonutrients than a basket of fruits and vegetables, plus Omega-3 essential fatty acids and selected herbs (see nutrition facts at www.livingfuel.com).

Living Fuel Rx is designed to be completely balanced, hypoal-lergenic and to have a low glycemic response. It is a blend of the earth's most potent organic, wildcrafted and all natural foods that have been optimized with the most bioavailable and usable nutrients and co-factors, including stabilized pro-biotics for healthy intestinal function, herbs to enhance major body systems, antioxidants to protect against free radical dam-age, vitamins and minerals to optimize the naturally occurring vitamin and mineral profile of the foods, amino acids to opti-mize the naturally occurring amino acid profile of the plant proteins and a custom enzyme complex to maximize the delivery of nutrients to the body. website: www.livingfuel.com

MINI-TRAMPOLINES (REBOUNDERS)

BounceWell 2003
P.O. Box 6245
Stateline, NV 89449-6245
877-541-7236
Web Site: www.bouncewell.com

NUTRITION

Price-Pottenger Nutrition Foundation
7890 Broadway
Lemon Grove, CA 91945
800-366-3748
fax: 619-433-3136
Web Site: www.price-pottenger.org

The Weston A. Price Foundation
4200 Wisconsin Ave., N.W.
Washington, DC 20007
202-333-HEAL
Web Site: www.westonaprice.org

SAUNAS (INFRARED)

High Tech Health, Inc.
2695 Linden Drive
Boulder, CO 80304-0450
303-413-8500 or 1-800-794-5355
Web Site: www.hightechhealth.com

TheraSauna™
1021 State St.
Bettendorf, IA 52722
Web Site: www.therasauna.com
1-888-729-7727

SLANT BOARDS

True Foods Market
877-274-5914
Web Site: www.truefoodsmarket.com/js249.html

HerbsFirst
501 W. 965 North, Suite 3
Orem, UT 84057
Fax: 1-801-437-3538
Web Site: www.herbsfirst.com/electronics/Slant6.html

SWEETENER (NATURAL)

SweetLife
Renew Life Formulas, Inc.
2076 Sunnydale Blvd.
Clearwater, FL 33765
1-800-830-4778, ext. 246
Web Site: www.renewlife.com

VITAMIN E

J.R. Carlson Laboratories, Inc.
15 College Drive
Arlington Heights, IL 60004-1985
847-255-1600
888-234-5656
Web Site: www.carlsonlabs.com

Endnotes

CHAPTER 1

[1] Steven R. Peikin, MD, *GastroIntestinal Health*, Quill, 1999, p. 17.

[2] M. Sara Rosenthal, *The Gastroinstestinal Sourcebook*, Lowell House, 1997, p. 2.

[3] Op. Cit., Peikin, p. 1.

[4] Tonia Reinhard, MS, RD, *Gastroinstestinal Disorders and Nutrition*, Contemporary Books, 2002, p. 17.

[5] *Dorland's Pocket Medical Dictionary*, 23rd edition, W. B. Saunders Company, 1982.

[6] Jordan S. Rubin, NMD, CNC, *Patient Heal Thyself*, Freedom Press, 2003, p.32.

[7] Michael D. Gershon, MD, *The Second Brain*, Harper Perennial, 1998, p. 70.

[8] Ibid., p.xiii.

[9] Ibid.

[10] Op.Cit., Rubin, p. 32

[11] Op. Cit., Rubin, p. 33.

CHAPTER 2

Barrett's Esophagus

[1] A.J. Cameron, et al., "The Incidence of Adenocarcinoma in Columnar-lined (Barrett's) Esophagus," *New England Journal of Medicine*, 1985; 313(14): 857-9.

[2] A.J. Cameron, et al., "Prevalence of Columnar-lined (Barrett's) Esophagus: Comparison of Population-Based Clinical and Autopsy Findings," *Gastroenterology*, 1990; 99(4):918-22

[3] http://health.yahoo.com/health/centers/digestive/104.html

[4] www.gicare.com/pated/ecdgs40.htm.

[5] Ibid.

[6] www.barrettsinfo.com

[7] Ibid.

[8] www.jamesline.com/output/barrett.htm.

[9] Op.Cit., http://health.yahoo.com

[10] A.J. Cameron and C.T. Lomboy, "Barrett's Esophagus: Age, Prevalence, Etiology, and Complications," *Gastroenterology*, 1992; 103(4):1241-5.

[11] Ibid.

[12] Op. Cit., www.jamesline.com.

[13] Op. Cit., www.barrettsinfo.com.

[14] Mark R. Dambro, *Griffith's 5-Minute Clinical Consult*, 2003, p. 430.

[15] Op. Cit., www.gicare.com

[16] R.E. Sampliner, "Practice Guidelines on the Diagnosis, Surveillance, and Therapy of Barrett's Esophagus: The Practice Parameters Committee of the American College of Gastroenterology. *The American Journal of Gastroenterology*, 1998; 93(7):1028-32.

[17] Op. Cit., www.barrettsinfo.com.

[18] Ibid.

[19] Op. Cit., http://health.yahoo.com

Esophagitis

[1] http://gastroresource.com/GITextbook/en/chapter5/5-8-pr.htm

[2] www.ecureme.com/emyhealth/data/Esophagitis.asp

[3] Op. Cit., http://gastrosource.com

[4] Ibid.

[5] Ibid.

[6] Tonia Reinhard, MS, RD, *Gastrointestinal Disorders and Nutrition*, Contemporary Books, 2002, p. 40.

[7] www.intelihealth.com/IH/ihtlH/WSlHW000/8293/25982/187000 /html?d=dmtHealthAZ

[8] Op. Cit., Reinhard.

[9] www.digitalnaturopath.com/cond/C341769.html

[10] Op. Cit., www.ecureme.com

[11] Op. Cit., http://gastroresource.com

GERD

[1] Jonathan V. Wright, MD and Lane Lenard, PhD, *Why Stomach Acid is Good for You*, M. Evans and Company, Inc., 2001, p. 135.

[2] Ibid.

[3] *The Merck Manual*, Eleventh Edition, Merck Sharp & Dohme Research Laboratories, 1966, p.531.

[4] Op. Cit., Wright Lenard,, p. 16.

[5] Ibid., p. 130.

[6] Judy Kitchen, "Hypochlorhydria: A Review – Part I," *Townsend Letter for Doctors and Patients*, October 2001, p. 56.

[7] Op. Cit., Wright and Lenard, p. 33.

[8] Raphael Kellman, MD, *Gut Reactions*, Broadway Books, 2002, p. 86.

[9] Michael Murray, ND & Joseph Pizzorno, ND, *Encyclopedia of Natural Medicine*, Prima Health, 1998, p. 135.

[10] Op. Cit., Wright, p. 40.

[11] Linda A. Ross (editor), *Gastrointestinal Diseases and Disorders Sourcebook*, Volume 16, Omnigraphics, Inc., 1996, p. 112.

[12] Ibid.

[13] Ibid., p. 43.

[14] M. Sara Rosenthal, *The Gastrointestinal Sourcebook*, Lowell House, 1997, p.61.

[15] Op. Cit., Wright, p. 22.

[16] John D. Kirschmann and Lavon J. Dunne, *Nutrition Almanac*, McGraw Hill Book Company, 1984, p. 171.

[17] Dr. John McKenna, *Hard to Stomach*, Newleaf, 2002, p. 78.

[18] Op. Cit., Wright and Lenard, p. 25-30.

[19] Op. Cit., Murray & Pizzorno, p. 134.

[20] Leonard Smith, "Ease the Burn – Promote Acid Production," *Complementary Therapies in Chronic Care*, January, 2001.

[21] Op. Cit., Wright and Lenard, p. 95.

[22] Ibid., p. 35.

[23] Op. Cit., Kellas and Dworkin.

[24] Op. Cit., Wright and Lenard, p. 35.

Heartburn

[1] National Heartburn Alliance, *Get Heartburn Smart*, Chicago, Il (www.heartburnalliance.org), p. 3.

[2] Steven R. Peikin, MD, *Gastrointestinal Health*, Quill, 2001, p. 43.

Hiatal Hernia

[1] Tonia Reinhard, MS, RD, *Gastrointestinal Disorders and Nutrition*, Contemporary Books, 2002, p. 52.

[2] Ibid.

[3] Raphael Kellman, *MD, Gut Reactions*, Broadway Books, 2002, p. 91.

[4] Jonathan V. Wright, MD, and Lane Lenard, PhD, *Why Stomach Acid is Good for You*, M. Evans and Company, Inc., 2001, p. 54.

[5] Ibid.

[6] Op. Cit., Reinhard, p. 54.

[7] Ibid., p. 52.

[8] Ibid.

[9] Ibid.

[10] Ibid.

General Recommendations for all Esophageal Problems

[1] Op. Cit. Wright and Lenard, p. 142, 143.

[2] Phyllis A. Balch, CNC and James F. Balch, MD, *Prescription for Nutritional Healing*, Third Edition, Avery, 2000, p. 423.

[3] Ibid.

[4] Op., Cit., Balch and Balch, p. 422.

[5] Op. Cit., Wright and Lenard, p. 144.

[6] Ibid., p. 152.

CHAPTER 3

Gastritis

[1] Tonia Reinhard, MS, RD, *Gastrointestinal Disorders and Nutrition*, Contemporary Books, 2002, p. 55.

[2] Ibid., p. 59.

[3] Raphael Kellman, MD, *Gut Reactions*, Broadway Books, 2002, p. 84.

[4] Op. Cit., Reinhard, p. 56.

[5] Ibid., p. 58.

[6] Ibid.

[7] Ibid.

[8] Ibid., p. 57.

[9] Ibid.

[10] Ibid.

[11] Steven R. Peikin, MD, *Gastrointestinal Health*, Quill, 2001, p. 52.

[12] Op. Cit., Reinhard, p. 60.

[13] Op. Cit., Kellman, p. 85.

[14] Elizabeth Lipski, MS, CCN, *Digestive Wellness*, Keats Publishing, Inc., 1996, p. 204.

[15] Jonathan V. Wright, MD and Lane Lenard, PhD, *Why Stomach Acid is Good for You*, M. Evans and Company, Inc., 2001, p. 92.

[16] Ibid, p. 93.

[17] Op. Cit., Reinhard, p. 62.

[18] Ibid.

[19] Ibid., p. 63.

Peptic Ulcers

[1] *Dorland's Pocket Medical Dictionary*, 23rd edition, W. B. Sanders Company, 1982, p. 527.

2 Michael Murray, ND and Joseph Pizzorno, ND, *Encyclopedia of Natural Medicine*, Revised 2nd Edition, Prima Health, 1998, p. 810.

3 Steven R. Peikin, MD, *Gastrointestinal Health*, Quill, 2001, p. 54.

4 Ibid.

5 Ibid.

6 Henry D. Janowitz, MD, *Indigestion*, Oxford University Press, 1992, p. 86.

7 Op. Cit. Janowitz, p. 62.

8 Raphael Kellman, MD, *Gut Reactions*, Broadway Books, 2002, p. 101.

9 Ibid.

10 Ibid.

11 Ibid., p. 101-102.

12 M. Sara Rosenthal, *The Gastrointestinal Sourcebook*, Lowell House, 1998, p.51.

13 Ibid., p. 47.

14 Op. Cit., Murray and Pizzorno, p. 811.

15 Linda M. Ross (editor), *Gastrointestinal Diseases and Disorders Sourcebook*, Volume 16, Omnigraphics, Inc., 1996, p. 140.

16 Op. Cit., Reinhard, p. 69.

17 Ibid., p. 812.

18 Dr. John McKenna, *Hard to Stomach*, Newleaf, 2002, p. 121.

19 Op. Cit., Murray and Pizzorno, p. 813.

20 Ibid.

21 D. Lindsey Berkson, *Healthy Digestion the Natural Way*, John Wiley and Sons, Inc., 2000, p. 117, 122.

22 Op. Cit. Murray and Pizzorno, p. 813.

23 Ibid.

24 Ibid., p. 812.

25 Ibid.

26 Op. Cit., Ross, p. 139.

27 Op. Cit., Reinhard, p. 64.

28 Op. Cit., Berkson, p. 113.

29 Op. Cit., Ross, p. 138.

30 Ibid., p. 141.

31 Op. Cit. Rosenthal, p. 40.

32 Op. Cit., Berkson, p. 114.

33 Op. Cit., Peikin, p. 53.

34 Op. Cit., Berkson.

35 Op. Cit. Janowitz, p. 68.

36 Op. Cit., Peikin, p. 57.

37 Op. Cit., Berkson, p. 119.

38 Op. Cit., Kellman, p. 102

39 Op. Cit., Murray and Pizzorno, p. 811.

41 Op. Cit., Peikin, p. 63.

CHAPTER 4

Appendix

1 www.ivillagehealth.com/library/onemed/content/0,,241012_245563.00.html

2 www.stayinginshape.com/30sfcorp/libv/i39.shtml

3 www.mothernature.com/Library/bookshelf/Books/62/7.cfm

4 Phyllis A. Balch, CNC and James F. Balch, MD, *Prescription for Nutritional Healing*, 3rd edition, Avery, 2000, p. 183.

5 Op. Cit., www.mothernature.com

6 www.netdoctor.co.uk/diseases/facts/appendicitis.htm

7 Op. Cit., www.stayinginshape.com

8 Op.Cit. www.netdoctor.co.uk

9 *Radiology*, October 2002; 225(1):131-6

Candidiasis

1 D. Lindsey Berkson, *Healthy Digestion the Natural Way*, John Wiley & Sons, Inc., 2000, p. 158.

2 Dr. William R. Kellas and Dr. Andrea Sharon Dworkin, *Surviving the Toxic Crisis*, Professional Preference, 1996, p. 184.

3 Ibid., p. 189

4 Michael Murray, ND and Joseph Pizzorno, ND, *Encyclopedia of Natural Medicine*, Revised 2nd edition, Prima Health, 1998, p. 300.

5 Op. Cit., Kellas and Dworkin, p. 438.

6 Phyllis A. Balch, CNC and James F. Balch, MD, *Prescription for Nutritional Healing*, Third Edition, Avery, 2000, p. 263.

7 Op. Cit., Murray and Pizzorno, p. 301.

8 Op. Cit., Kellas and Dworkin, p. 438.

9 Luc De Schepper, MD, PhD, CA, *Candida*, Second Edition, 1990, p. 6.

10 Op. Cit., Kellas and Dworkin, p. 437-438.

11 Op. Cit., Balch and Balch.

12 Op. Cit., Kellas and Dworkin, p. 437.

13 Op. Cit., Berkson, p. 159.

14 Op. Cit., Murray and Pizzorno, p. 304.

15 William Crook, MD, *The Yeast Connection*, Professional Books, Inc., p. 216.

Constipation

1 Andrew Gaeddert, *Healing Digestive Disorders*, North Atlantic Books, 1998, p. 130.

2 Linda M. Ross (editor), *Gastrointestinal Diseases and Disorders Sourcebook*, Omnigraphics, Inc., 1996, p.240-241.

3 Raphael Kellman, MD, *Gut Reactions*, Broadway Books, 2002, p. 74-75.

4 Steven R.Peikin, MD, *Gastrointestinal Health*, Revised edition, Quill, 1999, p. 93-94.

5 Henry D. Janowitz, MD, *Your Gut Feelings*, Consumer's Union, 1987, p. 95-96.

6 Phyllis A. Balch, CNC and James F. Balch, MD, *Prescription for Nutritional Healing*, Third edition, Avery, 2000, p. 301.

7 Elizabeth Lipski, MS, CCN, *Digestive Wellness*, Keats Publishing, Inc., 1996, p. 231.

8 Life Extension Media, *Disease Prevention and Treatment*, Expanded Third Edition, Life Extension Foundation, 2000, p. 213.

9 D. Lindsay Berkson, *Healthy Digestion the Natural Way*, John Wiley & Sons, Inc. 2000, p. 74.

10 "Constipation," *Nutri Notes*, Vol. 9, #1-02

11 www.wilsonsthyroidsyndrome.com

12 "The Thyroid as a Metabolic Regulator of the Colon," *Nutri Notes*, Vol. 9, #1-02.

13 Op. Cit., D. Lindsey Berkson, p. 12.

14 Op. Cit., Ross, p. 242.

15 Op. Cit., Kellman, p. 74.

16 Op. Cit., Lipski, p. 228.

17 Op. Cit., Balch and Balch.

18 Ibid.

19 Op. Cit., Berkson, p. 68.

20 Ibid, p. 69-70

21 Ibid, p. 70.

22 Ibid.

23 Op. Cit., Berkson, p. 12-13.

24 Op. Cit., Balch and Balch, p. 302.

25 Tonia Reinhard, MS, RD, *Gastrointestinal Disorders and Nutrition*, Contemporary Books, 2002, p. 104.

26 Dr. William R. Kellas and Dr. Andrea Sharon Dworkin, *Surviving the Toxic Crisis*, Professional Preference, 1996, p. 134.

27 Op. Cit., Life Extension Media, p. 212.

28 Ibid.

29 Jonathan V. Wright. MD and Lane Lenard, PhD., *Why Stomach Acid is Good for You*, M. Evans and Company, Inc., 2001, p. 28.

Diarrhea

1 D. Lindsey Berkson, *Healthy Digestion the Natural Way*, John Wiley & Sons, Inc., 2000, p. 81.

2 Ibid.

3 Michael Murray, ND and Joseph Pizzorno, ND, *Encyclopedia of Natural Medicine*, Prima Health, 1998, p. 433.

4 Steven R. Peikin, MD, *Gastrointestinal Health*, Quill, 1999, p. 108.

5 Raphael Kellman, MD, *Gut Reactions*, Broadway Books, 2002, p. 79.

6 Henry D. Janowitz, MD, *Your Gut Feelings*, Consumer's Union, 1987, p. 83.

7 Op. Cit., Murray and Pizzorno, p. 436.

8 Op. Cit., Janowitz, p. 80.

9 Ibid.

10 Ibid., p. 91.

11 Op. Cit., Janowitz, p. 80.

12 Ibid. p. 86.

13 Op. Cit., Peikin, p. 103.

14 Ibid., p. 100.

15 Linda M. Ross (editor), *Gastrointestinal Diseases and Disorders Sourcebook*, Volume 16, Omnigraphics, Inc., 1996, p. 236.

16 Michael D. Gershon, MD, *The Second Brain*, HarperPerennial, 1998, p. 150.

17 Op. Cit., Peikin, p. 104.

18 Andrew Gaeddert, *Healing Digestive Disorders*, North Atlantic Books, 1998, p. 141.

19 Ibid., p. 141-142.

Diverticular Disease

1 D. Lindsey Berkson, *Healthy Digestion the Natural Way*, John Wiley & Sons, Inc., 2000, p. 89.

2 Michael D. Gershon, MD, *The Second Brain*, Harper Perennial, 1998, p. 167.

3 Andrew Gaeddert, *Healing Digestive Disorders*, North Atlantic Books, 1998, p. 147.

4 Tonia Reinhard, MS, RD, *Gastrointestinal Disorders and Nutrition*, Contemporary Books, 2002, p. 111.

5 Phyllis A. Balch, CNC and James F. Balch, MD, *Prescription for Nutritional Healing*, Third Edition, Avery, 2000, p. 328.

6 Op. Cit., Reinhard, p. 109.

7 Op. Cit., Berkson, p. 88.

8 Op. Cit., Reinhard.

9 Linda A. Ross (editor), *Gastrointestinal Diseases and Disorders Sourcebook*, Omnigraphics, Inc., 1996, p. 186.

10 Elizabeth Lipski, MS, CCN, *Digestive Wellness*, Keats Publishing, Inc., 1996, p. 235.

11 Op. Cit., Balch and Balch.

12 Ibid.

13 Raphael Kellman, MD, *Gut Reactions*, Broadway Books, 2002, p. 82.

14 Steven R. Peikin, *Gastrointestinal Health*, Quill, 1999, p.107.

15 Ibid, p. 108.

16 Ibid.

17 Henry D. Janowitz, MD, *Your Gut Feelings*, Consumer's Union, 1987, p. 139.

18 Ibid.

19 Op. Cit., Berkson, p. 92.

20 Op. Cit., Renihard, p. 114.

21 Op. Cit., Janowitz, p. 139.

22 Op. Cit., Reinhard.

23 Ibid, p. 117

24 Op. Cit., Janowitz, p. 143

Gas

1 D. Lindsey Berkson, *Healthy Digestion the Natural Way*, John Wiley & Sons, Inc., 2000, p. 49.

2 Henry D. Janowitz, MD, *Your Gut Feelings*, Consumer's Union, 1987, p. 178.

3 Tonia Reinhard, MS, RD, *Gastrointestinal Disorders and Nutrition*, Contemporary Books, 2002, p. 89.

4 Steven R. Peikin, MD, *Gastrointestinal Health*, Quill, 1999, p. 89

5 Op. Cit., Berkson.

6 Susan Stockton, *The Terrain is Everything*, Power of One Publishing, 2000, p. 154.

7 Op. Cit., Peikin.

8 Linda M. Ross, editor, *Gastrointestinal Diseases and Disorders Sourcebook*, Omnigraphics, Inc., 1996, p. 53.

9 Op. Cit., Peikin.

10 Op. Cit., Berkson, p. 50.

11 Ibid., p. 54 and 51.

12 *The Merck Manual*, Seventeenth Edition, p. 317.

13 Ibid.

14 Op. Cit., Berkson, p. 52.

Gluten Sensitivity

1 John H. Dirckx, MD, editor, *Stedman's Concise Medical Dictionary for the Health Professions*, Lippincott Williams & Wilkins, 2001, p. 406.

2 Raphael Kellman, MD, *Gut Reactions*, Broadway Books, 2002, p.72.

3 Michael Murray, ND and Joseph Pizzorno, ND, *Encycopedia of Natural Medicine*, Prima Health, 1998, p. 325.

4 Op. Cit., Kellman.

5 Ibid., p. 73.

6 Op. Cit., Murray and Pizzorno, p. 325.

7 Ibid.

8 Elizabeth Lipski, MS, CCN, *Digestive Wellness*, Keats Publishing, Inc., 1996, p. 222.

9 Ibid.

10 Phyllis A. Balch, CNC and James F. Balch, MD, *Prescription for Nutritional Healing*, Third Edition, Avery, 2000, p. 279.

11 Op. Cit., Lipski.

12 Op. Cit., Murray and Pizzorno.

13 Ibid.

14 www.mercola.com/2000/Oct/9/gluten.htm

15 Op. Cit., Kellman, p. 73.

16 Tonia Reinhard, MS, RD, *Gastrointestinal Disorders and Nutrition*, Contemporary Books, 2002, p. 154.

17 Op. Cit., Balch and Balch.

18 Ibid.

19 Ibid.

20 Op. Cit., Murray and Pizzorno, p. 326.

21 Ibid.

22 Op. Cit., Reinhard, p. 157.

23 Ibid., p. 156.

24 Henry D. Janowitz, MD, *Your Gut Feelings*, Consumer's Union, 1987, p. 151.

25 Op. Cit., Murray and Pizzorno.

26 Op. Cit., Balch and Balch.

27 M. Sara Rosenthal, *The Gastrointestinal Sourcebook*, Lowell House, 1997, p. 25.

28 Op. Cit., Murray and Pizorno, p. 325.

29 Op. Cit., Balch and Balch, p. 281.

30 Op. Cit., Murray and Pizzorno, p. 327.

Hemmorrhoids

1 Michael Murray, ND and Joseph Pizzorno, ND, *Encyclopedia of Natural Medicine*, Revised 2nd edition, Prima Health, 1998, p. 507.

2 Ibid.

3 www.hemorrhoid.net

4 Phyllis A. Balch, CNC and James F. Balch, MD, *Prescription for Nutritional Healing*, Third Edition, Avery, 2000, p. 427.

5 Ibid.

6 Op. Cit., Murray and Pizzorno.

7 Op. Cit., Balch and Balch, p. 429.

Inflammatory Bowel Disease

1 Michael Murray, ND and Joseph Pizzorno, ND, *Encyclopedia of Natural Medicine*, Revised Second Edition, Prima Health, 1998, p. 594.

Ulcerative Colitis

1 Henry D. Janowitz, MD, *Your Gut Feelings*, Consumer's Union, 1987, p. 39.

2 Phylllis A. Balch, CNC and James F. Balch, MD, *Prescription for Nutritional Healing*, Third Edition, Avery, 2000, p. 666.

3 Ibid.

4 Michael Murray, ND and Joseph Pizzorno, ND, *Encyclopedia of Natural Medicine*, Revised Second Edition, Prima Health, 1998, p. 590.

5 Tonia Reinhard, MS, RD, *Gastrointestinal Disorders and Nutrition*, Contemporary Books, 2002, p. 146.

6 Ibid.

7 Op. Cit., Murray and Pizzorno, p. 588.

8 Op. Cit., Reinhard, p. 146.

9 Steven R. Peikin, MD, *Gastrointestinal Health*, Quill, 1999, p. 117.

10 Tonia Reinhard, MS, RD, *Gastrointestinal Disorders and Nutrition*, Contemporary Books, 2002, p. 148.

11 Linda M. Ross, editor, *Gastrointestinal Diseases and Disorders Sourcebook*, Omnigraphics, Inc., 1996, p. 206.

12 Op. Cit., Peikin, p. 122.

13 Ibid., p. 120.

14 Ibid.

15 Op. Cit., Ross, p. 208.

16 Ibid.

Irritable Bowel Syndrome

1 Steven R. Peikin, MD, *Gastrointestinal Health*, Quill, 1999, p. 81.

2 Raphael Kellman, MD, *Gut Reactions*, Broadway Books, 2002, p. 92.

3 Phyllis A. Balch, CNC and James F. Balch, MD, *Prescription for Nutritional Healing*, Third Edition,

Avery, 2000, p. 476-477.

4 Elizabeth Lipski, *Digestive Wellness*, Keats Publishing, Inc., 1996, p. 238.

5 Ibid.

6 Michael Murray, ND and Joseph Pizzorno, ND, *Encyclopedia of Natural Medicine*, Revised Second Edition, Prima Health, 1998, p. 611.

7 Op. Cit., Lipski, p. 239.

8 Dr. William R. Kellas and Dr. Andrea Sharon Dworkin, *Surviving the Toxic Crisis*, Professional Preference, 1996, p. 363.

9 Op. Cit., Balch and Balch, p. 476.

10 Op. Cit., Peikin, p. 82.

11 Op. Cit, Balch and Balch

12 Michael D. Gershon, MD, *The Second Brain*, Harper Perennial, 1998, p. 180.

13 Ibid, p. 179-180.

14 Tonia Reinhard, MS, RD, *Gastrointestinal Disorders and Nutrition*, Contemporary Books, 2002, p. 117.

15 Op. Cit., Gershon.

16 Ibid., p. 181.

17 Henry D. Janowitz, MD, *Your Gut Feelings*, Consumer's Union, 1987, p. 18.

18 Op. Cit., Peikin, p. 83.

19 Linda M. Ross, editor, *Gastrointestinal Diseases and Disorders Sourcebook*, Omnigraphics, Inc., 1996, p. 233.

20 Op. Cit., Peikin, p. 84.

21 Op. Cit., Murray and Pizzorno

22 Ibid., p. 612.

23 Ibid.

24 Ibid.

Lactose Intolerance

1 Tonia Reinhard, MS, RD, *Gastrointestinal Disorders and Nutrition*, Contemporary Books, 2002, p. 91.

2 Steven R. Peikin, MD, *Gastrointestinal Health*, Quill, 1999, p. 90-91.

3 D. Lindsey Berkson, *Healthy Digestion the Natural Way*, John Wiley & Sons, Inc., 2000, p. 140.

4 Andrew Gaeddert, *Healing Digestive Disorders*, North Atlantic Books, 1998, p. 182.

5 Phyllis A. Balch, CNC and James F. Balch, MD, *Prescription for Nutritional Healing*, Third Edition, Avery, 2000, p. 486.

6 James Scala, Ph.D., *The New Eating Right for a Bad Gut*, A Plume Book, 2000, p. 51.

7 Op. Cit., Reinhard, p. 90.

8 Raphael Kellman, MD, *Gut Reactions*, Broadway Books, 2002, p. 94.

9 Ibid.

10 Michael Murray, ND and Joseph Pizzorno, ND, *Encyclopedia of Natural Medicine*, Revised Second Edition, Prima Health, 1998, p. 435.

11 Op. Cit., Scala, p. 49.

12 Op. Cit., Kellman.

13 Op. Cit., Scala.

14 Op. Cit., Kellman.

15 Op. Cit., Balch and Balch.

16 Ibid, p. 487.

17 Ibid.

18 Op. Cit., Kellman.

19 Op. Cit., Scala.

20 Op. Cit., Reinhard, p. 94.

[21] Linda M. Ross, editor, *Gastrointestinal Diseases and Disorders Sourcebook*, Ominigraphics, Inc., 1996, p. 271.

[22] Ibid.

[23] Ibid.

[24] Op. Cit., Balch and Balch, p. 487.

[25] Op. Cit., Ross.

[26] Ibid.

Leaky Gut Syndrome

[1] Elizabeth Lipski, MS, CCN, *Digestive Wellness*, Keats Publishing, Inc., 1996, p. 78.

[2] Wendy Marson, "Gut Reactions," *Newsweek*, November 17, 1997, p. 95-99.

[3] http://www.health-n-energy.com/ronagut.htm

[4] Lynn Toohey, MS, PhD, "Leaky Gut – Detoxification," *Nutri Notes*, Vol. 5, #2, March-April, 1998.

[5] Dr. John McKenna, *Hard to Stomach*, NewLeaf, 2002, p. 10.

Parasitic Disease

[1] Timothy Kuss, Ph.D., *A Guidebook to Clinical Nutrition for the Health Professional*, Institute of Bioenergetic Research, 1992, p. 17.

[2] Ibid, p. 17-18

[3] www.genhealth.com/hupara.htm

[4] Michael Murray, ND and Joseph Pizzorno, ND, *Encyclopedia of Natural Medicine*, Revised 2nd edition, Prima Health, 1998, p. 144.

[5] Dr. Omar M. Amin, "Seasonal Prevalence of Intestinal Parasites in the United States During 2000," *Am J Trop Med Hyg*, 66(6), 2002, pp. 799-803.

[6] Ibid.

[7] Dr. William R. Kellas and Dr. Andrea Sharon Dworkin, *Surviving the Toxic Crisis*, Professional Preference, 1996, pp. 347, 359, 368 and 371.

[8] Ibid., p. 363.

[9] Ibid., p. 366.

[10] Op. Cit., Amin.

[11] Op. Cit., Kellas, p. 369.

[12] Op. Cit., Amin.

[13] Op. Cit., Kellas, p. 356.

[14] Ann Louise Gittleman, *Guess What Came to Dinner*, Avery Publishing Group, Inc., 1993, p. 97.

[15] Ibid., p. 357.

[16] Op. Cit., Gittleman, p. 97-100.

[17] www.freeyourself.com/html/aycop.htm

[18] Andrew Gaeddert

CHAPTER 5

Cirrhosis

[1] *Disease Prevention and Treatment, Expanded Fourth Edition*, Life Extension Media, 2003, p. 993.

[2] Linda M. Ross, editor, *Gastrointestinal Diseases and Disorders Handbook*, Omnigraphics, Inc., 1996, p. 332.

[3] Dr. William R. Kellas and Dr. Andrea Sharon Dworkin, *Surviving the Toxic Crisis*, Professional Preference, 1996, p. 54, 55.

[4] Ibid., p. 217 and 228.

[5] Rosenthal, M. Sara, *The Gastrointestinal Sourcebook*, Lowell House, 1997, p. 122.

[6] Op. Cit., *Disease Prevention and Treatment*, p. 989.

[7] Op. Cit., Kellas and Dworkin.

[8] Op. Cit., Ross.

[9] Op. Cit., *Disease Prevention and Treatment*.

[10] Op. Cit., Ross, p. 331.

[11] Op. Cit., *Disease Prevention and Treatment*, p. 991.

[12] Ibid.

[13] Ibid., p. 994.

[14] Ibid., p. 996.

Gallstones

[1] Henry D. Janowitz, MD, *Indigestion*, Oxford University Press, 1992, p. 117.

[2] Ibid.

[3] Linda M. Ross, *Gastrointestinal Diseases and Disorders Sourcebook*, Omnigraphics, Inc., 1996, p. 364.

[4] Steven R. Peikin, MD, *Gastrointestinal Health*, Quill, 1999, p. 76-77,

[5] Op. Cit., Ross, p. 365.

[6] Dr. William R. Kellas and Dr. Andrea Sharon Dworkin, *Surviving the Toxic Crisis*, Professional Preference, 1996, p. 66.

[7] Op. Cit., Peikin, p. 77.

[8] *Disease Preventon and Treatment*, expanded 4th edition, *Life Extension*, 2003, p. 990.

[9] Op. Cit., Ross.

[10] D. Lindsey Berkson, *Healthy Digestion the Natural Way*, John Wiley & Sons, Inc., 2000, p. 128.

[11] Michael Murray, ND and Joseph Pizzorno, ND, *Encyclopedia of Natural Medicine*, revised 2nd edition, Prima Health, 1998, p. 480.

[12] Phyllis A. Balch, CNC and James F. Balch, MD, *Prescription for Nutritional Healing*, third edition, Avery, 2000, p. 390.

[13] Op. Cit., Berkson, p. 127.

[14] Michael D. Gershon, MD, *The Second Brain*, Harper Perennial, 1998, p. 121.

[15] Elizabeth Lipski, MS, CCN, *Digestive Wellness*, Keats Publishing, Inc., 1996, p. 210.

[16] Op. Cit., Janowitz, p. 116.

[17] Op. Cit., Peikin, p. 76.

[18] Op. Cit., Janowitz.

[19] Op. Cit., Murray and Pizzorno, p. 479.

[20] Op. Cit., Lipski, p. 210.

[21] Op. Cit., Murray and Pizzorno, p. 476-477.

[22] Op. Cit., Ross, p. 366.

[23] Op. Cit., Peikin, p. 33.

[24] Ibid., p. 79

[25] Op. Cit., Janowitz, p. 131.

[26] Ibid.

[27] Andrew Gaeddert, *Healing Digestive Disorders*, North Atlantic Books, 1998, p.151.

[28] Op. Cit., Janowitz, p. 125-126.

[29] Ibid., p. 127

[30] Ibid., p. 128.

[31] *The Merck Manual*, Centennial Edition, Merck & Co., Inc., 1999, p. 402.

[32] Op. Cit., Janowitz, p. 122.

[33] Ibid., p. 124.

[34] Op. Cit., Lipski, p. 212.

Hepatitis

[1] Melissa Palmer, MD, *Hepatitis Liver Disease*, Avery Publishing Group, 2000, p. 72.

[2] Ibid., p. 73.

[3] Ibid., p. 78.

[4] Ibid., p. 180.

[5] Ibid., p. 381.

[6] Ibid., p. 382.

[7] www.immunize.or/catg.d/p4075abc.pdf

[8] Phyllis A. Balch, CNC and James F. Balch, MD, *Prescription for Nutritional Healing*, Avery, 2000, p. 430.

[9] Ibid.

[10] Elizabeth Lipski, *Digestive Wellness*, Keats Publishing, Inc., 1996, p. 120.

[11] Op. Cit., www.immunize.org

[12] www.mercola.com, "Hepatitis B Vaccine Continues to Kill Infants," #444.

[13] Michael Murray, ND and Joseph Pizzorno, ND, *Encyclopedia of Natural Medicine*, Revised 2nd Edition, Prima Health, 1998, p. 513.

[14] Ibid.

Pancreatitis

[1] Michael D. Gershon, MD, *The Second Brain*, HarperPerennial, 1998, p. 123.

[2] www.mamashealth.com/pancreatitis.asp

[3] Henry D. Janowitz, MD, *Your Gut Feelings*, Consumer's Union, 1987, p. 140.

[4] www.nlm.nih.gov/medlineplus/ency/article/001144.htm# visualContent

[5] Phyllis A. Balch, CNC and James F. Balch, MD, *Prescription for Nutritional Healing*, Third Edition, Avery, 2000, p. 556.

[6] Op. Cit., www.nlm.nih.gov

[7] Op. Cit., Janowitz, p. 138.

[8] Linda A. Ross, editor, *Gastrointestinal Diseases and Disorders Sourcebook*, Omnigraphics, Inc., 1996, p. 360.

[9] Ibid.

[10] Op. Cit., www.nlm.nih.gov

[11] Ibid.

APPENDIX

[1] www.gsdl.com/assessments/finsystems/metabolic.html

[2] Jonathan V. Wright, MD and Lane Lenard, PhD, *Why Stomach Acid is Good for You*, M. Evans and Company, Inc., 2001, p. 133.

[3] Elizabeth Lipski, MS, CNN, *Digestive Wellness*, Keats Publishing, Inc., 1996, p. 118.

[4] Omar M. Amin, "Seasonal Prevalence of Intestinal Parasites in the United Sates During 2002," *Am J. Trop Med. Hyg.*, 66(6), 2002, p. 799.

Index